GUIDE TO DRUG DOSAGES

THIRD EDITION

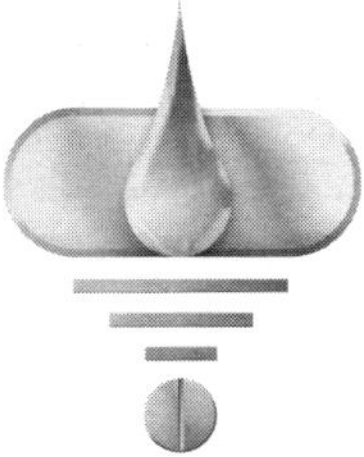

LIPPINCOTT WILLIAMS & WILKINS
A **Wolters Kluwer** Company
Philadelphia • Baltimore • New York • London
Buenos Aires • Hong Kong • Sydney • Tokyo

Staff

Editorial Director
William J. Kelly

Clinical Director
Marguerite S. Ambrose, RN, MSN, CS

Creative Director
Jake Smith

Art Director
Elaine Kasmer

Drug Information Editor
Melissa M. Devlin, PharmD

Senior Associate Editor
Ann E. Houska

Clinical Project Editor
Eileen Cassin Gallen, RN, BSN

Editor
Lynne Christensen

Clinical Editors
Christine M. Damico, RN, MSN, CPNP; Nancy Laplante, RN, BSN; Kimberly A. Zalewski, RN, MSN

Copy Editors
Dolores Connors Matthews, Jenifer F. Walker

Designers
Arlene Putterman (associate design director), Joseph John Clark, Jan Greenberg, Donald G. Knauss

Typographers
Diane Paluba (manager), Joyce Rossi Biletz

Manufacturing
Patricia K. Dorshaw (manager), Beth Janae Orr (book production manager)

Editorial Assistants
Danielle J. Barsky, Carol A. Caputo, Arlene P. Claffee

Indexer
Deborah K. Tourtlotte

The clinical procedures prescribed and recommended in this product are based on research and consultation with nursing, medical, pharmaceutical, and legal authorities. To the best of our knowledge, this information reflects currently accepted practice; nevertheless, it can't be considered absolute and universal. For individual application, all recommendations must be considered in light of the patient's clinical condition and, before the administration of new or infrequently used drugs, in light of the latest package-insert information. The publisher disclaims responsibility for adverse effects resulting directly or indirectly from the information presented, from undetected errors, or from the reader's misunderstanding of the text.

ISBN 1-58255-1286
NDHPGDD–D N O S A J J M A M F
03 02 01 00 10 9 8 7 6 5 4 3 2 1

Visit our Web site at NDHnow.com

Contents

Clinical consultants **iv**

How to use this book **v**

Guide to abbreviations **vi**

Generic drugs in alphabetical order 2

Appendices

Selected narcotic analgesic combination products **311**

Drugs that shouldn't be crushed **313**

Dangerous drug interactions **316**

Temperature conversions **319**

Infusion rates **320**

Index 325

Drug updates NDHnow.com

Clinical consultants

Steven R. Abel, RPh, PharmD
Professor and Head
Department of Pharmacy Practice
Purdue University
West Lafayette, Ind.

Lawrence Carey, PharmD
Clinical Pharmacist Supervisor
Jefferson Home Infusion Service
Philadelphia

Jennifer L. Defilippi, PharmD
Clinical Psychiatric Specialist
Central Texas Veteran's Health Care System
Waco, Tex.

Patricia L. Eltz, RN, MSN, CEN
Community Health Educator
Pottstown Memorial Medical Center
Pottstown, Pa.

Carmel A. Esposito, RN, MSN, EdD
Nurse Educator
Trinity Health System School of Nursing
Steubenville, Ohio

Ronald Greenberg, RPh, PharmD, BCPS
Clinical Pharmacy Coordinator
Fairview Ridges Hospital
Burnsville, Minn.

Tatyana Gurvich, PharmD
Clinical Pharmacologist
Glendale Adventist Family Practice
Residency Program
Glendale, Calif.

Michelle Kosich, PharmD
Clinical Pharmacist
Mercy Community Hospital
Havertown, Pa.

Thomas Lodise, PharmD
Infectious Diseases Pharmacotherapy and Outcomes Fellow
Wayne State University and Anti-Infective Research Laboratory
Detroit Receiving Hospital and UHC
Department of Pharmacy
Detroit

Randall A. Lynch, RPh, PharmD
Assistant Director, Pharmacy
Presbyterian Medical Center
University of Pennsylvania Health System
Philadelphia

Marie Maloney, PharmD
Clinical Pharmacist
University Medical Center
Tucson

George Melko, RPh, PharmD
Independent Consultant
West Chester, Pa.

William O'Hara, BS, PharmD
Clinical Team Leader
Thomas Jefferson University Hospital
Philadelphia

David Pipher, RPh, PharmD
Director of Pharmacy
Forbes Regional Hospital
Monroeville, Pa.

Ruthie Robinson, RN, MSN, CCRN, CEN
Nursing Instructor
Lamar University
Beaumont, Tex.

Joseph F. Steiner, RPh, PharmD
Professor and Director of Pharmacy Practice
University of Wyoming School of Pharmacy
Laramie

Barbara S. Wiggins, RPh, PharmD
Clinical Pharmacist, Cardiology
Clinical Instructor
University of Washington Medical Center
Seattle

How to use this book

NDH Pocket Guide to Drug Dosages, Third Edition, offers comprehensive dosage information in a unique, quick-scan format. The book opens with a list of abbreviations used in the entries. Then, organized alphabetically by generic name, each drug entry covers generic and common trade names, therapeutic class, pregnancy risk category, controlled substance schedule (where appropriate), common indications and dosages, and key nursing considerations. Information is divided into columns for quick reference.

The first column shows the generic name in boldface, followed by trade names. Canadian and Australian trade-names are indicated by a dagger (†) and a double-dagger (‡), respectively. After the list of trade names is the therapeutic class. Pregnancy risk category and, where applicable, controlled substance schedule are listed next.

Pregnancy risk categories parallel those assigned by the Food and Drug Administration to reflect a drug's potential to cause birth defects.

- A: Adequate studies in pregnant women have failed to show a risk to the fetus.
- B: Animal studies have not shown a risk to the fetus, but controlled studies have not been conducted in pregnant women; or animal studies have shown an adverse effect on the fetus, but adequate studies in pregnant women have not shown a fetal risk.
- C: Animal studies have shown an adverse effect on the fetus, but adequate studies have not been conducted in humans. The benefits may be acceptable despite potential risks.
- D: The drug may pose risks to the human fetus, but potential benefits may be acceptable despite the risks.
- X: Studies in animals or humans show fetal abnormalities, or reports of adverse reactions indicate evidence of fetal risk. The risks involved clearly outweigh the potential benefits.
- NR: Not rated.

Drugs regulated under the Controlled Substances Act of 1970 are divided into the following schedules:

- I: high abuse potential, no accepted medical use
- II: high abuse potential, severe dependence liability
- III: less abuse potential than schedule II drugs, moderate dependence liability
- IV: less abuse potential than schedule III drugs, limited dependence liability
- V: limited abuse potential.

The second column covers major indications and the most common dosages ordered for a particular drug. The third column lists the important nursing considerations, including those related to monitoring, drug administration, and patient teaching.

Appendices include selected narcotic analgesic combination products, drugs that shouldn't be crushed, dangerous drug interactions, a temperature conversion table, and infusion rate tables.

The index contains generic names, trade names, and indications.

Guide to abbreviations

ABG	arterial blood gas
ACE	angiotensin-converting enzyme
ADH	antidiuretic hormone
AIDS	acquired immunodeficiency syndrome
ALT	alanine aminotransferase
AST	aspartate aminotransferase
AV	atrioventricular
b.i.d.	twice a day
BP	blood pressure
BPH	benign prostatic hypertrophy
BUN	blood urea nitrogen
CABG	coronary artery bypass graft
CAD	coronary artery disease
CBC	complete blood count
CDC	Centers for Disease Control and Prevention
CK	creatinine kinase
cm	centimeter
CMV	cytomegalovirus
CNS	central nervous system
CO_2	carbon dioxide
COPD	chronic obstructive pulmonary disease
CrCl	creatinine clearance
CSF	cerebrospinal fluid
CV	cardiovascular
CVA	cerebrovascular accident
CVP	central venous pressure
D_5W	dextrose 5% in water
dl	deciliter
DTP	diphtheria, tetanus, and pertussis
ECG	electrocardiogram
EEG	electroencephalogram
ET	endotracheal
Fio_2	forced inspiratory oxygen
G	gauge
g	gram
GI	gastrointestinal
GU	genitourinary
H	histamine
Hct	hematocrit
HDL	high-density lipoprotein
Hgb	hemoglobin
HIV	human immunodeficiency virus
HR	heart rate
hr	hour
h.s.	at bedtime
I&O	intake and output
I.M.	intramuscular
INR	international normalized ratio
IOP	intraocular pressure
IPPB	intermittent positive-pressure breathing
IU	international unit
I.V.	intravenous
kg	kilogram
L	liter
lb	pound
LDL	low-density lipoprotein
LFT	liver function test

Guide to abbreviations

M	molar
m^2	square meter
MAC	*Mycobacterium avium* complex
MAO	monoamine oxidase
mcg	microgram
mEq	milliequivalent
mg	milligram
MI	myocardial infarction
min	minute
ml	milliliter
mm^3	cubic millimeter
mo	month
NaCl	sodium chloride
NG	nasogastric
NSAID	nonsteroidal anti-inflammatory drug
O_2	oxygen
OTC	over-the-counter
oz	ounce
$Paco_2$	partial pressure of arterial carbon dioxide
Pao_2	partial pressure of arterial oxygen
PAWP	pulmonary artery wedge pressure
P.O.	by mouth
P.R.	per rectum
p.r.n.	as needed
PSVT	paroxysmal supraventricular tachycardia
PT	prothrombin time
PTCA	percutaneous transluminal coronary angioplasty
PTT	partial thromboplastin time
PVC	premature ventricular contractions
PVD	peripheral vascular disease
q	every
q.d.	every day
q.i.d.	four times a day
RBC	red blood cell
RDA	recommended daily allowance
RSV	respiratory syncytial virus
SaO_2	oxygen saturation
S.C.	subcutaneous
sec	second
S.L.	sublingual
SSRI	selected serotonin reuptake inhibitor
T_3	triiodothyronine
T_4	thyroxine
TB	tuberculosis
TCA	tricyclic antidepressant
t.i.d.	three times a day
TPN	total parenteral nutrition
tsp	teaspoon
U	unit
USP	United States Pharmacopeia
UTI	urinary tract infection
w	with
WBC	white blood cell
wk	week
yr	year

DRUG & CLASS	INDICATIONS & DOSAGES	NURSING CONSIDERATIONS
abacavir sulfate Ziagen *Antiviral* Pregnancy Risk Category: C	*HIV type 1 infection* — **Adults:** 300 mg P.O. b.i.d. with other antiretrovirals. **Children 3 mo to 16 yr:** 8 mg/kg (maximum 300 mg) P.O. b.i.d. with other antiretrovirals.	▪ ***ALERT*** Always use with other antiretrovirals. Don't add as a single agent when antiretroviral regimens are changed because of loss of virologic response. ▪ May cause fatal hypersensitivity reactions.
abciximab ReoPro *Platelet aggregation inhibitor* Pregnancy Risk Category: C	*Adjunct to PTCA or atherectomy to prevent acute cardiac ischemic complications in patients at high risk for abrupt closure of treated coronary vessel* — **Adults:** 0.25 mg/kg I.V. bolus 10 to 60 min before start of PTCA or atherectomy; then continuous I.V. infusion of 10 mcg/min for 12 hr.	▪ Give in separate I.V. line; don't add other drug to solution. ▪ Institute bleeding precautions. Keep on bed rest for 6 to 8 hr after sheath removal or drug discontinuation, whichever is later. Minimize punctures and invasive procedures. ▪ Intended for use with aspirin and heparin.
acarbose Precose *Antidiabetic* Pregnancy Risk Category: B	*Adjunct to diet, insulin, sulfonylurea, or metformin to lower blood glucose in type 2 diabetes mellitus when hyperglycemia can't be managed by diet, diet plus a sulfonylurea, exercise, insulin, or metformin alone* — **Adults:** initially, 25 mg P.O. t.i.d. with 1st bite of each main meal. Adjust dose q 4 to 8 wk based on postprandial glucose levels and tolerance. Maintenance: 50 to 100 mg P.O. t.i.d. based on weight. Maximum 50 mg t.i.d. in patients < 60 kg (132 lb) or 100 mg t.i.d. in patients > 60 kg.	▪ May increase hypoglycemic potential of sulfonylureas. Closely monitor patient. ▪ Don't use in patients with severe liver impairment. ▪ Patient may need insulin during increased stress. Monitor for hyperglycemia. ▪ Monitor 1-hr postprandial plasma glucose.

acebutolol hydrochloride Sectral *Antihypertensive, antiarrhythmic* Pregnancy Risk Category: B	*Hypertension* — **Adults:** 400 mg P.O. as 1 daily dose or in divided doses b.i.d. to maximum 1,200 mg daily. *Ventricular arrhythmias* — **Adults:** 400 mg P.O. daily divided b.i.d.; increase p.r.n. Usual dose 600 to 1,200 mg. ***Adjust-a-dose:*** In patients with CrCl of 25 to 50 ml/min, reduce dose by 50%; if < 25 ml/min, reduce dose by 75%.	▪ Check apical pulse before giving; if < 60, withhold drug and call doctor. Monitor BP. ▪ Before surgery, tell anesthesiologist that patient is taking drug. ▪ Drug may mask hyperthyroidism signs. ▪ Don't discontinue drug abruptly.
acetaminophen (APAP, paracetamol) Acephen, Aceta, Anacin (aspirin free), Apacet, Dapacin, Feverall, Neopap, Panadol, Tempra, Tylenol *Nonnarcotic analgesic, antipyretic* Pregnancy Risk Category: B	*Mild pain or fever* — **Adults and children > 11 yr:** 325 to 650 mg P.O. q 4 to 6 hr; or 1 g P.O. t.i.d. or q.i.d., p.r.n. Or, 2 extended-release capsules P.O. q 8 hr. Maximim 4 g daily. For long-term use, maximum 2.6 g daily. **Children 11 yr:** 480 mg P.O. or P.R. q 4 to 6 hr. **Children 9 to 10 yr:** 400 mg P.O. or P.R. q 4 to 6 hr. **Children 6 to 8 yr:** 320 mg P.O. or P.R. q 4 to 6 hr. **Children 4 to 5 yr:** 240 mg P.O. or P.R. q 4 to 6 hr. **Children 2 to 3 yr:** 160 mg P.O. or P.R. q 4 to 6 hr. **Children 12 to 23 mo:** 120 mg P.O. q 4 to 6 hr. **Children 4 to 11 mo:** 80 mg P.O. q 4 to 6 hr. **Children ≤ 3 mo:** 40 mg P.O. q 4 to 6 hr.	▪ ***ALERT*** Warn that high doses or unsupervised long-term use can cause liver damage. ▪ Caution that excessive alcohol use may increase risk of liver toxicity. ▪ Warn not to take for marked fever (> 103.1° F [39.5° C]), fever lasting > 3 days, or recurrent fever, unless directed by doctor. ▪ May cause false-positive blood glucose decrease in home monitoring systems. ▪ Don't give to children < 2 yr without consulting doctor.
acetazolamide Acetazolam†, AK-Zol, Dazamide, Diamox, Diamox Sequels	*Secondary glaucoma and preoperative treatment of acute angle-closure glaucoma* — **Adults:** 250 mg P.O. q 4 hr; or 250 mg P.O. b.i.d. for short-term therapy. For extended-release capsules, 500 mg P.O. once daily or b.i.d. To rapidly lower IOP, 500 mg I.V.; then	▪ ***I.V. use:*** Inject 100 to 500 mg/min into large vein using 21G or 23G needle. ▪ Monitor I&O, glucose, and electrolytes. When drug used as diuretic, consult doctor and dietitian about high-potassium diet. *(continued)*

†Canadian, ‡Australian

DRUG & CLASS	INDICATIONS & DOSAGES	NURSING CONSIDERATIONS
acetazolamide *(continued)* **acetazolamide sodium** Diamox Parenteral *Antiglaucoma agent, diuretic* Pregnancy Risk Category: C	125 to 250 mg I.V. q 4 hr. *Edema in heart failure* — **Adults:** 250 to 375 mg P.O. or I.V. q morning. **Children:** 5 mg/kg P.O. or I.V. q morning. *Chronic open-angle glaucoma* — **Adults:** 250 mg to 1 g P.O. daily in divided doses q.i.d., or 500 mg (extended-release) P.O. b.i.d. **Children:** 8 to 30 mg/kg P.O. in 3 divided doses.	▪ Weigh patient daily; rapid fluid loss may cause weight loss and hypotension. ▪ Elderly patients are especially susceptible to excessive diuresis; monitor closely.
acetylcysteine Airbron†, Mucomyst, Mucomyst 10, Mucosil-10, Mucosil-20 *Mucolytic agent, antidote for acetaminophen overdose* Pregnancy Risk Category: B	*Adjunct therapy for abnormal viscid or inspissated mucus secretions in pneumonia, bronchitis, TB, cystic fibrosis, emphysema, atelectasis, pulmonary complications of thoracic and CV surgery* — **Adults and children:** 1 to 2 ml of 10% or 20% solution by direct instillation into trachea up to q hr; or 1 to 10 ml of 20% solution or 2 to 20 ml of 10% solution by nebulization q 2 to 6 hr, p.r.n. *Acetaminophen toxicity* — **Adults and children:** initially, 140 mg/kg P.O.; then 70 mg/kg P.O. q 4 hr for 17 doses.	▪ ***ALERT*** Start treatment immediately; don't wait for blood drug levels. Drug can't be given if > 24 hr has elapsed since ingestion. ▪ To use orally for acetaminophen overdose, dilute with cola, juice, or water. Add 3 ml diluent to each ml acetylcysteine. Use diluted oral solutions within 1 hr. If given by NG tube, water may be used as diluent. ▪ Repeat dose if patient vomits within 1 hr of loading or maintenance dose. ▪ Use plastic, glass, stainless steel, or other nonreactive metal when giving by nebulization. Don't use hand-bulb nebulizer.
activated charcoal Actidose, Actidose-Aqua, Charcoaid, Charcocaps, Liqui-Char *Antidote, antidiarrheal,*	*Flatulence, dyspepsia* — **Adults:** 600 mg to 5 g P.O. as single dose or 0.975 to 3.9 g P.O. t.i.d. after meals. *Poisoning* — **Adults and children:** initially, 1 to 2 g/kg (30 to 100 g) P.O. or 10 times	▪ Inactivates ipecac syrup; give after emesis. ▪ Mix powder form with water to form thick consistency. May add small amount of juice. Give by large-bore NG tube after lavage, p.r.n.

antiflatulent Pregnancy Risk Category: C	amount of poison ingested, given as suspension in 120 to 240 ml of water. Check with poison control center for specific uses in poisonings or overdoses.	▪ Space doses ≥ 1 hr apart from other drugs when giving for indications other than poisoning.
acyclovir Zovirax *Antiviral* Pregnancy Risk Category: C	*Initial herpes genitalis; limited, non–life-threatening mucocutaneous herpes simplex virus infections in immunocompromised patients* — **Adults and children:** cover all lesions q 3 hr, 6 times daily for 7 days.	▪ As ordered, start therapy as soon as possible after symptom onset. ▪ Apply with finger cot or rubber glove. ▪ For cutaneous use only; don't apply to eye.
acyclovir sodium Avirax†, Zovirax *Antiviral* Pregnancy Risk Category: C	*Mucocutaneous herpes simplex virus infections in immunocompromised patients; genital herpes in immunocompetent patients* — **Adults and children ≥ 12 yr:** 5 mg/kg I.V. q 8 hr for 7 to 14 days (5 to 7 days for severe initial genital episode). **Children < 12 yr:** 250 mg/m^2 I.V. q 8 hr for 7 days. *Initial genital herpes* — **Adults:** 200 mg P.O. q 4 hr while awake (total 5 capsules daily); or 400 mg P.O. q 8 hr. Continue 7 to 10 days. *Chronic suppression therapy for recurrent genital herpes* — **Adults:** 400 mg P.O. b.i.d. for up to 12 mo. *Varicella (chickenpox) infections in immunocompromised patients* — **Adults and children ≥ 12 yr:** 10 mg/kg I.V. q 8 hr for 7 days. **Children < 12 yr:** 500 mg/m^2 I.V. q 8 hr for 7 to 10 days. *Varicella (chickenpox) infections in immunocompetent patients* — **Adults and children**	▪ ***I.V. use:*** Give infusion over ≥ 1 hr. ▪ Don't give by bolus, I.M., or S.C. injection. ▪ Start therapy as soon as possible after symptom onset. ▪ Encourage adequate fluid intake. ▪ Encephalopathic changes more likely in neurologic disorders and in history of neurologic reactions to cytotoxic drugs. ▪ Dosage for obese patients based on ideal weight.

(continued)

†Canadian, ‡Australian

DRUG & CLASS	INDICATIONS & DOSAGES	NURSING CONSIDERATIONS
acyclovir sodium *(continued)*	**> 40 kg:** 800 mg P.O. q.i.d for 5 days. **Children ≥ 2 yr ≤ 40 kg:** 20 mg/kg P.O. q.i.d. for 5 days. Maximum daily dose is 80 mg/kg. ***Adjust-a-dose:*** Adjust dosage in patients with renal failure.	
adenosine Adenocard *Antiarrhythmic* Pregnancy Risk Category: C	*Conversion of PSVT to sinus rhythm* — **Adults:** 6 mg rapid I.V. push over 1 to 2 sec. If PSVT persists after 1 to 2 min, give 12 mg by rapid I.V. push and repeat p.r.n. Don't give > 12 mg in single dose.	▪ Use cautiously in asthma. ▪ ***I.V. use:*** Give directly into vein if possible; use port closest to patient and flush immediately and rapidly with 0.9% NaCl. ▪ Monitor ECG for arrhythmias.
albumin 5% Albuminar 5, Albutein 5% **albumin 25%** Albuminar 25, Albutein 25% *Plasma protein* Pregnancy Risk Category: C	*Hypovolemic shock* — **Adults:** initially, 500 to 750 ml of 5% solution by I.V. infusion; repeat q 30 min, p.r.n. Or, 100 to 200 ml I.V. of 25% solution; repeat in 10 to 30 min, p.r.n. **Children:** 12 to 20 ml 5% solution/kg by I.V. infusion; repeat in 15 to 30 min if response inadequate. Or, 2.5 to 5 ml I.V. of 25% solution/kg; repeat in 10 to 30 min, p.r.n. *Hypoproteinemia* — **Adults:** 200 to 300 ml of 25% albumin. *Hyperbilirubinemia* — **Infants:** 1 g/kg albumin (4 ml/kg of 25% solution) 1 to 2 hr before transfusion.	▪ Ensure proper hydration before infusion. ▪ ***I.V. use:*** Specific dosage and rate vary with condition. 5% albumin infused undiluted; 25% albumin infused undiluted or diluted with 0.9% NaCl or D_5W. Don't give > 250 g in 48 hr. ▪ Watch for hemorrhage or shock after surgery or injury. ▪ Watch for signs of vascular overload. ▪ Monitor I&O, Hgb, Hct, serum protein, and electrolytes.
albuterol (salbutamol) Asmol‡, Proventil, Ventolin	*To prevent or treat bronchospasm in reversible obstructive airway disease or to prevent exercise-induced bronchospasm* — **Adults > 65 yr:** 2 mg P.O. t.i.d. or q.i.d.	▪ Use extended-release tablets cautiously in preexisting GI narrowing. ▪ Pleasant-tasting syrup may be taken by children as young as 2 yr. Contains no al-

		cohol or sugar.
albuterol sulfate (salbutamol sulfate) Proventil, Proventil Repetabs, Respolin Inhaler‡, Respolin Respirator Solution‡, Ventolin, Volmax *Bronchodilator* Pregnancy Risk Category: C	**Adults and children ≥ 12 yr:** *Oral solution:* 2 to 4 mg (1 to 2 tsp) t.i.d. or q.i.d. *Solution for inhalation:* 2.5 mg t.i.d. or q.i.d. by nebulizer. *Oral tablet:* 2 to 4 mg P.O. t.i.d. or q.i.d.; maximum 8 mg q.i.d. *Extended-release tablet:* 4 to 8 mg P.O. q 12 hr; maximum 16 mg b.i.d. **Children 6 to 11 yr:** *Extended-release tablet:* 4 mg q 12 hr. Oral solution or solution for inhalation: 0.1 mg/kg t.i.d. or q.i.d., up to 2 mg (1 tsp) q.i.d. **Children 2 to 5 yr:** 0.1 mg/kg P.O. t.i.d., up to 2 mg (1 tsp) t.i.d. **Adults and children ≥ 4 yr:** *Aerosol inhalation:* 1 to 2 inhalations q 4 to 6 hr. *Capsule for inhalation:* 200 to 400 mcg inhaled q 4 to 6 hr using Rotahaler. *Prevention of exercise-induced bronchospasm* — **Adults and children ≥ 4 yr:** 1 to 2 inhalations 15 min before exercise.	▪ Aerosol form may be used 15 min before exercise. ▪ ***ALERT*** May use tablets and aerosol together. Monitor closely for toxicity. ▪ If doctor orders > 1 inhalation, instruct patient to wait ≥ 2 min between inhalations. ▪ If patient also uses steroid inhaler, advise him to use steroid 5 min after taking albuterol.
aldesleukin (interleukin-2, IL-2) Proleukin *Immunoregulatory agent* Pregnancy Risk Category: C	*Metastatic renal cell carcinoma* — **Adults:** 600,000 IU/kg (0.037 mg/kg) I.V. q 8 hr for 5 days (total of 14 doses). After 9-day rest, repeat sequence for another 14 doses. May repeat courses after resting ≥ 7 wk.	▪ Monitor CBC, serum electrolytes, and renal and LFTs. ▪ Monitor vital signs closely. ▪ Withhold dose if moderate lethargy occurs. ▪ Add ordered dose of reconstituted drug to 50 ml D_5W and infuse over 15 min. Don't use in-line filter.
alendronate sodium Fosamax	*Osteoporosis in men and postmenopausal women* — **Adults:** 10 mg P.O. q.d. or 70 mg P.O. once weekly.	▪ Correct hypocalcemia and other disturbances of mineral metabolism before therapy begins. *(continued)*

†Canadian, ‡Australian

DRUG & CLASS	INDICATIONS & DOSAGES	NURSING CONSIDERATIONS
alendronate sodium *(continued)* *Antiosteoporotic* Pregnancy Risk Category: C	*Prevention of osteoporosis in postmenopausal women* — **Adults:** 5 mg P.O. q.d. or 35 mg P.O. q wk. *Glucocorticoid-induced osteoporosis* — **Adults:** 5 mg P.O. q.d. Postmenopausal women *not* receiving estrogen should receive 10 mg q.d. *Paget's disease of bone* — **Adults:** 40 mg P.O. q.d. for 6 mo.	▪ Patients should remain upright for ≥ 30 min after ingesting drug. ▪ ***ALERT*** Drug should be taken with a full glass of water, ≥ 30 min before first food, beverage, or medication of day.
alitretinoin Panretin *Antineoplastic* Pregnancy Risk Category: D	*Cutaneous lesions in patients with Kaposi's sarcoma related to AIDS* — **Adults:** initially, apply generous coating of gel b.i.d. to lesions only. May increase to t.i.d. to q.i.d. If site toxicity occurs, may reduce frequency. If severe irritation occurs, may stop drug for a few days.	▪ Use enough gel to cover lesion with generous coating. Allow to dry for 3 to 5 min before covering with clothing. ▪ Don't apply gel to normal skin around lesions on or near mucosal surfaces of body. ▪ Don't use occlusive dressings.
allopurinol Lopurin, Purinol†, Zyloprim *Antigout agent* Pregnancy Risk Category: C	*Gout* — Dosage varies with disease severity; divide doses > 300 mg. **Adults:** mild gout, 200 to 300 mg P.O. q.d.; severe gout, 400 to 600 mg P.O. q.d. *Hyperuricemia secondary to malignancies* — **Adults:** 200 to 800 mg P.O. q.d. **Children 6 to 10 yr:** 300 mg P.O. once daily or divided t.i.d. **Children < 6 yr:** 50 mg P.O. t.i.d. *Prevention of acute gout* — **Adults:** 100 mg P.O. q.d.; increase q wk by 100 mg up to maximum of 800 mg until serum uric acid ≤ 6 mg/dl.	▪ Monitor serum uric acid. ▪ Monitor I&O; daily output of ≥ 2 L and maintenance of neutral or slightly alkaline urine desirable. ▪ Periodically monitor CBC and hepatic and renal function. ▪ If renal insufficiency occurs, may reduce dosage. ▪ Optimal benefits may require 2 to 6 wk of therapy. Concurrent colchicine may be prescribed prophylactically for acute gout.

alprazolam Apo-Alpraz†, Novo-Alprazol†, Nu-Alpraz†, Xanax *Anxiolytic* Pregnancy Risk Category: D Controlled Substance Schedule: IV	*Anxiety* — **Adults:** initially, 0.25 to 0.5 mg P.O. t.i.d., to maximum of 4 mg q.d. in divided doses. For elderly or debilitated patients or those with advanced liver disease, initially, 0.25 mg P.O. b.i.d. or t.i.d., to maximum of 4 mg q.d. in divided doses. *Panic disorders* — **Adults:** 0.5 mg P.O. t.i.d., increased q 3 to 4 days ≤ 1 mg. Maximum 10 mg q.d. in divided doses.	▪ Not to be used for everyday stress or for longer than 4 mo. ▪ ***ALERT*** Warn not to withdraw abruptly after long-term use; withdrawal symptoms may occur. Abuse or addiction possible. ▪ In repeated or prolonged therapy, monitor liver, renal, and blood studies periodically as ordered.
alprostadil Caverject *Corrective agent for impotence* Pregnancy Risk Category: NR	*Erectile dysfunction of vasculogenic, psychogenic, or mixed etiology* — **Adults:** dosages highly individualized, with 1st dose of 2.5 mcg intracavernously. If partial response occurs, give 2nd dose of 2.5 mcg; then increase in increments of 5 to 10 mcg until suitable erection. If no response to 1st dose, may increase 2nd dose to 7.5 mcg within 1 hr; then increase in increments of 5 to 10 mcg until suitable erection. *Erectile dysfunction of neurologic etiology* — **Adults:** dosage individualized, with 1st dose of 1.25 mcg intracavernously. If partial response occurs, give 2nd dose of 1.25 mcg, followed by increments of 2.5 mcg, to dose of 5 mcg, and then in increments of 5 mcg until suitable erection. If no initial response, may give next higher dose within 1 hr.	▪ Regular follow-up care with thorough exam of penis strongly recommended to detect penile fibrosis. ▪ Erection should occur 5 to 20 min after treatment and should last preferably ≤ 1 hr. Erection > 6 hr requires immediate medical intervention. With initial dose, patient must stay in doctor's office until complete detumescence. ▪ Should not be used > 3 times/wk. Wait ≥ 24 hr between uses. ▪ Monitor for adverse reactions, such as penile redness, swelling, tenderness, curvature, unusual pain, nodules, or priapism. ▪ Bleeding at injection site may increase risk of transmitting blood-borne disease to sexual partner.

†Canadian, ‡Australian

DRUG & CLASS	INDICATIONS & DOSAGES	NURSING CONSIDERATIONS
alprostadil Prostin VR Pediatric *Adjunct for ductus arteriosus patency* Pregnancy Risk Category: NR	*Palliative therapy for maintenance of patency of ductus arteriosus until surgery* — **Infants:** 0.05 to 0.1 mcg/kg/min I.V. infusion. When response achieved, reduce rate to lowest dosage that will maintain response; maximum 0.4 mcg/kg/min. Or, give through umbilical artery catheter placed at ductal opening.	▪ ***ALERT*** Not for use in neonatal respiratory distress syndrome. ▪ Don't use diluents with benzyl alcohol. ▪ If apnea and bradycardia occur, stop infusion immediately. ▪ In restricted pulmonary blood flow, monitor blood oxygenation. In restricted systemic blood flow, monitor systemic BP and blood pH.
alteplase (tissue plasminogen activator, recombinant; t-PA) Actilyse‡, Activase *Thrombolytic enzyme* Pregnancy Risk Category: C	*Lysis of thrombi obstructing coronary arteries in acute MI* — **Adults:** 100 mg I.V. infusion over 3 hr as follows: 60 mg in 1st hr, of which 6 to 10 mg given as bolus over 1st 1 to 2 min. Then 20 mg/hr infusion for 2 hr. Smaller adults (< 65 kg [143 lb]) should receive 1.25 mg/kg in similar fashion (60% in 1st hr, 10% as bolus; then 20% of total dose per hr for 2 hr). *Management of acute massive pulmonary embolism* — **Adults:** 100 mg I.V. infusion over 2 hr. Begin heparin at end of infusion when PTT or thrombin time returns to twice normal or less. Don't exceed 100-mg dose. *Acute ischemic stroke* — **Adults:** 0.9 mg/kg I.V. infusion over 1 hr with 10% of total dose given as initial I.V. bolus over 1 min. Maximum 90 mg total. *Note:* Give within 3 hr after symptoms occur and only when intracranial bleeding has been ruled out.	▪ ***I.V. use:*** Check manufacturer's labeling for specific reconstitution information. ▪ Must be started as soon as possible after symptom onset when used to recanalize occluded coronary arteries. ▪ Monitor vital signs and neurologic status carefully. Keep patient on strict bed rest. ▪ Have antiarrhythmics readily available, and carefully monitor ECG. ▪ Avoid invasive procedures. Carefully monitor for signs of internal bleeding, and frequently check all puncture sites. ▪ If uncontrollable bleeding occurs, stop infusion (and concomitant heparin), apply pressure to site if possible, and notify doctor.

aluminum carbonate Basaljel *Antacid, hypophosphatemic* Pregnancy Risk Category: B	*Antacid* — **Adults:** 5 to 10 ml of oral suspension P.O. q 2 hr, p.r.n.; or 1 to 2 tablets or capsules P.O. q 2 hr, p.r.n. Maximum 24 capsules, tablets, or tsp per 24 hr. *To prevent urinary phosphate stones* — **Adults:** 15 to 30 ml oral suspension in water or juice P.O. 1 hr after meals and h.s.; or 2 to 6 tablets or capsules 1 hr after meals and h.s.	▪ When giving drug through NG tube, ensure correct tube placement and patency; after instilling, flush tube with water. ▪ Monitor long-term, high-dose use in patients on restricted sodium intake. ▪ Watch for hypophosphatemia symptoms with prolonged use.
aluminum hydroxide AlternaGEL, Alu-Cap, Alu-tab, Amphojel, Dialume, Nephrox *Antacid, hypophosphatemic, adsorbent* Pregnancy Risk Category: C	*Antacid* — **Adults:** 500 to 1,500 mg P.O. (5 to 30 ml of most suspension products) 3 to 6 times a day between meals and h.s.; or, 300-mg or 600-mg tablets (chewed before swallowing) taken with milk or water 5 to 6 times daily after meals and h.s.	▪ When giving drug through NG tube, ensure correct tube placement and patency; after instilling, flush tube with water. ▪ Monitor long-term, high-dose use in patients on restricted sodium intake. ▪ Watch for hypophosphatemia symptoms with prolonged use.
amantadine hydrochloride Symadine, Symmetrel *Antiviral, antiparkinsonian* Pregnancy Risk Category: C	*Prophylaxis or symptomatic treatment of influenza type A virus, respiratory tract illnesses* — **Adults ≤ 65 yr with normal renal function and children > 9 yr > 45 kg (99 lb):** 200 mg P.O. q.d. in single dose or divided b.i.d. **Children 1 to 9 yr or < 45 kg:** 4.4 to 8.8 mg/kg P.O. q.d. as single dose or divided b.i.d., up to 150 mg q.d. **Adults > 65 yr with normal renal function:** 100 mg P.O. q.d. Start treatment within 24 to 48 hr after symptoms appear and continue for 24 to 48 hr after they disappear. Start as soon as possible after initial exposure.	▪ Elderly patients are more susceptible to adverse neurologic effects. ▪ If insomnia occurs, advise taking drug several hr before bedtime. ▪ Use cautiously in elderly patients and in those with seizure disorders, heart failure, peripheral edema, hepatic disease, mental illness, eczematoid rash, renal impairment, orthostatic hypotension, or CV disease. ▪ ***ALERT*** In patient taking anticholinergic, may reduce dosage of anticholinergic before starting amantidine. *(continued)*

DRUG & CLASS	INDICATIONS & DOSAGES	NURSING CONSIDERATIONS
amantadine hydrochloride *(continued)*	*Parkinson's disease* — **Adults:** 100 mg P.O. b.i.d. In patients receiving other antiparkinsonians or those who are seriously ill, 100 mg P.O. once daily for 1 wk; then 100 mg P.O. b.i.d. May increase to 400 mg/day. ***Adjust-a-dose:*** Patients with renal dysfunction should have maintenance dose based on CrCl.	▪ Don't discontinue abruptly in patients with Parkinson's disease. ▪ If orthostatic hypotension occurs, instruct patient to stand or change position slowly. ▪ Observe for adverse reactions, especially dizziness, depression, anxiety, nausea, and urine retention.
amifostine Ethyol *Cytoprotective agent* Pregnancy Risk Category: C	*Reduction of cumulative renal toxicity from repeated cisplatin administration in patients with advanced ovarian or non–small-cell lung cancer* — **Adults:** 910 mg/m^2 q.d. as 15-min I.V. infusion, starting 30 min before chemotherapy. If hypotension occurs and BP doesn't return to normal within 5 min after treatment stops, use 740 mg/m^2 for subsequent cycles. *Reduction of incidence of xerostomia in patients undergoing postoperative radiation treatment for head and neck cancer, including the parotid glands* — **Adults:** 200 mg/m^2 q.d. as 3-min I.V. infusion, starting 15 to 30 min before standard fraction radiation therapy.	▪ Should stop antihypertensive therapy 24 hr before giving amifostine. ▪ Antiemetics, including dexamethasone 20 mg and a serotonin-receptor antagonist, should be given before and in conjunction with amifostine. ▪ Patient should be adequately hydrated before treatment. Keep supine during infusion. Monitor I&O. ▪ Monitor BP q 5 min during infusion. ▪ ***ALERT*** Don't infuse drug for > 15 min. Longer infusion has been associated with higher incidence of adverse reactions.
amikacin sulfate Amikin *Antibiotic* Pregnancy Risk Category: D	*Serious infections caused by sensitive strains of susceptible organisms* — **Adults and children:** 15 mg/kg/day divided q 8 to 12 hr by I.M. or I.V. infusion. **Neonates:** loading dose	▪ Obtain specimen for culture and sensitivity tests before 1st dose. ▪ Evaluate weight, hearing, and renal function before and during therapy.

	of 10 mg/kg I.V.; then 7.5 mg/kg q 12 hr. *Uncomplicated UTI* — **Adults:** 250 mg I.M. or I.V. b.i.d. ***Adjust-a-dose:*** Adults with renal dysfunction, initially 7.5 mg/kg I.V. or I.M. Subsequent doses and frequency based on blood levels and renal function studies.	▪ ***ALERT*** Peak levels > 35 mcg/ml and trough levels > 10 mcg/ml may indicate toxicity. ▪ Give I.V. infusions in 100 to 200 ml D_5W or 0.9% NaCl over 30 to 60 min.
amiloride hydrochloride Kaluril‡, Midamor *Diuretic, antihypertensive* Pregnancy Risk Category: B	*Hypertension; edema from heart failure, usually in patients also taking thiazide or other potassium-wasting diuretics* — **Adults:** initial dose 5 mg P.O. q.d. Increase to 10 mg q.d. if necessary. Maximum 20 mg daily.	▪ To prevent nausea, give with meals. ▪ ***ALERT*** Monitor serum potassium. Alert doctor immediately if level is > 5.5 mEq/L, and expect to discontinue.
amino acid infusions Aminosyn, Aminosyn II in Dextrose, Aminosyn II with Electrolytes in Dextrose, Aminosyn-HBC, Aminosyn-RF, FreAmine III, Hepat-Amine, Novamine, Travasol with Electrolytes, TrophAmine *Parenteral nutritional therapy, caloric agent* Pregnancy Risk Category: C	*TPN in patients who can't or won't eat* — **Adults:** 1 to 1.5 g/kg I.V. q.d. **Children > 10 kg (22 lb):** 2 to 2.5 g/kg I.V. q.d. for first 10 kg; then 1 to 1.25 g/kg I.V. q.d for each kg over 10 kg. **Children ≤ 10 kg (22 lb):** 2 to 4 g/kg I.V. q.d. *Nutritional support in cirrhosis, hepatitis, and hepatic encephalopathy* — **Adults:** 80 to 120 g of amino acids I.V. q.d. (hepatic failure form). *Nutritional support in high metabolic stress* — **Adults:** 1.5 g/kg I.V. q.d. (high metabolic stress form). *Nutritional support in renal failure* — **Adults:** 0.3 to 0.5 g/kg I.V. q.d. (maximum 26 g q.d.). Dialysis patients may require 1 to 1.2 g/kg q.d.	▪ Obtain baseline serum electrolyte, glucose, BUN, calcium, and phosphorus levels before therapy, as ordered. Monitor periodically throughout therapy. ▪ Limit peripheral infusions to 2.5% amino acids and dextrose 10%. Check infusion site frequently. Change peripheral sites routinely. If subclavian catheter is used, give solution into midsuperior vena cava. ▪ ***ALERT*** Assess body temperature q 4 hr. If chills, fever, or other signs of sepsis occur, replace I.V. tubing and bottle and send to lab for culture. ▪ Give cautiously to diabetics and to patients with cardiac insufficiency.

†Canadian, ‡Australian

DRUG & CLASS	INDICATIONS & DOSAGES	NURSING CONSIDERATIONS
aminophylline (theophylline ethylenediamine) Phyllocontin, Truphylline *Bronchodilator* Pregnancy Risk Category: C	*Acute bronchospasm* — **Patients not taking theophylline:** loading dose 6 mg/kg (equivalent to 4.7 mg/kg anhydrous theophylline) I.V.; then maintenance infusion. **Adults (nonsmokers) not taking theophylline:** 0.7 mg/kg/hr I.V. for 12 hr; then 0.5 mg/kg/hr. **Otherwise healthy adult smokers not taking theophylline:** 1 mg/kg/hr I.V. for 12 hr; then 0.8 mg/kg/hr. **Children 9 to 16 yr not taking theophylline:** 1 mg/kg/hr I.V. for 12 hr; then 0.8 mg/kg/hr. **Children 6 mo to 9 yr not taking theophylline:** 1.2 mg/kg/hr for 12 hr; then 1 mg/kg/hr. **Patients taking theophylline:** Determine time, amount, route, and form of last dose. Infusions of 0.63 mg/kg (0.5 mg/kg anhydrous theophylline) increase plasma drug level by 1 mcg/ml. If no signs of toxicity, 3.1 mg/kg (2.5 mg/kg anhydrous theophylline). *Chronic bronchial asthma* — **Adults and children:** 16 mg/kg or 400 mg (whichever is less) P.O. q.d. in divided doses q 6 to 8 hr (for rapidly absorbed forms). May increase by 25% q 2 to 3 days. Or, 12 mg/kg or 400 mg (whichever is less) P.O. q.d. in divided doses q 8 to 12 hr (for extended-release forms). May increase by 2 to 3 mg/kg q.d. q 3 days.	▪ ***I.V. use:*** Giving I.V. can cause burning; dilute with compatible I.V. solution and inject ≤ 25 mg/min. ▪ ***ALERT*** Before loading dose, ensure that patient has recently had theophylline. ▪ Relieve GI symptoms by giving oral drug with full glass of water at meals (although food in stomach delays absorption). ▪ Monitor serum theophylline. Desirable level is 10 to 20 mcg/ml; toxicity reported at > 20 mcg/ml. ▪ Tell elderly patient that dizziness is common. ▪ Caution patient not to switch brands. ▪ Tell patient to check with doctor or pharmacist before taking with other drugs. ▪ Rectal dosage same as oral dosage.

amiodarone hydrochloride Aratac‡, Cordarone, Cordarone X‡, Pacerone *Antiarrhythmic* Pregnancy Risk Category: D	*Recurrent ventricular fibrillation and recurrent hemodynamically unstable ventricular tachycardia refractory to other antiarrhythmics* — **Adults:** loading dose 800 to 1,600 mg P.O. q.d. for 1 to 3 wk until initial response; then 600 to 800 mg/day P.O. for 1 mo and maintenance of 200 to 600 mg P.O. q.d. Or, loading dose 150 mg I.V. over 10 min (15 mg/min); then 360 mg I.V. over next 6 hr (1 mg/min); then 540 mg I.V. over next 18 hr (0.5 mg/min). After 1st 24 hr, continue maintenance infusion of 720 mg/24 hr (0.5 mg/min).	▪ Obtain baseline thyroid test and LFT results. ▪ Continuously monitor cardiac status of patient receiving drug I.V. ▪ High incidence of adverse reactions limits use. ▪ ***ALERT*** Monitor carefully for pulmonary toxicity, which can be fatal. Incidence increases with doses > 400 mg/day. ▪ Methylcellulose ophthalmic solution during therapy minimizes corneal microdeposits.
amitriptyline hydrochloride Apo-Amitriptyline†, Elavil *Antidepressant* Pregnancy Risk Category: C	*Depression* — **Adults:** initially, 50 to 100 mg P.O. h.s., increased to 150 mg q.d.; maximum 300 mg q.d., if needed. Maintenance: 50 to 100 mg/day P.O. or 20 to 30 mg I.M. q.i.d. **Elderly and adolescents:** 10 mg P.O. t.i.d. and 20 mg h.s. q.d.	▪ ***ALERT*** Parenteral form for I.M. use only. ▪ Has strong anticholinergic effects and is one of the most sedating tricyclic antidepressants. ▪ If signs of psychosis occur or worsen, expect to reduce dosage. ▪ Don't withdraw abruptly.
amlodipine besylate Norvasc *Antianginal, antihypertensive* Pregnancy Risk Category: C	*Chronic stable angina; vasospastic angina* — **Adults:** initially, 5 to 10 mg P.O. q.d. *Hypertension* — **Adults:** initially, 2.5 to 5 mg P.O. q.d. **Elderly:** 2.5 mg P.O. q.d. With small or frail patients, those receiving other antihypertensives, or those with hepatic insufficiency, begin at 2.5 mg q.d. Adjust according to response. Maximum 10 mg/day. Adjust over 7 to 14 days.	▪ Monitor carefully for increased frequency, duration, or severity of angina or acute MI. ▪ Monitor BP frequently when therapy begins. ▪ Notify doctor if patient has signs of heart failure (shortness of breath, swelling of hands and feet).

†Canadian, ‡Australian

DRUG & CLASS	INDICATIONS & DOSAGES	NURSING CONSIDERATIONS
amoxapine Asendin *Antidepressant* Pregnancy Risk Category: C	*Depression* — **Adults:** 50 mg P.O. b.i.d. or t.i.d., increased to 100 mg b.i.d or t.i.d. by end of 1st wk if tolerated. Increase > 300 mg q.d. only if this dose ineffective during trial of ≥ 2 wk. Maximum for outpatients, 400 mg q.d. When effective dose established, entire dose (≤ 300 mg) may be given h.s. **Elderly:** 25 mg b.i.d or t.i.d. If tolerated by end of 1st wk, increase to 50 mg b.i.d. or t.i.d. Carefully increase up to 300 mg q.d.	▪ ***ALERT*** Use with extreme caution in patients with seizure disorders. ▪ Full effect may take ≥ 4 wk. ▪ If signs of psychosis occur or worsen, expect to reduce dosage. ▪ Monitor for tardive dyskinesia, especially in elderly women. ▪ Drug has been linked to neuroleptic malignant syndrome.
amoxicillin/clavulanate potassium (amoxycillin/clavulanate potassium) Augmentin, Clavulin† *Antibiotic* Pregnancy Risk Category: B	*Lower respiratory tract infections, otitis media, sinusitis, skin infections, and UTIs caused by susceptible gram-positive and -negative organisms* — **Adults and children ≥ 40 kg (88 lb) (dosages based on amoxicillin component):** 250 to 500 mg P.O. q 8 hr. For more severe infections, 875 mg P.O. q 12 hr. **Children < 40 kg (dosage based on amoxicillin component):** 20 to 40 mg/kg P.O. daily in divided doses q 8 hr.	▪ Assess history of drug allergies. ▪ Obtain specimen for culture and sensitivity tests before 1st dose. ▪ ***ALERT*** Two 250-mg tablets are not equivalent to one 500-mg tablet. ▪ Give ≥ 1 hr before bacteriostatic antibiotics. ▪ Advise patient to take with food. ▪ Instruct to call doctor if rash occurs.
amoxicillin trihydrate (amoxycillin trihydrate) Amoxil, Cilamox‡, Larotid, Polymox, Trimox, Wymox *Antibiotic* Pregnancy Risk Category: B	*Systemic infections, acute and chronic UTIs caused by susceptible strains of gram-positive and -negative organisms* — **Adults and children ≥ 20 kg (44 lb):** 250 to 500 mg P.O. q 8 hr. **Children < 20 kg:** 20 mg/kg P.O. q.d. in divided doses q 8 hr; in severe infection, 40 mg/kg P.O. q.d. in divided dos-	▪ Assess history of allergic reactions to penicillin. (However, negative history doesn't preclude future reactions.) ▪ Obtain specimen for culture and sensitivity tests before 1st dose. ▪ With prolonged therapy, observe for fungal or bacterial superinfection, especially

es q 8 hr or 500 mg to 1 g/m^2 P.O. in divided doses q 8 hr.

Uncomplicated gonorrhea — **Adults and children > 2 yr > 45 kg (99 lb):** 3 g P.O. with 1 g probenecid as single dose.

Endocarditis prophylaxis for dental procedures — **Adults:** 2 g P.O. as single dose 1 hr before procedure. **Children > 2 yr:** 50 mg/kg P.O. as single dose 1 hr before procedure.

in elderly, debilitated, or immunosuppressed patients.

- Give ≥ 1 hr before bacteriostatic antibiotics.
- Advise patient taking oral suspension form that drug can be stored at room temperature for up to 2 wk, but should be refrigerated.
- Don't give to children < 2 yr.

---

amphotericin B
Amphocin, Amphotericin B for Injection, Fungilin Oral‡, Fungizone Intravenous
amphotericin B Liposome for injection
AmBisome
Antifungal
Pregnancy Risk Category: B

Systemic fungal infections; meningitis — **Adults:** test dose of 1 mg in 20 ml D_5W infused I.V. over 20 to 30 min. If tolerated, start as 0.25 to 0.3 mg/kg q.d. by slow I.V. infusion (0.1 mg/ml) over 2 to 6 hr. Increase dosage gradually up to 1 mg/kg q.d. If stopped for ≥ 1 wk, resume with test dose and increase gradually.

GI tract infections caused by Candida albicans — **Adults:** 100 mg P.O. q.i.d. for 2 wk.

Oral and perioral candidal infections — **Adults:** 1 lozenge q.i.d. for 7 to 14 days. Lozenge should dissolve slowly. Or, 1 ml (100 mg) of oral suspension P.O. q.i.d.

Cryptococcal meningitis in HIV-infected patients — **Adults and children:** 6 mg/kg q.d. I.V. infusion over 2 hr. Infusion time may be reduced to 1 hr if well tolerated or increased if discomfort occurs.

- ***I.V. use:*** Monitor pulse, respiratory rate, temperature, and BP for ≥ 4 hr after test dose.
- Monitor vital signs q 30 min; fever, shaking chills, and hypotension may appear 1 to 2 hr after I.V. infusion starts and should subside within 4 hr of stopping drug.
- Report change in urine appearance or volume. Monitor BUN and creatinine q wk.
- Use infusion pump and in-line filter with mean pore diameter > 1 micron.
- For severe reactions, discontinue and notify doctor.

DRUG & CLASS	INDICATIONS & DOSAGES	NURSING CONSIDERATIONS
amphotericin B cholesteryl sulfate complex Amphotec *Antifungal* Pregnancy Risk Category: B	*Invasive aspergillosis in patients who can't use amphotericin B deoxycholate because of renal impairment, toxicity, or previous treatment failure* — **Adults and children:** 3 to 4 mg/kg/day I.V. Dilute in D_5W and give by continuous infusion at 1 mg/kg/hr. Give test dose before new treatment course, infuse small amount of drug (10 ml of final preparation containing 1.6 to 8.3 mg of drug) over 15 to 30 min and monitor for next 30 min. Can shorten infusion time to 2 hr or lengthen based on patient tolerance.	▪ ***I.V. use:*** Reconstitute with sterile water for injection only and dilute in D_5W. Drug is incompatible with saline, electrolyte solutions, and bacteriostatic agents. ▪ Monitor I&O; report changes in urine appearance or volume. ▪ Monitor renal function tests, LFTs, serum electrolyte levels, CBC, and PT. ▪ Pretreating with antihistamines and corticosteroids and reducing infusion may reduce acute infusion-related reactions. ▪ Monitor vital signs every 30 min during initial therapy. Acute infusion-related reactions usually occur 1 to 3 hr after starting I.V. infusion.
ampicillin sodium/ sulbactam sodium Unasyn *Antibiotic* Pregnancy Risk Category: B	*Intra-abdominal, gynecologic, and skin-structure infections caused by susceptible strains* — **Adults and children ≥ 40 kg (88 lb):** dosage expressed as total drug (each 1.5-g vial contains 1 g ampicillin sodium and 0.5 g sulbactam sodium) — 1.5 to 3 g I.M. or I.V. q 6 hr. Maximum daily dose 4 g sulbactam and 8 g ampicillin (12 g of combined drugs). **Children ≥ 1 yr and < 40 kg:** 300 mg/kg/day I.V. divided equally q 6 hr. ***Adjust-a-dose:*** Dose adjustment necessary in patients with renal insufficiency.	▪ ***I.V. use:*** Give I.V. over 10 to 15 min, or dilute in 50 to 100 ml of compatible diluent and infuse over 15 to 30 min. If permitted, give intermittently. Change site every 48 hr. ▪ Assess history of allergy to penicillin. (Negative history doesn't preclude future reactions.) ▪ Obtain specimen for culture and sensitivity tests before 1st dose. ▪ For I.M. injection, reconstitute with sterile water for injection or 0.5% or 2% lidocaine.

amprenavir Agenerase *Antiretroviral* Pregnancy Risk Category: C	*HIV-1 infection, with other antiretrovirals* — **Adults and children 13 to 16 yr weighing ≥ 50 kg (110 lb):** 1,200 mg P.O. b.i.d. **Children 4 to 12 yr or 13 to 16 yr and weighing < 50 kg:** *Capsules:* 20 mg/kg P.O. b.i.d. or 15 mg/kg P.O. t.i.d. (to maximum of 2,400 mg q.d.). *Oral solution:* 22.5 mg/kg P.O. (1.5 ml/kg) b.i.d. or 17 mg/kg P.O. (1.1 ml/kg) t.i.d. (to maximum of 2,800 mg q.d.). ***Adjust-a-dose:*** Use with caution in patients with moderate or severe hepatic impairment. In those with Child-Pugh score of 5 to 8, reduce capsule dose to 450 mg b.i.d.; with score of 9 to 12, reduce capsule dose to 300 mg b.i.d.	▪ ***ALERT*** Don't give with astemizole, bepridil, cisapride, dihydroergotamine, midazolam, rifampin, sildenafil, triazolam, or vitamin E. Obtain a thorough drug history. ▪ Always use with other antiretroviral agents. ▪ ***ALERT*** Capsules and oral solution are not interchangeable on a mg-per-mg basis. ▪ Use cautiously in patients with sulfonamide allergy. ▪ Instruct patients receiving hormonal contraceptives to use alternative contraceptives during therapy. ▪ High-fat meals may decrease absorption of drug.
anagrelide hydrochloride Agrylin *Anticoagulant* Pregnancy Risk Category: C	*To reduce elevated platelet count and risk of thrombosis and to improve symptoms of essential thrombocythemia* — **Adults:** 0.5 mg P.O. q.i.d. or 1 mg P.O. b.i.d. for ≥ 1 wk; then lowest effective dose to maintain platelet count < 600,000/mm^3 and, ideally, to normal range. Don't increase dosage by > 0.5 mg/day in any 1 wk; maximum 10 mg/day or 2.5 mg in single dose.	▪ Use cautiously in patients with CV disease or serum creatinine > 2 mg/dl and in those with LFT results > 1.5 times the upper normal limits. ▪ Use cautiously in breast-feeding women. ▪ During first 2 wk of treatment, monitor blood counts, LFTs, and renal function tests. ▪ Monitor patient for bleeding, bruising, and cardiac symptoms. ▪ Give drug 1 hr before or 2 hr after meals.
anastrozole Arimidex *Antineoplastic*	*Advanced breast cancer in postmenopausal women with disease progression after tamoxifen therapy* — **Adults:** 1 mg P.O. q.d.	▪ Use cautiously in breast-feeding women.

(continued)

DRUG & CLASS	INDICATIONS & DOSAGES	NURSING CONSIDERATIONS
anastrozole *(continued)* Pregnancy Risk Category: D	*Locally advanced or metastatic breast cancer in postmenopausal women* — **Adults:** 1 mg P.O. q.d. until tumor progression is evident.	▪ Give under supervision of qualified doctor experienced in use of anticancer drugs.
asparaginase (L-asparaginase) Elspar, Kidrolase† *Antineoplastic* Pregnancy Risk Category: C	*Acute lymphocytic leukemia (combined with other drugs)* — **Adults and children:** 1,000 IU/kg I.V. q.d.over 30 min for 10 days; or 6,000 IU/m^2 I.M. at intervals specified in protocol. *Sole induction agent for acute lymphocytic leukemia* — **Adults:** 200 IU/kg I.V. q.d. for 28 days.	▪ ***I.V. use:*** Give through side port of I.V. tubing of infusion of normal saline or D_5W. ▪ Hypersensitivity risk rises with repeated doses. Intradermal skin test needed. ▪ Monitor CBC, bleeding studies, glucose and serum amylase levels. ▪ If drug contacts skin, flush with copious amounts of water for ≥ 15 min. ▪ Limit I.M. injection to 2 ml.
aspirin (acetylsalicylic acid) A.S.A., Ascriptin, Aspergum, Bayer Timed-Release, Bufferin, Ecotrin, Empirin, Halfprin *Nonnarcotic analgesic, anti-inflammatory, antipyretic, antiplatelet agent* Pregnancy Risk Category: C (D in 3rd trimester)	*Rheumatoid arthritis; other inflammatory conditions* — **Adults:** initially, 2.4 to 3.6 g P.O. q.d. in divided doses. Maintenance: 3.2 to 6 g P.O. q.d. in divided doses. *Mild pain or fever* — **Adults and children > 11 yr:** 325 to 650 mg P.O. or P.R. q 4 hr, p.r.n. **Children 2 to 11 yr** : 10 to 15 mg/kg P.O. or P.R. q 4 hr up to 60 to 80 mg/kg/day. *MI prophylaxis; reduction of MI risk in patients with previous MI or unstable angina* — **Adults:** 160 to 325 mg P.O. q.d.	▪ ***ALERT*** Don't give to children or teenagers with chickenpox or flulike illness; always use cautiously. ▪ Give on schedule for inflammatory conditions, rheumatic fever, and thrombosis. ▪ Monitor blood drug levels. Tinnitus may occur at ≥ 30 mg/100 ml. ▪ During prolonged therapy, periodically assess Hct, Hgb, PT, and renal function. ▪ Instruct patient to discontinue aspirin 5 to 7 days before elective surgery.
atenolol Apo-Atenolol†, Noten‡, Nu-Atenol†, Tenormin *Antihypertensive, anti-*	*Hypertension* — **Adults:** initially, 50 mg P.O. q.d. as single dose, increased to 100 mg q.d. after 1 to 2 wk. *Angina pectoris* — **Adults:** 50 mg P.O. q.d.,	▪ If apical pulse < 60, withhold drug and call doctor. ▪ ***I.V. use:*** Give by slow I.V. injection, ≤ 1 mg/min.

anginal Pregnancy Risk Category: D	increased to 100 mg q.d. after 1 wk for optimal effect. Maximum 200 mg q.d. *To reduce CV mortality and risk of reinfarction in acute MI* — **Adults:** 5 mg I.V.; repeat 10 min later. After additional 10 min, 50 mg P.O.; then 50 mg P.O. in 12 hr. Then, 100 mg P.O. q.d. (or 50 mg b.i.d.) for ≥ 1 wk. ***Adjust-a-dose:*** Adjust dosage in patients with CrCl < 35 ml/min.	▪ Monitor BP. ▪ Caution not to increase dosage without consulting doctor. High dosages may lead to arrhythmias. ▪ Instruct patient to take on empty stomach ≥ 2 hr after meals and avoid eating for ≥ 1 hr after taking. ▪ Withdraw gradually over 2 wk.
atorvastatin calcium Lipitor *Antilipemic* Pregnancy Risk Category: X	*Adjunct to diet in primary hypercholesterolemia and mixed dyslipidemia, in elevated serum triglyceride levels, and in primary dysbetalipoproteinemia in patients who don't respond to diet alone* — **Adults:** 10 mg P.O. q.d.; increase p.r.n. to maximum of 80 mg q.d. Dosage based on blood lipid levels drawn 2 to 4 wk after therapy starts. *Alone or as adjunct to lipid-lowering treatments in homozygous familial hypercholesterolemia* — **Adults:** 10 to 80 mg P.O. q.d.	▪ Give only after diet and other nonpharmacologic treatments prove ineffective. ▪ Obtain periodic LFTs and lipid levels before initiating drug, 6 and 12 wk after initiation or after dosage increase, and periodically thereafter. ▪ Watch for signs of myositis.
atovaquone Mepron *Antiprotozoal* Pregnancy Risk Category: C	*Acute, mild to moderate* Pneumocystis carinii *pneumonia in patients who can't tolerate co-trimoxazole* — **Adults:** 750 mg P.O. b.i.d. with food for 21 days. *Prevention of* Pneumocystis carinii *pneumonia in patients who can't tolerate co-trimoxazole* — **Adults and adolescents age 13 to 16:** 1,500 mg (10 ml) P.O. q.d. with food.	▪ Risk of concurrent pulmonary infections; monitor patient closely during therapy. ▪ Instruct patient to take with meals.

†Canadian, ‡Australian

DRUG & CLASS	INDICATIONS & DOSAGES	NURSING CONSIDERATIONS
atropine sulfate (ophthalmic) Atropisol, Atropt‡, BufOpto Atropine, Isopto Atropine *Cycloplegic, mydriatic* Pregnancy Risk Category: C	*Acute iritis, uveitis* — **Adults:** 1 to 2 drops of 1% solution instilled in eyes up to t.i.d., or small strip of ointment applied to conjunctival sac up to t.i.d. **Children:** 1 to 2 drops of 0.5% solution instilled in eyes up to t.i.d., or 0.3 to 0.5 cm of ointment applied to conjunctival sac up to t.i.d. *Cycloplegic refraction* — **Adults:** 1 to 2 drops of 1% solution instilled in eyes 1 hr before refraction. **Children:** 1 to 2 drops of 0.5% solution instilled in eyes b.i.d. for 1 to 3 days before eye exam and 1 hr before refraction.	▪ ***ALERT*** Not for internal use; signs of poisoning are disorientation and confusion. Antidote is physostigmine salicylate. ▪ Watch for signs of glaucoma: increased IOP (ocular pain, headache, progressive blurring of vision). ▪ Apply light pressure on lacrimal sac for 1 min after instillation. ▪ Excessive use in children and in susceptible patients may cause atropine poisoning.
atropine sulfate (systemic) *Antiarrhythmic, vagolytic* Pregnancy Risk Category: C	*Symptomatic bradycardia, bradyarrhythmia* — **Adults:** usually 0.5 to 1 mg I.V. push; repeat q 3 to 5 min to maximum of 2 mg p.r.n. **Children:** 0.01 mg/kg I.V.; may repeat q 4 to 6 hr; maximum of 0.4 mg or 0.3 mg/m^2. *Preoperatively to diminish secretions and block cardiac vagal reflexes* — **Adults and children ≥ 20 kg (44 lb):** 0.4 to 0.6 mg I.M. or S.C. 30 to 60 min before anesthesia. **Children < 20 kg:** 0.01 mg/kg I.M. or S.C. (maximum 0.4 mg) 30 to 60 min before anesthesia.	▪ May give by ET tube. Dose is 2 to 2½ times I.V. dose, diluted with 10 ml 0.9% NaCl or sterile water. ▪ ***I.V. use:*** Give by direct I.V. into large vein or I.V. tubing over ≥ 1 min. ▪ Monitor for paradoxical initial bradycardia (usually disappears within 2 min). ▪ Monitor I&O. Watch for urine retention and urinary hesitancy. ▪ ***ALERT*** Doses < 0.5 mg can cause bradycardia.
attapulgite Children's Kaopectate, Diasorb, Donnagel, Fowler's†, Kaopectate Advanced	*Acute, nonspecific diarrhea* — **Adults and adolescents:** 1.2 to 1.5 g (up to 3 g of Diasorb) P.O. after each loose bowel movement, up to 9 g/24 hr. **Children 6 to 12 yr:** 600 mg	▪ Don't give if diarrhea accompanied by fever or by blood or mucus in stool. ▪ Instruct to take after each loose bowel movement until diarrhea controlled.

Formula, Parepectolin, Rheaban Maximum Strength *Antidiarrheal* Pregnancy Risk Category: NR	(suspension) or 750 mg (tablets) P.O. after each loose bowel movement, up to 4.2 g (suspension) or 4.5 g (tablets) per 24 hr. **Children 3 to 6 yr:** 300 mg P.O. after each loose bowel movement, up to 2.1 g/24 hr.	▪ Tell patient to notify doctor if diarrhea not controlled in 48 hr or if fever develops. ▪ Tell patient to chew tablets well before swallowing or to shake liquid well before measuring dose.
auranofin Ridaura *Antarthritic* Pregnancy Risk Category: C	*Rheumatoid arthritis* — **Adults:** 6 mg P.O. q.d., either as 3 mg b.i.d. or 6 mg q.d. After 6 mo, may increase to 9 mg q.d.	▪ ***ALERT*** Stop drug if monthly platelet count < 100,000/mm^3, if Hgb drops suddenly, if granulocytes < 1,500/mm^3, or if patient develops leukopenia or eosinophilia. ▪ Monitor urinalysis for proteinuria or hematuria.
aurothioglucose Gold-50‡, Solganal **gold sodium thiomalate** Aurolate *Antarthritic* Pregnancy Risk Category: C	*Rheumatoid arthritis* — ***Aurothioglucose:*** **Adults:** 10 mg I.M.; then 25 mg for 2nd and 3rd doses at weekly intervals. Then, 50 mg q wk until 800 mg to 1 g given. If improvement occurs without toxicity, 25 to 50 mg q 3 to 4 wk indefinitely. **Children 6 to 12 yr:** 25% of usual adult dosage. Don't exceed 25 mg/dose. ***Gold sodium thiomalate:*** **Adults:** 10 mg I.M.; then 25 mg in 1 wk. Then, 25 to 50 mg q wk to total dose of 1 g. If improvement occurs without toxicity, 25 to 50 mg q 2 wk for 2 to 20 wk; then, 25 to 50 mg q 3 to 4 wk as maintenance. If relapse occurs, resume injections q wk. **Children:** 10 mg I.M.; then 1 mg/kg I.M. q wk. Follow adult dose intervals.	▪ Watch for anaphylactoid reaction for 30 min after giving. ▪ ***ALERT*** Keep dimercaprol on hand to treat acute toxicity. ▪ Give I.M., as ordered, preferably intragluteally. Drug is pale yellow; don't use if it darkens. ▪ Immerse aurothioglucose vial in warm water; shake vigorously before injecting. ▪ When injecting gold sodium thiomalate, have patient lie down for 10 to 20 min to minimize hypotension. ▪ Analyze urine for protein and sediment changes before each injection. Monitor CBC, platelet count, and LFT results.

†Canadian, ‡Australian

DRUG & CLASS	INDICATIONS & DOSAGES	NURSING CONSIDERATIONS
azathioprine Imuran, Thioprine‡ *Immunosuppressive* Pregnancy Risk Category: D	*Immunosuppression in kidney transplant* — **Adults and children:** initially, 3 to 5 mg/kg P.O. or I.V. q.d., usually starting on day of transplant. Maintain at 1 to 3 mg/kg daily (dosage depends on patient response). *Severe, refractory rheumatoid arthritis* — **Adults:** initially, 1 mg/kg P.O. as single dose or divided b.i.d. If response not satisfactory after 6 to 8 wk, may increase by 0.5 mg/kg q.d. (to maximum of 2.5 mg/kg q.d.) at 4-wk intervals.	▪ ***I.V. use:*** Reconstitute 100-mg vial with 10 ml sterile water for injection. May give by direct I.V. injection or further dilute in 0.9% NaCl for injection or D_5W, and infuse over 30 to 60 min. Use only in patients who can't tolerate oral medications. ▪ Give after meals. ▪ Monitor Hgb and WBC and platelet counts at least q mo, as ordered, more often at beginning of treatment. ▪ Watch for early signs of hepatotoxicity and for increased alkaline phosphatase, bilirubin, AST, and ALT levels. ▪ Reduce dose of azathioprine to 25% to 33% of usual dose when used with allopurinol.
azithromycin Zithromax *Antibiotic* Pregnancy Risk Category: B	*Acute bacterial exacerbations of COPD; mild community-acquired pneumonia; second-line therapy of pharyngitis or tonsillitis caused by susceptible organisms* — **Adults and adolescents ≥ 16 yr:** 500 mg P.O. on day 1; then 250 mg q.d. on days 2 through 5. Total dose 1.5 g. *Otitis media; community-acquired pneumonia* — **Children ≥ 6 mo:** 10 mg/kg P.O. (up to 500 mg) on day 1; then 5 mg/kg (up to 250 mg) on days 2 to 5. *Community-acquired pneumonia in patients requiring initial I.V. therapy* — **Adults and adolescents ≥ 16 yr:** 500 mg I.V. q.d. for 2	▪ ***I.V. use:*** Reconstitute drug in 500-mg vial with 4.8 ml of sterile water for injection. Dilute solution further in ≥ 250 ml of NSS, ½ NSS, D_5W, or lactated Ringer's to yield a concentration range of 1 to 2 mg/ml. ▪ Obtain specimen for culture and sensitivity tests before 1st dose. ▪ Give capsules and multidose suspension 1 hr before or 2 hr after meals. Tablets and single-dose packets for oral suspension can be taken with or without food. ▪ Reduce GI distress by giving with food or milk; don't give with antacids.

Drug	Indications and dosages	Key considerations
	days. Then 500 mg P.O. q.d. to complete a 7- to 10-day course. *Nongonococcal urethritis or cervicitis caused by* C. trachomatis; *chancroid* — **Adults and adolescents ≥ 16 yr:** 1 g P.O. as single dose. *Gonococcal urethritis or cervicitis* — **Adults:** 2 g P.O. as single dose. *Prevention of disseminated MAC disease in advanced HIV infection* — **Adults:** 1,200 mg P.O. q wk, as indicated.	▪ Caution to avoid alcohol and activities requiring alertness until CNS effects known. ▪ Suspension doesn't require refrigeration. ▪ Monitor blood counts (including platelets) during long-term therapy. Watch for signs of blood dyscrasia. ▪ Monitor for superinfection. ▪ ***ALERT*** Infuse a 500-mg dose of azithromycin I.V. over ≥ 1 hr. Never give as bolus or I.M.
aztreonam Azactam *Antibiotic* Pregnancy Risk Category: B	*UTIs, lower respiratory tract infections, septicemia and skin and skin-structure, intra-abdominal, surgical, and gynecologic infections from susceptible gram-negative aerobic organisms; respiratory infections from* H. influenzae — **Adults ≥ 12 yr:** 500 mg to 2 g I.V. or I.M. q 8 to 12 hr. For severe systemic or life-threatening infections, may give 2 g q 6 to 8 hr, up to 8 g q.d. **Children 1 mo to 11 yr:** 30 mg/kg I.V. q 6 to 8 hr, up to 120 mg/kg q.d. ***Adjust-a-dose:*** Reduce dose in patients with impaired renal function or alcoholic cirrhosis.	▪ Obtain culture and sensitivity tests before 1st dose. ▪ ***I.V. use:*** Inject bolus dose slowly (over 3 to 5 min) directly into vein or I.V. tubing. Give infusions over 20 min to 1 hr. ▪ Give I.M. deep into large muscle. Give doses > 1 g I.V. ▪ Don't give I.M. to children.
bacitracin (ophthalmic) AK-Tracin *Ophthalmic antibiotic* Pregnancy Risk Category: NR	*Surface bacterial infections involving conjunctiva and cornea* — **Adults and children:** small amount of ointment applied into conjunctival sac q.d. or p.r.n. until favorable response.	▪ Clean eye area of excessive exudate before application. ▪ Ophthalmic ointment may be stored at room temperature. ▪ Don't touch tip of tube to eye.

DRUG & CLASS	INDICATIONS & DOSAGES	NURSING CONSIDERATIONS
bacitracin (systemic) Baciguent, Baci-IM, Bacitin† *Systemic antibiotic* Pregnancy Risk Category: C	*Pneumonia or empyema from susceptible staphylococci* — **Infants > 2.5 kg (5.5 lb):** 1,000 U/kg I.M. q.d., divided q 8 to 12 hr. **Infants < 2.5 kg:** 900 U/kg q.d., divided q 8 to 12 hr.	▪ Obtain culture and sensitivity tests before 1st dose. ▪ Assess baseline renal function studies before and during therapy; monitor urine output. ▪ Maintain urine pH > 6.0.
bacitracin (topical) Baciguent, Bacitin† *Topical antibiotic* Pregnancy Risk Category: C	*Topical infections, abrasions, cuts, minor burns or wounds* — **Adults and children:** clean area and apply thin film once daily to t.i.d., depending on severity of condition. Don't use for > 1 wk.	▪ Anticipate alternative treatment for burns covering > 20% of body surface. ▪ Prolonged use may result in overgrowth of nonsusceptible organisms. ▪ May cover drug with sterile bandage.
baclofen Clofen‡, Lioresal, Lioresal Intrathecal *Skeletal muscle relaxant* Pregnancy Risk Category: C	*Spasticity in multiple sclerosis, spinal cord injury* — **Adults:** 5 mg P.O. t.i.d. for 3 days, then 10 mg t.i.d. for 3 days, 15 mg t.i.d. for 3 days, 20 mg t.i.d. for 3 days. Increase p.r.n. to maximum of 80 mg q.d. *Management of severe spasticity in patients who can't tolerate or don't respond to oral therapy* — **Adults:** *Test dose:* 1 ml of 50-mcg/ml dilution into intrathecal space by barbotage over ≥ 1 min. If poor response, give 2nd test dose (75 mcg/1.5 ml) 24 hr after 1st. If poor response, give test dose (100 mcg/2 ml) 24 hr later. Patients unresponsive to final test dose shouldn't have implantable pump. Initial maintenance dose titrated based on test-dose response. Effective dose doubled and given over 24 hr. If test-dose	▪ With test dose, markedly decreased severity or frequency of spasms or reduced muscle tone should appear within 4 to 8 hr. ▪ After test dose, give maintenance dose by implantable infusion pump. Most patients need 300 to 800 mcg daily. ▪ Don't give orally to treat muscle spasm caused by rheumatic disorders, cerebral palsy, Parkinson's disease, or CVA; efficacy not established. ▪ Watch for sensitivity reactions, such as skin eruptions and respiratory distress. ▪ Observe for increased risk of seizures in patients with seizure disorder. ▪ Amount of relief determines whether dosage can be reduced. ▪ ***ALERT*** Don't withdraw abruptly after

	efficacy maintained for ≥ 12 hr, don't double dose. After 1st 24 hr, increase dose slowly, p.r.n. and as tolerated, by 10% to 30% q.d.	long-term use unless required by severe adverse reactions; doing so may trigger hallucinations or rebound spasticity.
basiliximab Simulect *Immunosuppressant* Pregnancy Risk Category: B	*To prevent acute organ rejection in renal transplant patients when part of immunosuppressive regimen that includes cyclosporine and corticosteroids* — Used only under the supervision of a doctor qualified and experienced in immunosuppression therapy and management of organ transplant. **Adults ≥ 16 yr:** 20 mg I.V. given within 2 hr before transplant, and 20 mg I.V. given 4 days after transplantation. **Children 2 to 15 yr:** 12 mg/m^2 (up to 20 mg) I.V. given within 2 hr before transplant, and 12 mg/m^2 (up to 20 mg) I.V. given 4 days after transplant.	▪ Reconstitute with 5 ml sterile water for injection. Shake gently to dissolve. Dilute to volume of 50 ml with 0.9% NaCl or dextrose 5% for infusion. When mixing, gently invert bag to avoid foaming. Don't shake. Infuse over 20 to 30 min via central or peripheral vein. Don't add or infuse other drugs through same I.V. line. Use solution immediately. ▪ Use with caution in elderly patients. ▪ Anaphylactoid reactions may occur. ▪ Monitor for electrolyte imbalances and acidosis during therapy. ▪ Monitor I&O, vital signs, Hgb, and Hct.
becaplermin Regranex Gel *Wound repair enhancer* Pregnancy Risk Category: C	*Diabetic neuropathic leg ulcers that extend into or beyond subcutaneous tissue and have adequate blood supply* — **Adults:** apply daily in 1⁄16" thickness to entire surface of wound. If tube size is 2 g, find length of gel to apply by taking wound length (inches) × wound width × 1.3, or wound length (cm) × wound width ÷ 2. If tube size is 7.5 or 15 g, find length of gel to apply by taking wound length (inches) × wound width × 0.6, or wound length (cm) × wound width ÷ 4.	▪ Use as an adjunct to good ulcer care practices (initial sharp debridement, infection control, pressure relief). ▪ Measure ulcer's greatest length and width. Squeeze calculated length of gel onto clean measuring surface, such as waxed paper. Use cotton swab or other applicator to transfer and spread drug over entire ulcer area. Place saline-moistened dressing over site and leave in place for 12 hr. Then remove dressing and rinse away residual gel with 0.9% NaCl or water; *(continued)*

DRUG & CLASS	INDICATIONS & DOSAGES	NURSING CONSIDERATIONS
becaplermin *(continued)*		apply fresh, moist dressing without becaplermin for rest of day. Recalculate dose at least q wk. ▪ Monitor for application site reactions.
beclomethasone dipropionate (nasal) Beconase AQ Nasal Spray, Beconase Nasal Inhaler, Vancenase AQ Double Strength, Vancenase AQ Nasal Spray, Vancenase Nasal Inhaler *Anti-inflammatory* Pregnancy Risk Category: C	*Seasonal or perennial rhinitis, prevention of nasal polyps recurrence after surgical removal* — **Adults and children > 12 yr:** usual dosage 1 or 2 sprays in each nostril b.i.d. to q.i.d. **Children 6 to 12 yr:** 1 spray in each nostril t.i.d. ***Double-strength form*** — **Adults and children > 6 yr:** 1 or 2 sprays in each nostril once daily.	▪ Observe for fungal infections. ▪ Not effective for acute rhinitis exacerbations. Decongestants or antihistamines may be needed. ▪ Don't use longer than 3 wk if no improvement noted.
beclomethasone dipropionate (oral inhalant) Becloforte Inhaler‡, Beclovent, Vanceril, Vanceril Double Strength *Anti-inflammatory, antiasthmatic* Pregnancy Risk Category: C	*Steroid-dependent asthma* — **Adults and children ≥ 12 yr:** 2 inhalations t.i.d. or q.i.d. or 4 inhalations b.i.d., up to 20 inhalations (840 mcg) q.d. Or, 2 inhalations of double-strength formulation (168 mcg) b.i.d., to a maximum of 10 inhalations q.d. **Children 6 to 12 yr:** 1 to 2 inhalations t.i.d. or q.i.d. or 2 to 4 inhalations b.i.d., up to 10 inhalations (420 mcg) q.d. Or, 2 inhalations of double-strength formulation (168 mcg) b.i.d. up to a maximum of 5 inhalations q.d.	▪ ***ALERT*** Taper P.O. therapy slowly. Acute adrenal insufficiency and death have occurred in asthmatics who changed abruptly from P.O. corticosteroids to beclomethasone. ▪ Spacer device may ensure proper dose and decrease local (oral) adverse effects. ▪ Rinse mouth with water after each use. ▪ ***ALERT*** Check package labeling carefully; different strengths are available.

benazepril hydrochloride Lotensin *Antihypertensive* Pregnancy Risk Category: C (D in 2nd and 3rd trimesters)	*Hypertension* — **Adults:** in patients not receiving diuretics, 10 mg P.O. q.d. initially. Most patients receive 20 to 40 mg q.d. in 1 or 2 doses; patient receiving diuretic, 5 mg P.O. q.d. ***Adjust-a-dose:*** Give patients with CrCl < 30 ml/min 5 mg P.O. q.d.; may increase to 40 mg q.d.	▪ Measure BP 2 to 6 hr after dose and just before next dose. Monitor for hypotension. ▪ Assess renal and hepatic function before and during therapy. Monitor serum potassium levels. ▪ Safety and efficacy of doses over 80 mg have not been established.
benzonatate Tessalon *Nonnarcotic antitussive* Pregnancy Risk Category: C	*Symptomatic relief of cough* — **Adults and children > 10 yr:** 100 mg P.O. t.i.d.; may increase to 600 mg q.d., p.r.n.	▪ Don't give when cough is valuable diagnostic sign or is beneficial. ▪ Don't crush capsules. ▪ Monitor cough type and frequency. ▪ Use with percussion and chest vibration.
benztropine mesylate Apo-Benztropine†, Cogentin, PMS-Benztropine† *Antiparkinsonian* Pregnancy Risk Category: C	*Drug-induced extrapyramidal disorders (except tardive dyskinesia)* — **Adults:** 1 to 4 mg P.O. or I.M. once daily or b.i.d. *Acute dystonic reaction* — **Adults:** 1 to 2 mg I.V. or I.M.; then 1 to 2 mg P.O. b.i.d. *Parkinsonism* — **Adults:** 0.5 to 6 mg P.O. or I.M. daily. Initial dose 0.5 mg to 1 mg, increased by 0.5 mg q 5 to 6 days. Adjust dosage to meet individual requirements.	▪ Give initial dose h.s. ▪ Never discontinue abruptly. ▪ Monitor vital signs carefully. Watch for adverse reactions, especially in elderly or debilitated patients. ▪ May aggravate tardive dyskinesia. ▪ Watch for intermittent constipation and abdominal distention and pain; may indicate onset of paralytic ileus.
bepridil hydrochloride Bepadin‡, Vascor *Antianginal* Pregnancy Risk Category: C	*Chronic stable angina in patients who can't tolerate or don't respond to other agents* — **Adults:** initially, 200 mg P.O. q.d. After 10 days, increase dosage based on response. Maintenance dosage in most patients 300 mg q.d. Maximum 400 mg q.d.	▪ Use cautiously in left bundle-branch block, sinus bradycardia, impaired renal or hepatic function, or heart failure. ▪ ***ALERT*** Can cause severe ventricular arrhythmias. ▪ Don't adjust dosage more often than q 10 to 14 days.

†Canadian ‡Australian

DRUG & CLASS	INDICATIONS & DOSAGES	NURSING CONSIDERATIONS
beractant (natural lung surfactant) Survanta *Lung surfactant* Pregnancy Risk Category: NR	*Prevention of respiratory distress syndrome (RDS) in premature neonates ≤ 1,250 g at birth or having symptoms of surfactant deficiency* — **Neonates:** 4 ml/kg intratracheally; give each dose in 4 quarter-doses; in between, use handheld resuscitation bag at rate of 60 breaths/min and sufficient oxygen to prevent cyanosis. Give within 15 min of birth, if possible. Repeat in 6 hr if respiratory distress continues. Give no more than 4 doses in 48 hr. *Rescue treatment of RDS in premature neonates* — **Neonates:** 4 ml/kg intratracheally; before giving, increase ventilator rate to 60 with inspiratory time of 0.5 sec and FiO_2 of 1. Give each dose in 4 quarter-doses; in between, continue ventilation for 30 sec or until stable. Give dose as soon as RDS confirmed. Repeat in 6 hr if distress continues. Give no more than 4 doses in 48 hr.	▪ Continuous monitoring of ECG and SaO_2 essential; frequent arterial BP monitoring and frequent ABG sampling highly desirable. ▪ Accurate weight determination essential to proper dosage measurements. ▪ ***ALERT*** Can rapidly affect oxygenation and lung compliance. May need to adjust peak ventilator inspiratory pressures if chest expansion improves markedly after administration. Notify doctor and adjust immediately as directed.
betamethasone Betnesol†, Celestone **betamethasone acetate and betamethasone sodium phosphate** Celestone Soluspan **betamethasone sodium phosphate**	*Conditions with severe inflammation, conditions requiring immunosuppression* — **Adults:** 0.6 to 7.2 mg P.O. q.d.; or 0.5 to 9 mg I.M., I.V., or into joint or soft tissue q.d. Betamethasone sodium phosphate-acetate suspension 6 to 12 mg injected into large joints or 1.5 to 6 mg injected into smaller joints. May give both injections q 1 to 2 wk, p.r.n. *Note:* Betamethasone sodium phos-	▪ Don't use for alternate-day therapy. ▪ Obtain baseline weight before starting therapy and weigh daily; report sudden gain. ▪ ***ALERT*** For better results and less toxicity, give once-daily dose in morning. ▪ To reduce GI irritation, give with milk or food. ▪ Monitor blood glucose and serum potassi-

Celestone Phosphate *Anti-inflammatory* Pregnancy Risk Category: C	phate and betamethasone acetate suspension combination product should *not* be given I.V.	um regularly, as ordered. Diabetics may require insulin dosage adjustments.
betamethasone dipropionate Alphatrex, Diprolene, Diprolene AF, Diprosone, Maxivate **betamethasone valerate** Betatrex, Beta-Val, Betnovate†‡, Luxiq, Valisone *Anti-inflammatory* Pregnancy Risk Category: C	*Inflammation from corticosteroid-responsive dermatoses* — **Adults and children:** clean area; apply cream, ointment, lotion, or aerosol spray sparingly. Give dipropionate once daily or b.i.d.; valerate once daily to q.i.d. Maximum dosage 45 g/wk for Diprolene cream, 50 ml/wk for Diprolene lotion.	▪ Gently wash skin before applying. Rub in gently, leaving thin coat. When treating hairy sites, part hair and apply directly to lesions. For eczematous dermatitis, hold dressing in place with gauze, elastic bandage, stocking, or stockinette. ▪ Don't apply near eyes or mucous membranes or in ear canal. ▪ Notify doctor and remove occlusive dressing if fever, infection, striae, or atrophy occurs. ▪ Don't discontinue abruptly.
betaxolol hydrochloride (ophthalmic) Betoptic, Betoptic S, *Antiglaucoma agent* Pregnancy Risk Category: C	*Chronic open-angle glaucoma and ocular hypertension* — **Adults:** 1 or 2 drops of 0.5% solution or 0.25% suspension b.i.d.	▪ Shake suspension well before instilling. ▪ Wash hands before and after instilling. Apply light finger pressure on lacrimal sac for 1 min after instillation. Don't touch dropper tip to eye or surrounding tissue. ▪ Patient may need several weeks of treatment to stabilize IOP-lowering response. Determine IOP after 4 wk.
betaxolol hydrochloride (oral) Kerlone *Antihypertensive* Pregnancy Risk Category: C	*Hypertension (used alone or with other antihypertensives)* — **Adults:** initially, 10 mg P.O. q.d.; if necessary, 20 mg P.O. q.d. if desired response not achieved in 7 to 14 days. For elderly patients, consider 5 mg P.O. initially.	▪ May mask tachycardia associated with hyperthyroidism. In suspected thyrotoxicosis, withdraw gradually, as ordered. ▪ Abrupt discontinuation may trigger angina pectoris in unrecognized CAD. ▪ Monitor BP closely.

†Canadian ‡Australian

DRUG & CLASS	INDICATIONS & DOSAGES	NURSING CONSIDERATIONS
bethanechol chloride Duvoid, Myotonachol, Urecholine, Urocarb Tablets‡ *Urinary tract and GI tract stimulant* Pregnancy Risk Category: C	*Acute postoperative and postpartum nonobstructive urine retention; neurogenic atony of urinary bladder with urine retention* — **Adults:** 10 to 50 mg P.O. t.i.d. to q.i.d. Or 2.5 to 5 mg S.C. Never give I.M. or I.V. For urine retention, may require 50 to 100 mg P.O. per dose. Use such doses with extreme caution. *Test dose:* 2.5 mg S.C., repeated at 15- to 30-min intervals to total of 4 doses to determine minimal effective dose; then use minimal effective dose q 6 to 8 hr. All doses adjusted individually.	▪ Never give I.M. or I.V. ▪ Give on empty stomach; otherwise, may cause nausea and vomiting. ▪ Monitor vital signs frequently, especially respirations. Always have atropine injection available. ▪ ***ALERT*** Watch for toxicity. Edrophonium ineffective against muscle relaxation caused by bethanechol. ▪ Inform patient that drug is usually effective within 30 to 90 min after oral dose and 5 to 15 min after S.C. dose.
bexarotene Targretin *Tumor cell growth inhibitor* Pregnancy Risk Category: X	*Cutaneous T-cell lymphoma refractory to previous systemic therapy* — **Adults:** 300 mg/m²/day P.O. as single dose with meal. If no response after 8 wk, and 1st dose was tolerated, increase to 400 mg/m²/day. ***Adjust-a-dose:*** Lower dose for patients with hepatic insufficiency. If toxicity occurs, may adjust dose to 200 mg/m²/day, then to 100 mg/m²/day; or temporarily stop drug. When toxicity is controlled, doses may be carefully readjusted upward.	▪ ***ALERT*** Women of childbearing age should use effective contraception ≥ 1 mo before therapy starts, during therapy, and for ≥ 1 mo after therapy stops. During therapy, two reliable forms of contraception should be used simultaneously, unless abstinence is chosen. Pregnancy test result must be negative 1 wk before starting therapy and monthly during therapy. ▪ Start therapy on the 2nd or 3rd day of a normal menstrual period. ▪ Check total cholesterol, HDL cholesterol, and triglyceride levels when therapy starts; repeat weekly until lipid response is established (2 to 4 wk) and q 8 wk thereafter. If triglyceride levels increase during

		therapy, patient should receive antilipemics, and bexarotene dose may be reduced or suspended p.r.n. ▪ Monitor LFT results at baseline and after 1, 2, and 4 wk of treatment. If stable, monitor every 8 wk during treatment. Consider suspending treatment if LFT results reach 3 times the upper limit of normal.
bisacodyl Bisac-Evac, Bisacodyl Uniserts, Dacodyl, Deficol, Dulcagen, Dulcolax, Durolax‡, Fleet Bisacodyl, Fleet Bisacodyl Prep, Fleet Laxative, Theralax *Stimulant laxative* Pregnancy Risk Category: B	*Chronic constipation; preparation for delivery, surgery, or rectal or bowel examination* — **Adults and children > 12 yr:** 10 to 15 mg P.O. h.s. or before breakfast. May give up to 30 mg P.O. or 10 mg P.R. for evacuation before examination or surgery. **Children 6 to 12 yr:** 5 mg P.O. or P.R. h.s. or before breakfast. Oral form not recommended if unable to swallow tablet whole.	▪ Soft, formed stools usually produced 15 to 60 min after giving P.R. ▪ For constipation, ask if patient has adequate fluid intake, exercise, and diet. ▪ Avoid embedding suppositories in fecal material; may delay drug onset. ▪ Don't crush tablets; they must be swallowed whole. ▪ Don't give within 1 hr of milk or antacid. ▪ Discourage excessive use.
bismuth subsalicylate Bismatrol, Pepto-Bismol, Pink Bismuth *Antidiarrheal* Pregnancy Risk Category: C	*Mild, nonspecific diarrhea* — **Adults:** 30 ml or 2 tablets P.O. q ½ to 1 hr, to maximum of 8 doses for ≤ 2 days. **Children 9 to 12 yr:** 15 ml or 1 tablet P.O. **Children 6 to 9 yr:** 10 ml or ⅔ tablet P.O. **Children 3 to 6 yr:** 5 ml or ⅓ tablet P.O. *Note:* Give children's doses q ½ to 1 hr, to maximum of 8 doses for ≤ 2 days.	▪ Use cautiously in patients taking aspirin. ▪ ***ALERT*** Don't use in children with chickenpox or flu. ▪ Shake suspension well before use. ▪ Tell patient that drug may darken stools. ▪ Avoid use before GI radiologic procedures.
bisoprolol fumarate Zebeta	*Hypertension (drug used alone or in combination)* — **Adults:** 5 mg P.O. q.d. If response inadequate, increase to 10 to 20	▪ Use cautiously in bronchospastic disease, diabetes, PVD, or thyroid disease and in history of heart failure. *(continued)*

†Canadian ‡Australian

DRUG & CLASS	INDICATIONS & DOSAGES	NURSING CONSIDERATIONS
bisoprolol fumarate *(continued)* *Antihypertensive* Pregnancy Risk Category: C	mg P.O. q.d. Maximum dose 20 mg q.d. ***Adjust-a-dose:*** In patients with hepatic insufficiency or CrCl < 40 ml/min, start dose at 2.5 mg q.d.	▪ Monitor BP frequently. ▪ May mask hypoglycemia signs.
bleomycin sulfate Blenoxane *Antineoplastic* Pregnancy Risk Category: D	*Squamous cell carcinoma; lymphosarcoma; reticulum cell carcinoma; testicular carcinoma* — **Adults:** 10 to 20 U/m² I.V., I.M., or S.C. once or twice q wk to total of 300 to 400 U. *Hodgkin's disease* — **Adults:** 10 to 20 U/m² I.V., I.M., or S.C. once or twice/wk. After 50% response, maintenance dosage is 1 U I.M. or I.V. q.d. or 5 U I.M. or I.V./wk. *Malignant pleural effusion; prevention of recurrent pleural effusions* — **Adults:** 60 U in 50 to 100 ml 0.9% NaCl as single-dose bolus intrapleural injection.	▪ Dosage and indications may vary. ▪ Obtain pulmonary function tests as ordered. Pulmonary toxicity may increase in patients receiving radiation therapy. ▪ Watch for hypersensitivity reactions. May need to give test dose. Monitor for fever, which may be treated with antipyretics. ▪ Reconstitute per manufacturer's labeling. Give I.V. infusion over 10 min. ▪ ***ALERT*** Pulmonary toxicity increases dramatically when total dose is > 400 U and in patients > 70 yr.
bretylium tosylate Bretylate†, Bretylol *Antiarrhythmic* Pregnancy Risk Category: C	*Ventricular fibrillation or hemodynamically unstable ventricular tachycardia unresponsive to other antiarrhythmics* — **Adults:** 5 mg/kg I.V. push over 1 min. If necessary, increase dose to 10 mg/kg and repeat q 15 to 30 min until 30 mg/kg given. For continuous suppression, diluted solution given at 1 to 2 mg/min continuously or 5 to 10 mg/kg diluted and given over > 8 min q 6 hr.	▪ To prevent nausea and vomiting, follow dosage directions carefully. ▪ Keep patient supine until tolerance to hypotension develops. ▪ ***ALERT*** Monitor patient closely for transient hypertension and arrhythmias. ▪ Monitor BP and HR continuously. ▪ Observe susceptible patients for increased angina.

bromocriptine mesylate Parlodel *Antiparkinsonian, inhibitor of prolactin release, inhibitor of growth hormone release* Pregnancy Risk Category: B	*Amenorrhea and galactorrhea from hyperprolactinemia; female infertility* — **Adults:** 1.25 to 2.5 mg P.O. q.d., increased by 2.5 mg q.d. at 3- to 7-day intervals until response achieved. Therapeutic dosage range 2.5 to 15 mg/q.d. *Parkinson's disease* — **Adults:** 1.25 mg P.O. b.i.d. with meals. Increase dose q 14 to 28 days, up to 100 mg q.d., p.r.n. *Acromegaly* — **Adults:** 1.25 to 2.5 mg P.O. with snack h.s. for 3 days. Additional 1.25 to 2.5 mg may be added q 3 to 7 days until benefit obtained. Maximum 100 mg/q.d.	▪ Monitor for adverse reactions. Incidence of such reactions high, especially at start of therapy; however, most are mild to moderate, with nausea being most common. ▪ For Parkinson's disease, usually given in conjunction with levodopa or levodopa-carbidopa. ▪ Give with meals. ▪ May lead to early postpartum conception. Test for pregnancy q 4 wk or whenever period missed after menses resumes.
brompheniramine maleate Bromphen, Chlorphed, Codimal-A, Dimetane, Veltane *Antihistamine (H_1-receptor antagonist)* Pregnancy Risk Category: C	*Rhinitis, allergy symptoms* — **Adults:** 4 to 8 mg P.O. t.i.d. or q.i.d.; or 8 to 12 mg extended-release P.O. b.i.d. or t.i.d. Maximum P.O. dose 24 mg/day. Or, 5 to 20 mg q 6 to 12 hr I.M., I.V., or S.C. Maximum parenteral dose 40 mg/day. **Children 6 to 12 yr:** 2 to 4 mg P.O. t.i.d. or q.i.d.; or 8 to 12 mg extended-release P.O. q 12 hr; or 0.5 mg/kg I.M., I.V., or S.C. q.d. divided t.i.d. or q.i.d. **Children < 6 yr:** 0.5 mg/kg P.O., I.M., I.V., or S.C. q.d. divided t.i.d. or q.i.d.	▪ ***I.V. use:*** Can give injectable form containing 10 mg/ml diluted or undiluted very slowly I.V. ▪ Don't give 100 mg/ml injection I.V. ▪ Monitor blood count during long-term therapy, as ordered; observe for blood dyscrasia. ▪ Children < 12 yr should use only as directed by doctor.
budesonide (nasal) Rhinocort *Anti-inflammatory* Pregnancy Risk Category: C	*Symptoms of seasonal or perennial allergic rhinitis* — **Adults and children ≥ 6 yr:** 2 sprays in each nostril in a.m. and p.m., or 4 sprays in each nostril in a.m. Maintenance dose is fewest sprays needed.	▪ Shake well before use. ▪ Instruct patient to avoid exposure to chickenpox or measles. ▪ Don't break or incinerate canister or store in extreme heat.

†Canadian ‡Australian

DRUG & CLASS	INDICATIONS & DOSAGES	NURSING CONSIDERATIONS
budesonide (oral inhalant) Pulmicort Turbuhaler, Pulmicort Respules *Anti-inflammatory* Pregnancy Risk Category: C	Turbuhaler — *Prophylactic therapy in asthma maintenance* — **Adults previously on bronchodilators alone:** initially, 200 to 400 mcg inhaled b.i.d., to maximum 400 mcg b.i.d. **Adults previously on inhaled corticosteroids:** initially, 200 to 400 mcg inhaled b.i.d., to maximum 800 mcg b.i.d. **Adults previously on oral corticosteroids:** initially, 400 to 800 mcg inhaled b.i.d., to maximum 800 mcg b.i.d. **Children > 6 yr previously on bronchodilators alone or inhaled corticosteroids:** initially, 200 mcg inhaled b.i.d., to maximum 400 mcg b.i.d. **Children > 6 yr previously on oral corticosteroids:** maximum dose 400 mcg inhaled b.i.d. *Note:* In all patients, use lowest effective dose after patient stabilizes. Respules — *Prophylactic therapy in asthma maintenance* — **Children 1 to 8 yr previously on bronchodilators alone:** 0.5 mg inhaled once daily or 0.25 mg b.i.d. **Children 1 to 8 yr previously on inhaled corticosteroids:** 0.5 mg once daily or b.i.d. **Children 1 to 8 yr previously on oral corticosteroids:** 0.5 mg b.i.d. or 1 mg once daily.	▪ Use cautiously, if at all, in patients with TB of the respiratory tract; untreated systemic fungal, bacterial, viral, or parasitic infections; or ocular herpes. ▪ Use caution when transferring from systemic steroid to budesonide; gradually decrease steroid dose to prevent adrenal insufficiency. ▪ If bronchospasm occurs after giving drug, stop therapy and treat with bronchodilator. ▪ Lung function may improve within 24 hr of starting treatment, although full benefit may not occur for ≥ 1 to 2 wk. ▪ Watch for *Candida* infections of mouth or pharynx. ▪ ***ALERT*** Corticosteroid use may increase risk of developing serious or fatal infections in patients exposed to viral illnesses, such as chickenpox or measles. ▪ Respules are inhaled using a jet nebulizer connected to an air compressor. ▪ Don't mix Respules with other medications that can be nebulized.

bumetanide Bumex, Burinex‡ *Diuretic* Pregnancy Risk Category: C	*Edema in heart failure or hepatic or renal disease* — **Adults:** 0.5 to 2 mg P.O. q.d. as single dose. If diuretic response inadequate, may give 2nd or 3rd dose at 4- to 5-hr intervals. Maximum 10 mg/day. May be given I.V. if P.O. not feasible. Usual initial dose 0.5 to 1 mg, given I.V. or I.M. If response inadequate, may give 2nd or 3rd dose at 2- to 3-hr intervals. Maximum 10 mg/day.	▪ ***I.V. use:*** Give direct I.V. doses over 1 to 2 min. For intermittent infusion, give diluted at ordered rate. ▪ Intermittent dosage is safest and most effective way to control edema. ▪ Monitor I&O, weight, BP, pulse, oxygen, and serum electrolyte, BUN, creatinine, glucose, and uric acid levels. ▪ Watch for signs of hypokalemia.
bupropion hydrochloride (antidepressant) Wellbutrin, Wellbutrin SR *Antidepressant* Pregnancy Risk Category: B	*Depression* — **Adults:** initially, 100 mg P.O. b.i.d., increased after 3 days to 100 mg P.O. t.i.d., if needed. If no response after several weeks of therapy, increase to 150 mg t.i.d. No single dose should exceed 150 mg. For sustained-release tablets, initially 150 mg P.O. q.d. Increase to 150 mg P.O. b.i.d. as early as day 4 of dosing.	▪ May cause agitation, insomnia, or anxiety. ▪ To minimize risk of seizure, don't exceed 450 mg/day, and give daily dosage in 3 to 4 equally divided doses. ▪ Closely monitor patients with history of bipolar disorders.
bupropion hydrochloride (nicotine replacement) Zyban *Nicotine replacement, antidepressant* Pregnancy Risk Category: B	*Aid to smoking cessation* — **Adults:** 150 mg P.O. daily for 3 days; increased to maximum of 300 mg P.O. daily given in 2 divided doses at least 8 hr apart. Tapering dose is not required.	▪ Start therapy while patient is still smoking; about 1 wk is required to achieve steady-state plasma drug levels. ▪ ***ALERT*** To reduce seizure risk, don't exceed daily dose of 300 mg. Divide dose (150 mg b.i.d.) so that no single dose exceeds 150 mg. ▪ Stop therapy if patient hasn't made progress by wk 7 of therapy.

DRUG & CLASS	INDICATIONS & DOSAGES	NURSING CONSIDERATIONS
buspirone hydrochloride BuSpar *Anxiolytic* Pregnancy Risk Category: B	*Short-term relief of anxiety* — **Adults:** initially, 5 mg P.O. t.i.d., increased at 3-day intervals in 5-mg increments. Usual maintenance dosage 20 to 30 mg daily in divided doses. Don't exceed 60 mg daily.	▪ Monitor closely for adverse CNS reactions. ▪ Less sedating than other anxiolytics. ▪ Drug has no potential for abuse. ▪ Warn patient taking benzodiazepine against stopping that drug abruptly.
busulfan Myleran *Antineoplastic* Pregnancy Risk Category: D	*Palliative treatment of chronic myelocytic leukemia* — **Adults:** 4 to 8 mg P.O. q.d., up to 12 mg P.O. q.d., until WBC $\leq$ 15,000/mm^3; drug stopped until WBC $\geq$ 50,000/mm^3, and then resumed as before; or 4 to 8 mg P.O. q.d. until WBC $\leq$ 10,000 to 20,000/mm^3; then daily dose reduced p.r.n. to maintain WBC at this level (usually 1 to 3 mg q.d.). **Children:** 0.06 to 0.12 mg/kg/day or 1.8 to 4.6 mg/m^2/day P.O.; adjust dosage to maintain WBC count at 20,000/mm^3 but never $<$ 10,000/mm^3.	▪ To prevent bleeding, avoid all I.M. injections when platelet count $<$ 100,000/mm^3. ▪ Give drug at same time each day. ▪ Monitor patient response (increased appetite and sense of well-being, decreased total WBC count, reduced spleen size), which usually begins within 1 to 2 wk. ▪ Monitor serum uric acid. To prevent hyperuricemia, allopurinol may be ordered. Keep patient adequately hydrated. ▪ Anticipate possible blood transfusion. ▪ Toxicity can accompany therapeutic effects.
butorphanol tartrate Stadol, Stadol NS *Analgesic, adjunct to anesthesia* Pregnancy Risk Category: C	*Moderate to severe pain* — **Adults:** 1 to 4 mg I.M. q 3 to 4 hr, p.r.n. or around the clock; or 0.5 to 2 mg I.V. q 3 to 4 hr, p.r.n. or around the clock. Not to exceed 4 mg per dose. Or, 1 mg intranasally q 3 to 4 hr (1 spray in 1 nostril); repeated in 60 to 90 min if pain relief inadequate. *Preoperative anesthesia or preanesthesia* — **Adults:** 2 mg I.M. 60 to 90 min before surgery.	▪ Periodically monitor postoperative vital signs and bladder function. ▪ Respiratory depression apparently doesn't increase with larger dose. ▪ Psychological and physical addiction may occur.

calcitonin (human)
Cibacalcin
calcitonin (salmon)
Calcimar, Miacalcin, Miacalcin Nasal Spray, Osteocalcin, Salmonine
Hypocalcemic
Pregnancy Risk Category: C

Paget's disease of bone (osteitis deformans) — **Adults:** 100 IU of calcitonin (salmon) q.d. S.C. or I.M.; maintenance dose is 50 to 100 IU q.d. or every other day. Or, calcitonin (human) 0.5 mg 2 or 3 times weekly or 0.25 mg q.d., up to 0.5 mg b.i.d.
Hypercalcemia — **Adults:** 4 IU/kg of calcitonin (salmon) q 12 hr I.M. If poor response after 1 or 2 days, increase to 8 IU/kg I.M. q 12 hr. If response remains poor after 2 more days, increase to maximum 8 IU/kg I.M. q 6 hr.
Postmenopausal osteoporosis — **Adults:** 100 IU of calcitonin (salmon) q.d. I.M. or S.C. Or, 200 IU (1 activation) of calcitonin (salmon) q.d. intranasally, alternating nostrils q.d.

- Skin test usually done before therapy.
- ***ALERT*** Systemic allergic reactions possible. Keep epinephrine handy.
- Use reconstituted solution within 2 hr.
- Observe for signs of hypocalcemic tetany.
- Facial flushing and warmth may occur within minutes of injection and usually last about 1 hr.
- Monitor serum calcium, alkaline phosphatase, and 24-hr urine hydroxyproline levels closely.
- Store calcitonin (human) at room temperature; refrigerate calcitonin (salmon).

---

calcitriol (1,25-dihydroxycholecalciferol)
Calcijex, Rocaltrol
Antihypocalcemic
Pregnancy Risk Category: A (D if given in doses above RDA)

Hypocalcemia in patients undergoing chronic dialysis — **Adults:** 0.25 mcg P.O. q.d. Increased by 0.25 mcg q.d. q 4 to 8 wk. Maintenance is 0.25 mcg every other day, up to 1.25 mcg q.d.
Hypoparathyroidism and pseudohypoparathyroidism — **Adults and children > 6 yr:** 0.25 mcg P.O. q.d. May be increased q 2 to 4 wk. Maintenance, 0.25 to 2 mcg q.d.
Hypoparathyroidism — **Children 1 to 6 yr:** 0.25 to 0.75 mcg P.O. q.d.
Management of secondary hyperparathyroidism and resultant metabolic bone disease in predialysis patients (moderate to se-

- Monitor serum calcium level. Stop drug and notify doctor if hypercalcemia occurs.
- Protect from heat and light.
- Tell patient to immediately report weakness, nausea, vomiting, dry mouth, constipation, muscle or bone pain, or metallic taste.
- Drug shouldn't be taken without a prescription for it.

(continued)

DRUG & CLASS	INDICATIONS & DOSAGES	NURSING CONSIDERATIONS
calcitriol *(continued)*	*vere chronic renal failure with CrCl of 15 to 55 ml/min)* — **Adults and children ≥ 3:** initially, 0.25 mcg P.O. q.d. May be increased to 0.5 mcg/q.d., p.r.n. **Children < 3:** initially, 10 to 15 ng/kg P.O. q.d.	
calcium acetate Phos-Lo **calcium chloride** Calciject† **calcium citrate** Citracal, Cal-citrate 250 **calcium glubionate** Neo-Calglucon **calcium gluceptate** **calcium gluconate** **calcium lactate** **calcium phosphate, tribasic** Posture *Therapeutic agent for electrolyte balance, cardiotonic* Pregnancy Risk Category: C	*Hypocalcemic emergency* — **Adults:** 7 to 14 mEq calcium I.V. (as 10% gluconate solution, 2% to 10% chloride solution, or 22% gluceptate solution). **Children:** 1 to 7 mEq calcium I.V. **Infants:** up to 1 mEq calcium I.V. *Hypocalcemic tetany* — **Adults:** 4.5 to 16 mEq calcium I.V. Repeat until controlled. **Children:** 0.5 to 0.7 mEq/kg calcium I.V. t.i.d. to q.i.d. until controlled. **Neonates:** 2.4 mEq/kg I.V. q.d. in divided doses. *Adjunct treatment for cardiac arrest* — **Adults:** 0.027 to 0.054 mEq/kg calcium chloride I.V., 4.5 to 6.3 mEq calcium gluceptate I.V., or 2.3 to 3.7 mEq calcium gluconate I.V. **Children:** 0.27 mEq/kg calcium chloride I.V. May repeat in 10 min; check serum calcium levels before giving further doses. *Adjunct treatment for magnesium intoxication* — **Adults:** initially, 7 mEq I.V. Subsequent doses based on response. *During exchange transfusions* — **Adults:** 1.35 mEq I.V. concurrently with each 100 ml citrated blood. **Neonates:** 0.45 mEq I.V. af-	▪ Use all calcium products with extreme caution in patients with sarcoidosis and renal or cardiac disease, and in digitalized patients. ▪ ***I.V. use (direct injection):*** Give slowly through small needle into large vein or I.V. line with free-flowing, compatible solution at maximum 1 ml/min (1.5 mEq/min) for chloride, 1.5 to 5 ml/min for gluconate, and 2 ml/min for gluceptate. Don't use scalp veins. ***(Intermittent infusion):*** Infuse diluted solution through I.V. line with compatible solution at maximum rate of 200 mg/min for gluceptate and gluconate. ▪ ***ALERT*** Give chloride and gluconate I.V. only. Use in-line filter. ▪ ***ALERT*** Drug will precipitate if given I.V. with alkaline drugs. ▪ Monitor ECG when giving calcium I.V. Stop for complaints of discomfort, and notify doctor. Following I.V. injection, patient should remain recumbent for 15 min. ▪ Ensure that doctor specifies form of calci-

	ter each 100 ml citrated blood. *Hyperphosphatemia* — **Adults:** 1,334 to 2,000 mg P.O. acetate t.i.d. with meals. Dialysis patients need 3 to 4 tablets with meals.	um to be used. ▪ Monitor blood calcium levels frequently. ▪ Severe necrosis and tissue sloughing can occur after extravasation.
calcium carbonate Alka-Mints, CalCarb-HD, Calcarb 600, Calci-Chew, Caltrate 600, Chooz, Os-Cal 500, Rolaids Calcium Rich, Tums *Therapeutic agent for electrolyte balance* Pregnancy Risk Category: NR	*Antacid* — **Adults:** 350 mg to 1.5 g P.O., or 2 pieces of chewing gum 1 hr after meals and h.s., p.r.n. *Dietary supplement* — **Adults:** 500 mg to 2 g P.O. b.i.d. to q.i.d.	▪ Watch for nausea, vomiting, headache, mental confusion, and anorexia. ▪ Monitor serum calcium level. ▪ Record amount and consistency of stools. ▪ Tell patient to shake suspension and take with small amount of water.
calcium polycarbophil Equalactin, Fiberall, Fiber-Con, Fiber-Lax, FiberNorm, Mitrolan *Bulk laxative, antidiarrheal* Pregnancy Risk Category: NR	*Constipation; diarrhea from irritable bowel syndrome; acute nonspecific diarrhea* — **Adults:** 1 g P.O. q.i.d., p.r.n. Maximum 6 g in 24-hr period. **Children 6 to 12 yr:** 500 mg P.O. once daily to t.i.d., p.r.n. Maximum 3 g in 24-hr period. **Children 2 to 6 yr:** as directed by doctor. 500 mg P.O. b.i.d., p.r.n. Maximum 1.5 g in 24-hr period.	▪ Before giving for constipation, ask if patient has adequate fluid intake, exercise, and diet. ▪ For diarrhea, may repeat dose q 30 min. ▪ If given as laxative, tell patient to drink 8 oz water with each dose. ▪ Rectal bleeding or failure to respond to therapy may indicate need for surgery.
candesartan cilexetil Atacand *Antihypertensive* Pregnancy Risk Category: C (1st trimester); D (2nd and 3rd trimesters)	*Hypertension (alone or with other antihypertensives)* — **Adults:** initially, 16 mg P.O. q.d. when used as monotherapy; usual dosage range is 8 to 32 mg P.O. q.d. as single dose or divided b.i.d.	▪ Use cautiously in patients (such as those with heart failure) whose renal function depends on the renin-angiotensin-aldosterone system because of potential for oliguria and progressive azotemia with acute renal failure or death. ▪ Use cautiously in patients who are volume- or salt-depleted because *(continued)*

†Canadian ‡Australian

DRUG & CLASS	INDICATIONS & DOSAGES	NURSING CONSIDERATIONS
candesartan cilexetil *(continued)*		of potential for symptomatic hypotension. Start therapy with a lower dosage range, as ordered, and monitor BP carefully. ▪ ***ALERT*** Drug can cause fetal and neonatal morbidity and death when given to pregnant women, especially after 1st trimester. If pregnancy is suspected, notify doctor because drug should be stopped ▪ If hypotension occurs after dose, place patient supine and give an I.V. infusion of 0.9% NaCl, as ordered. ▪ Monitor therapeutic response and occurrence of adverse reactions carefully in elderly patients and in those with renal disease.
capecitabine Xeloda *Antineoplastic* Pregnancy Risk Category: D	*Metastatic breast cancer resistant to both paclitaxel and an anthracycline-containing chemotherapy regimen or resistant to paclitaxel and for which further anthracycline therapy isn't indicated* — **Adults:** 2,500 mg/m^2 P.O. q.d. in 2 divided doses (about 12 hr apart) after meals for 2 wk, followed by 1-wk rest period; given as 3-wk cycles. ***Adjust-a-dose:*** National Cancer Institute of Canada (NCIC) Common Toxicity Criteria: NCIC grade 2: 1st appearance, stop treatment until resolved to grade 0 to 1, and use 100% of starting dose for next cycle; 2nd appearance, stop treatment until resolved to	▪ Use cautiously in patients with history of CAD, mild-to-moderate hepatic dysfunction caused by liver metastases, hyperbilirubinemia, or renal insufficiency, and in elderly patients. ▪ Patients $\geq$ 80 yr may experience greater incidence of GI adverse effects. ▪ For severe diarrhea, notify doctor. If patient becomes dehydrated, give fluid and electrolyte replacement, as ordered. May need to stop drug immediately until diarrhea resolves or decreases. ▪ ***ALERT*** Adjust treatment immediately if patient has symptoms of hand-and-foot

grade 0 to 1 and use 75% of starting dose for next cycle; 3rd appearance, stop treatment until resolved to grade 0 to 1 and use 50% of starting dose for next cycle; 4th appearance, stop treatment permanently.

NCIC grade 3: 1st appearance, stop treatment until resolved to grade 0 to 1 and use 75% of starting dose for next cycle; 2nd appearance, stop treatment until resolved to grade 0 to 1 and use 50% of starting dose for next cycle; 3rd appearance, stop treatment permanently.

NCIC grade 4: 1st appearance, stop treatment permanently or until resolved to grade 0 to 1, then use 50% of starting dose for next cycle.

syndrome (numbness, paresthesia, tingling, painless or painful swelling, erythema, desquamation, blistering and severe pain of hands or feet), hyperbilirubinemia, or severe nausea.

- Hyperbilirubinemia may require stopping drug.
- ***ALERT*** Toxicity criteria relate to degrees of severity of diarrhea, nausea, vomiting, stomatitis, and hand-and-foot syndrome. Refer to package insert for specific toxicity definitions.
- Monitor patient carefully for toxicity. Toxicity may be managed by symptomatic treatment, dose interruptions, and dosage adjustments.

---

capsaicin
Dolorac, Zostrix, Zostrix-HP 0.075%
Topical analgesic
Pregnancy Risk Category: NR

Temporary relief from pain from herpes zoster infections; neuralgias; osteoarthritis or rheumatoid arthritis — **Adults and children > 2 yr:** apply to affected areas not more than q.i.d.

- For external use only.
- Warn patient to avoid getting drug in eyes or on broken skin.
- Advise patient not to bandage area tightly after application.
- Wash hands thoroughly after use.

---

captopril
Apo-Capto†, Capoten, Novo-Captoril†
Antihypertensive, adjunct treatment for heart failure
Pregnancy Risk Category: C (D in 2nd and 3rd trimesters)

Hypertension — **Adults:** initially, 25 mg P.O. b.i.d. or t.i.d. If BP not controlled in 1 to 2 wk, increase to 50 mg b.i.d. or t.i.d. If BP not controlled after another 1 to 2 wk, expect to add diuretic. If further BP reduction needed, may increase dosage to 150 mg t.i.d. while continuing diuretic. Maximum 450 mg q.d.

- Monitor BP and HR frequently.
- Elderly patients may be more sensitive to hypotensive effects.
- In renal impairment or collagen vascular disease, monitor WBC and differential before treatment starts and q 2 wk for first 3 mo of therapy.

(continued)

†Canadian ‡Australian

DRUG & CLASS	INDICATIONS & DOSAGES	NURSING CONSIDERATIONS
captopril *(continued)*	*Heart failure; to reduce risk of death and to slow development of heart failure after MI* — **Adults:** initially, 6.25 to 12.5 mg P.O. t.i.d. Gradually increase to 50 mg t.i.d., p.r.n. Maximum 450 mg q.d.	▪ Give tablet 1 hr before meals because food in GI tract may reduce absorption. ▪ Inform patient that dizziness may occur during first few days of therapy.
carbamazepine Apo-Carbamazepine†, Carbatrol, Epitol, Novo-Carbamaz†, Tegretol *Anticonvulsant, analgesic* Pregnancy Risk Category: C	*Generalized tonic-clonic and complex partial seizures; mixed seizure patterns* — **Adults and children > 12 yr:** 200 mg P.O. b.i.d. (tablets) or 1 tsp (suspension) P.O. q.i.d. Increase q wk by 200 mg P.O. q.d., in divided doses q 6 to 8 hr. Adjust to minimum effective level. Maximum 1 g q.d. in ages 12 to 15 or 1.2 g q.d. in patients > 15 yr. **Children 6 to 12 yr:** 100 mg P.O. b.i.d. or ½ tsp of suspension P.O. q.i.d. Increase q wk by 100 mg P.O. q.d. Maximum 1 g q.d. **Children < 6 yr:** 10 to 20 mg/kg/day P.O. b.i.d. or t.i.d. (tablets) or q.i.d. (suspension). Maximum 35 mg/kg/day.	▪ Therapeutic blood level is 4 to 12 mcg/ml. ▪ Observe for appetite changes. ▪ Monitor urinalysis, BUN, LFTs, CBC, platelet and reticulocyte counts, and serum iron level. ▪ Institute seizure precautions. ▪ When giving by NG tube, mix with equal volume water, 0.9% NaCl, or D_5W. Then flush with 100 ml diluent. ▪ Tell patient not to stop drug suddenly and to notify doctor immediately if adverse reactions occur.
carbamide peroxide Auro Ear Wax Removal Aid, Debrox, Murine Ear Drops *Ceruminolytic, topical antiseptic* Pregnancy Risk Category: NR	*Impacted cerumen* — **Adults and children:** 5 to 10 drops into ear canal b.i.d. for up to 4 days. Allow to remain in ear canal for 15 to 30 min; remove with warm water.	▪ Use in children < 12 years only under a doctor's direction. ▪ Tell patient to flush ear gently with warm water, using a rubber bulb syringe. ▪ Tell patient to call doctor if redness, pain, or swelling persists.

carboplatin Paraplatin, Paraplatin-AQ† *Antineoplastic* Pregnancy Risk Category: D	*Palliative treatment of ovarian cancer* — **Adults:** 360 mg/m² I.V. on day 1 q 4 wk; doses not repeated until platelet count > 100,000/mm³ and neutrophil count > 2,000/mm³. Subsequent doses based on blood counts. ***Adjust-a-dose:*** Adjust dosage in renal impairment and for CrCl < 60 ml/min. Don't give if CrCl ≤ 15 ml/min.	▪ Check serum electrolytes, creatinine, BUN, CBC, and CrCl before 1st infusion and each course of treatment. ▪ I.V. form has mutagenic, teratogenic, and carcinogenic risks for personnel. ▪ Have emergency drugs available when giving drug. ▪ Don't use needles or I.V. sets containing aluminum to give drug. ▪ Monitor vital signs during infusion.
carisoprodol Soma *Skeletal muscle relaxant* Pregnancy Risk Category: NR	*Adjunct in acute, painful musculoskeletal conditions* — **Adults**: 350 mg P.O. t.i.d. and h.s.	▪ ***ALERT*** Watch for idiosyncratic reactions (weakness, ataxia, visual and speech difficulties, fever, skin eruptions, and mental changes) after 1st to 4th dose and for severe reactions (including bronchospasm, hypotension, and anaphylactic shock). ▪ Record amount of relief to help determine whether dosage can be reduced. ▪ Don't stop drug abruptly.
carmustine (BCNU) BiCNU *Antineoplastic* Pregnancy Risk Category: D	*Brain tumor; Hodgkin's disease; malignant lymphoma; multiple myeloma* — **Adults:** 75 to 100 mg/m² I.V. by slow infusion q.d. for 2 days; repeated q 6 wk if platelet count > 100,000/mm³ and WBC count > 4,000/mm³. ***Adjust-a-dose:*** Reduce dosage when WBC count < 4,000/mm³. Reduce dosage by 30% when WBCs 2,000 to 3,000/mm³ and	▪ Parenteral form poses carcinogenic, mutagenic, and teratogenic risks for personnel. ▪ Dilute solution with 27 ml sterile water for injection. Resultant solution contains 3.3 mg carmustine/ml in 10% alcohol. Dilute in 0.9% NaCl or D_5W for I.V. infusion. Give ≥ 250 ml over 1 to 2 hr. ▪ Monitor CBC, uric acid, LFTs, and renal and pulmonary function tests periodically.

(continued)

†Canadian ‡Australian

DRUG & CLASS	INDICATIONS & DOSAGES	NURSING CONSIDERATIONS
carmustine *(continued)*	platelet count falls. Or, 150 to 200 mg/m^2 I.V. by slow infusion as single dose, repeated q 6 wk.	
carteolol hydrochloride (ophthalmic) Ocupress Ophthalmic Solution, 1% *Antihypertensive* Pregnancy Risk Category: C	*Chronic open-angle glaucoma, intraocular hypertension* — **Adults:** 1 drop b.i.d. in conjunctival sac of affected eye.	▪ ***ALERT*** Stop drug at 1st sign of heart failure and notify doctor. ▪ If signs of serious adverse reactions or hypersensitivity occur, tell patient to stop drug and notify doctor immediately.
carteolol hydrochloride (oral) Cartrol *Antihypertensive* Pregnancy Risk Category: C	*Hypertension* — **Adults:** initially, 2.5 mg P.O. q.d.; increase gradually to 5 or 10 mg p.r.n. Doses > 10 mg q.d. don't produce greater response (may actually decrease response). ***Adjust-a-dose:*** In patients with CrCl from 20 to 60 ml/min, dosage interval is 48 hr. In those with CrCl < 20 ml/min, interval is 72 hr.	▪ Monitor BP frequently. ▪ May inhibit glycogenolysis and hypoglycemia signs and symptoms. ▪ May mask tachycardia from hyperthyroidism. ▪ Patients with unrecognized CAD may have angina pectoris on withdrawal.
carvedilol Coreg *Vasodilator, antihypertensive* Pregnancy Risk Category: C	*Hypertension* — **Adults:** dosage highly individualized. Initially, 6.25 mg P.O. b.i.d. Obtain a standing BP 1 hr after initial dose. If tolerated, continue dosage for 7 to 14 days. May increase to 12.5 mg P.O. b.i.d. for 7 to 14 days, following BP monitoring protocol noted above. Maximum dose 25 mg P.O. b.i.d., as tolerated. *Heart failure* — **Adults:** dosage highly indi-	▪ Before starting drug, dosages of digoxin, diuretics, or ACE inhibitors should be stabilized. ▪ ***ALERT*** Patients on beta-blocker therapy with history of severe anaphylactic reaction to several allergens may be more reactive to repeated challenge and may not respond to epinephrine typically used to treat allergic reactions.

Drug	Indications & dosages	Nursing considerations
	vidualized. Initially, 3.125 mg P.O. b.i.d. for 2 wk; if tolerated, increase to 6.25 mg P.O. b.i.d. Dosage may be doubled q 2 wk, as tolerated. Maximum for patients < 85 kg (187 lb) 25 mg P.O. b.i.d.; for those > 85 kg, 50 mg P.O. b.i.d. **Children:** Safety and efficacy in patients < 18 yr have not been established. ***Adjust-a-dose:*** If patient has bradycardia with pulse rate < 55 beats/min, use reduced dose.	▪ If drug is to be stopped, do so gradually over 1 to 2 wk. ▪ Monitor patient with heart failure for worsened condition, renal dysfunction, or fluid retention; diuretics may need to be increased. ▪ Observe patient for dizziness or lightheadedness for 1 hr after giving each new dose.
cascara sagrada *Laxative* Pregnancy Risk Category: C	*Acute constipation; preparation for bowel or rectal exam* — **Adults and children ≥ 12 yr:** one 325-mg tablet P.O. q.d. h.s. **Children 2 to 11 yr:** ½ adult dosage. **Children < 2 yr:** ¼ adult dosage.	▪ Before giving for constipation, determine if fluid intake, exercise, and diet are adequate. ▪ Give with full glass of water. ▪ Monitor serum electrolytes.
cefaclor Ceclor *Antibiotic* Pregnancy Risk Category: B	*Respiratory, urinary tract, skin, or soft-tissue infections and otitis media caused by susceptible organisms* — **Adults:** 250 to 500 mg P.O. q 8 hr. For pharyngitis or otitis media, may give in 2 equally divided doses q 12 hr. **Children:** 20 mg/kg/day P.O. in divided doses q 8 hr. For pharyngitis or otitis media, may give in 2 equally divided doses q 12 hr. In more serious infections, give 40 mg/kg/day; maximum 1 g/day.	▪ Obtain specimen for culture and sensitivity tests before 1st dose. ▪ With large doses or prolonged therapy, monitor for superinfection, especially in high-risk patients. ▪ Store reconstituted suspension in refrigerator for up to 14 days. Shake well before using. ▪ Tell patient to call doctor if rash occurs.
cefadroxil monohydrate Duricef *Antibiotic* Pregnancy Risk Category: B	*UTIs, skin and soft-tissue infections, and pharyngitis or tonsillitis caused by susceptible organisms* — **Adults:** 1 to 2 g P.O. q.d., depending on infection type. Usually given once daily or b.i.d. **Children:** 30 mg/kg P.O.	▪ Obtain specimen for culture and sensitivity tests before 1st dose. ▪ With large doses or prolonged therapy, monitor for superinfection, especially in high-risk patients. *(continued)*

†Canadian ‡Australian

DRUG & CLASS	INDICATIONS & DOSAGES	NURSING CONSIDERATIONS
cefadroxil monohydrate *(continued)*	q.d. in 2 divided doses q 12 hr. ***Adjust-a-dose:*** In patients with CrCl < 50 ml/min, reduce dosage.	▪ Instruct patient to take with food or milk. ▪ Advise patient to call doctor if rash occurs.
cefazolin sodium Ancef, Kefzol, Zolicef *Antibiotic* Pregnancy Risk Category: B	*Prophylaxis in contaminated surgery* — **Adults:** 1 g I.M. or I.V. 30 to 60 min before surgery; then 0.5 to 1 g I.M. or I.V. q 6 to 8 hr for 24 hr. In operations > 2 hr, may give another 0.5 to 1 g I.M. intraoperatively. Where infection would be devastating, prophylaxis may continue for 3 to 5 days. *Respiratory, biliary, GU, skin, soft-tissue, bone and joint infections; septicemia; endocarditis caused by susceptible organisms* — **Adults:** 250 mg I.M. or I.V. q 8 hr to 1.5 g P.O. q 6 hr. Maximum 12 g/day in life-threatening situations. **Infants > 1 mo:** 25 to 50 mg/kg or 1.25 g/m² q.d. I.M. or I.V. in 3 or 4 divided doses. May increase to 100 mg/kg/day. Don't exceed adult dose. ***Adjust-a-dose:*** If CrCl 11 to 34 ml/min, give 50% usual dose q 12 hr; if CrCl < 10 ml/min, give 50% usual dose q 18 to 24 hr.	▪ Obtain specimen for culture and sensitivity tests before 1st dose. ▪ ***I.V. use:*** Reconstitute with diluent: 2 ml to 500-mg vial; 2.5 ml to 1-g vial. Shake until dissolved. Resultant concentration: 225 mg/ml or 330 mg/ml, respectively. ▪ For direct injection, dilute Ancef with 5 ml or Kefzol with 10 ml of sterile water for injection. Inject into large vein or tubing of free-flowing I.V. solution over 3 to 5 min. For intermittent infusion, add reconstituted drug to 50 to 100 ml of compatible solution or use premixed solution. ▪ With large doses or prolonged therapy, monitor for superinfection.
cefdinir Omnicef *Antibiotic* Pregnancy Risk Category: B	*Community-acquired pneumonia; acute exacerbations of chronic bronchitis; acute maxillary sinusitis; acute bacterial otitis media; uncomplicated skin and skin-structure infections* — **Adults and children ≥ 13 yr:** 300 mg	▪ Use cautiously in patients hypersensitive to penicillin because of possible cross-sensitivity with other beta-lactam antibiotics and in those with history of colitis and renal insufficiency.

P.O. q 12 hr or 600 mg P.O. q 24 hr for 10 days. (Use q-12-hr doses for pneumonia and skin infections.) **Children 6 mo to 12 yr:** 7 mg/kg P.O. q 12 hr or 14 mg/kg P.O. q 24 hr for 10 days, up to 600 mg q.d. (Use q-12-hr doses for skin infections.)

Pharyngitis and tonsillitis — **Adults and children ≥ 13 yr:** 300 mg P.O. q 12 hr for 5 to 10 days or 600 mg P.O. q 24 hr for 10 days. **Children 6 mo to 12 yr:** 7 mg/kg P.O. q 12 hr for 5 to 10 days or 14 mg/kg P.O. q 24 hr for 10 days.

Adjust-a-dose: If CrCl < 30 ml/min, reduce dosage to 300 mg P.O. q.d. for adults and 7 mg/kg (up to 300 mg) P.O. q.d. for children. In patients receiving chronic hemodialysis, 300 mg or 7 mg/kg P.O. at end of each dialysis session and subsequently every other day.

- Prolonged drug treatment may result in possible emergence and overgrowth of resistant organisms. Monitor for symptoms of superinfection.
- Pseudomembranous colitis has been reported with cefdinir and should be considered in patients with diarrhea after antibiotic therapy or in those with history of colitis.
- Tell diabetic patients that each tsp of suspension contains 2.86 g of sucrose.
- Antacids, iron supplements, and multivitamins containing iron reduce rate of absorption and bioavailability; give these types of preparations 2 hr before or after cefdinir.
- Cephalosporins may induce a positive Coombs' test result.

---

cefepime hydrochloride
Maxipime
Antibiotic
Pregnancy Risk Category: B

Mild to moderate UTI from susceptible organisms — **Adults and children ≥ 12 yr:** 0.5 to 1 g I.M. (I.M. used only for infections from *E. coli*) or I.V infused over 30 min q 12 hr for 7 to 10 days.

Severe UTI — **Adults and children ≥ 12 yr:** 2 g I.V. infused over 30 min q 12 hr for 10 days.

Moderate to severe pneumonia — **Adults and children ≥ 12 yr:** 1 to 2 g I.V. infused over 30 min q 12 hr for 10 days.

Adjust-a-dose: Reduce dose in patients with renal failure.

- Obtain specimens for culture and sensitivity tests before 1st dose, if appropriate.
- ***I.V. use:*** Give resulting solution over about 30 min.
- Monitor PT, as ordered. Give exogenous vitamin K, as ordered.
- Monitor patient for superinfection.
- Instruct patient to report adverse reactions promptly.

(continued)

DRUG & CLASS	INDICATIONS & DOSAGES	NURSING CONSIDERATIONS
cefepime hydrochloride *(continued)*	*Moderate to severe uncomplicated skin and skin-structure infections; complicated intra-abdominal infections* — **Adults:** 2 g I.V. q 12 hr for 10 days. *Empiric therapy for febrile neutropenic patients* — **Adults:** 2 q I.V. q 8 hr for 7 days.	
cefmetazole sodium (cefmetazone) Zefazone *Antibiotic* Pregnancy Risk Category: B	*Lower respiratory tract, intra-abdominal, skin, and skin-structure infections caused by susceptible organisms* — **Adults:** 2 g I.V. q 6 to 12 hr for 5 to 14 days. *UTIs caused by* E. coli — **Adults:** 2 g I.V. q 12 hr. ***Adjust-a-dose:*** Patients with renal failure may receive reduced dose, longer dosing interval, or both.	▪ Obtain specimen for culture and sensitivity tests before 1st dose. ▪ Monitor patient for superinfection. ▪ Monitor PT in patients at risk from renal or hepatic impairment, malnutrition, or prolonged therapy. ▪ Tell patient to report adverse reactions promptly.
cefonicid sodium Monocid *Antibiotic* Pregnancy Risk Category: B	*Perioperative prophylaxis in contaminated surgery* — **Adults:** 1 g I.M. or I.V. 30 to 60 min before surgery; then 1 g I.M. or I.V. q.d. for 2 days after surgery. If used for prophylaxis in cesarean section, 1 g I.M. or I.V. after umbilical cord is clamped. *Serious infections of lower respiratory and urinary tracts; skin and skin-structure infections; septicemia; bone and joint infections; preoperative prophylaxis* — **Adults:** usual dose 1 g I.V. or I.M. q 24 hr; in life-threatening infections, 2 g q 24 hr.	▪ Obtain specimen for culture and sensitivity tests before 1st dose. ▪ With large doses or prolonged therapy, monitor for superinfection. ▪ When giving 2-g I.M. doses q.d., divide dose equally and inject deeply into large muscle, such as gluteus maximus or lateral aspect of thigh.

	Adjust-a-dose: Adjust dosage in patients with CrCl < 80 ml/min.	
cefoperazone sodium Cefobid *Antibiotic* Pregnancy Risk Category: B	*Serious respiratory tract infections; intra-abdominal, gynecologic, and skin infections; bacteremia; septicemia from susceptible organisms* — **Adults:** 1 to 2 g q 12 hr I.M. or I.V. In severe infections or infections from less-sensitive organisms, may increase dosage to 16 g/day. ***Adjust-a-dose:*** In patients with hepatic and biliary obstruction, dose shouldn't exceed 4 g/day.	▪ Obtain specimen for culture and sensitivity tests before 1st dose. ▪ Give doses of 4 g/day cautiously in hepatic disease or biliary obstruction. ▪ With large doses or prolonged therapy, monitor for superinfection. ▪ Monitor PT regularly. Give vitamin K promptly to reverse bleeding. ▪ For I.M. use, inject deeply into large muscle.
cefotaxime sodium Claforan *Antibiotic* Pregnancy Risk Category: B	*Perioperative prophylaxis in contaminated surgery* — **Adults:** 1 g I.M. or I.V. 30 to 60 min before surgery. For cesarean section, 1 g I.M. or I.V. when umbilical cord clamped; then 1 g I.M. or I.V. 6 and 12 hr later. *Serious lower respiratory tract, urinary tract, CNS, skin, bone, and joint infections; gynecologic and intra-abdominal infections; bacteremia; septicemia from susceptible organisms* — **Adults:** usually 1 g I.V. or I.M. q 6 to 8 hr; up to 12 g q.d. in life-threatening infections. **Children ≥ 50 kg (110 lb):** usual adult dose, but don't exceed 12 g q.d. **Children 1 mo to 12 yr weighing < 50 kg:** 50 to 180 mg/kg/day I.M. or I.V. in 4 to 6 divided doses. **Neonates 1 to 4 wk:** 50 mg/kg I.V. q 8 hr.	▪ Obtain specimen for culture and sensitivity tests before 1st dose. ▪ ***I.V. use:*** Inject into large vein or into tubing of free-flowing I.V. solution over 3 to 5 min. For infusion, infuse over 20 to 30 min. ▪ For I.M. use, inject deeply into large muscle, such as gluteus maximus or lateral aspect of thigh. ▪ With large doses or prolonged therapy, monitor for superinfection. ▪ Tell patient to report adverse reactions promptly.

(continued)

DRUG & CLASS	INDICATIONS & DOSAGES	NURSING CONSIDERATIONS
cefotaxime sodium *(continued)*	**Neonates ≤ 1 wk:** 50 mg/kg I.V. q 12 hr. ***Adjust-a-dose:*** If CrCl < 20 ml/min, give ½ usual dose at usual interval.	
cefotetan disodium Cefotan *Antibiotic* Pregnancy Risk Category: B	*Serious urinary tract, lower respiratory tract, gynecologic, skin and skin-structure, intra-abdominal, and bone and joint infections caused by susceptible organisms* — **Adults:** 1 to 2 g I.V. or I.M. q 12 hr for 5 to 10 days. Up to 6 g q.d. in life-threatening infections. *Perioperative prophylaxis* — **Adults:** 1 to 2 g I.V. given once 30 to 60 min before surgery. In cesarean section, give dose as soon as umbilical cord clamped. ***Adjust-a-dose:*** If CrCl 10 to 30 ml/min, give usual dose q 24 hr. If < 10 ml/min, give usual dose q 48 hr.	▪ Obtain specimen for culture and sensitivity tests before 1st dose. ▪ ***I.V. use:*** Reconstitute with sterile water for injection. Then drug may be mixed with 50 to 100 ml D_5W or 0.9% NaCl. ▪ With large doses or prolonged therapy, monitor for superinfection.
cefoxitin sodium Mefoxin *Antibiotic* Pregnancy Risk Category: B	*Serious respiratory and GU tract; skin, soft-tissue, bone, and joint; and bloodstream and intra-abdominal infections from susceptible organisms; perioperative prophylaxis* — **Adults:** 1 to 2 g q 6 to 8 hr in uncomplicated infections. Up to 12 g q.d. in life-threatening infections. **Children > 3 mo:** 80 to 160 mg/kg q.d. in 4 to 6 equally divided doses. Maximum 12 g q.d. *Prophylactic use in surgery* — **Adults:** 2 g I.M. or I.V. 30 to 60 min before surgery; then	▪ Obtain specimen for culture and sensitivity tests before 1st dose. ▪ ***I.V. use:*** For direct injection, inject into large vein or into tubing of free-flowing ▪ I.V. solution over 3 to 5 min. For intermittent infusion, add reconstituted drug to 50 or 100 ml D_5W, $D_{10}W$, or 0.9% NaCl injection. Interrupt flow of primary I.V. solution during infusion. ▪ Assess I.V. site frequently. I.V. use linked to thrombophlebitis.

	2 g I.M. or I.V. q 6 hr for 24 hr (72 hr after prosthetic arthroplasty). **Children > 3 mo:** 30 to 40 mg/kg I.M. or I.V. 30 to 60 min before surgery; then 30 to 40 mg/kg q 6 hr for 24 hr (72 hr after prosthetic arthroplasty). ***Adjust-a-dose:*** If CrCl < 50 ml/min, reduce dosage.	▪ ***ALERT*** For I.M. use, reconstitute I.M. injection with 0.5% or 1% lidocaine hydrochloride (without epinephrine) to minimize pain. Inject deeply into large muscle. ▪ With large doses or prolonged therapy, monitor for superinfection.
cefpodoxime proxetil Vantin *Antibiotic* Pregnancy Risk Category: B	*Acute, community-acquired pneumonia from susceptible organisms* — **Adults and children ≥ 13 yr:** 200 mg P.O. q 12 hr for 14 days. *Acute bacterial exacerbation of chronic bronchitis caused by susceptible organisms* — **Adults and children ≥ 13 yr:** 200 mg P.O. q 12 hr for 10 days. *Uncomplicated UTI from* E. coli, K. pneumoniae, P. mirabilis, *or* S. saprophyticus — **Adults:** 100 mg P.O. q 12 hr for 7 days. *Mild to moderate acute maxillary sinusitis from* H. influenzae, S. pneumoniae, *and* M. catarrhalis — **Adults and adolescents ≥ 12 yr:** 200 mg P.O. q 12 hr for 10 days. **Children ages 2 mo to 11 yr:** 5 mg/kg P.O. q 12 hr for 10 days; maximum dosage 200 mg/dose. ***Adjust-a-dose:*** If CrCl < 30 ml/min, give q 24 hr. *Acute otitis media* — **Children 2 mo to 12 yr:** 5 mg/kg (up to 200 mg) P.O. q 12 hr for 5 days.	▪ Obtain specimen for culture and sensitivity tests before 1st dose. ▪ Keep oral suspension refrigerated. Shake well before measuring dose. ▪ Give tablets with food to enhance absorption. ▪ Monitor for superinfection. ▪ May cause false-positive urine glucose results with copper sulfate tests (Clinitest). Glucose enzymatic tests (Diastix) not affected.

(continued)

DRUG & CLASS	INDICATIONS & DOSAGES	NURSING CONSIDERATIONS
cefpodoxime proxetil *(continued)*	*Pharyngitis or tonsillitis from* S. pyogenes — **Adults:** 100 mg P.O. q 12 hr for 7 to 10 days. **Children 2 mo to 12 yr:** 5 mg/kg (up to 100 mg) P.O. q 12 hr for 5 to 10 days.	
cefprozil Cefzil *Antibiotic* Pregnancy Risk Category: B	*Pharyngitis or tonsillitis from* S. pyogenes — **Adults and children ≥ 13 yr:** 500 mg P.O. q.d. for ≥ 10 days. *Otitis media from* S. pneumoniae, H. influenzae, *or* M. (Branhamella) catarrhalis — **Infants and children 6 mo to 12 yr:** 15 mg/kg P.O. q 12 hr for 10 days. *Acute sinusitis from susceptible organisms* — **Adults and children ≥ 13 yr:** 250 to 500 mg P.O. q 12 hr for 10 days. **Children 6 mo to 12 yr:** 7.5 to 15 mg/kg P.O. q 12 hr for 10 days. *Uncomplicated skin and skin-structure infections from susceptible organisms* — **Adults and children ≥ 13 yr:** 250 mg or 500 mg P.O. q 12 hr or 500 mg P.O. q.d. for 10 days. **Children 2 to 12 yr:** 20 mg/kg P.O. q.d. for 10 days. ***Adjust-a-dose:*** If CrCl < 30 ml/min, give 50% of usual dose.	▪ Obtain specimen for culture and sensitivity tests before 1st dose. ▪ Removed by hemodialysis; give after hemodialysis treatment is completed. ▪ Monitor patient for superinfection. ▪ Tell patient to shake suspension well before measuring dose. ▪ Instruct patient to notify doctor if rash develops.
ceftazidime Ceptaz, Fortaz, Tazicef, Tazidime *Antibiotic*	*Serious lower respiratory and urinary tract, gynecologic, intra-abdominal, CNS, and skin infections; bacteremia; septicemia* — **Adults and children ≥ 12 yr:** 1 g I.V. or I.M. q 8 to	▪ Obtain specimen for culture and sensitivity tests before 1st dose. ▪ ***I.V. use:*** Read and carefully follow instructions for reconstitution.

Pregnancy Risk Category: B	12 hr; up to 6 g q.d. in life-threatening infections. **Children 1 mo to 11 yr:** 25 to 50 mg/kg I.V. q 8 hr (sodium carbonate formulation). **Neonates 0 to 4 wk:** 30 mg/kg I.V. q 12 hr (sodium carbonate formulation). ***Adjust-a-dose:*** Adjust dosage in patients with CrCl < 50 ml/min.	▪ Removed by hemodialysis; give supplemental dose after each dialysis period, as ordered. ▪ For I.M. use, inject deeply into large muscle. ▪ With large doses or prolonged therapy, monitor for superinfection.
ceftibuten Cedax *Antibiotic* Pregnancy Risk Category: B	*Acute bacterial exacerbation of chronic bronchitis from susceptible organisms* — **Adults and children ≥ age 12:** 400 mg P.O. q.d. for 10 days. *Pharyngitis and tonsillitis from* S. pyogenes; *acute bacterial otitis media from* H. influenzae, M. catarrhalis, *or* S. pyogenes — **Adults and children ≥ age 12:** 400 mg P.O. q.d. for 10 days. **Children < age 12:** 9 mg/kg P.O. q.d. for 10 days. **Children > 45 kg:** ≥ 400 mg P.O. q.d. for 10 days. ***Adjust-a-dose:*** Patients with renal impairment and those undergoing hemodialysis require dosage adjustment.	▪ Obtain specimen for culture and sensitivity tests before 1st dose. ▪ Discontinue if allergic reaction suspected. Emergency treatment may be required. ▪ Consider possibility of pseudomembranous colitis in patients who develop diarrhea secondary to therapy. Obtain specimens for *C. difficile*. ▪ Monitor patient for superinfection. ▪ Suspension must be administered ≥ 2 hr before or 1 hr after a meal.
ceftizoxime sodium Cefizox *Antibiotic* Pregnancy Risk Category: B	*Serious infections of lower respiratory and urinary tracts; gynecologic, intra-abdominal, bone, joint, and skin infections; bacteremia; septicemia; meningitis from susceptible microorganisms* — **Adults:** usual dose 1 to 2 g I.V. or I.M. q 8 to 12 hr. In life-threatening infections, up to 2 g q 4 hr. **Children > 6 mo:** 33 to 50 mg/kg I.V. q 6 to 8 hr. Serious in-	▪ Obtain specimen for culture and sensitivity tests before 1st dose. ▪ ***I.V. use:*** To reconstitute powder, add 5 ml sterile water to 500-mg vial, 10 ml to 1-g vial, or 20 ml to 2-g vial. Reconstitute piggyback vials with 50 to 100 ml 0.9% NaCl or D_5W. Shake well.

(continued)

†Canadian ‡Australian

DRUG & CLASS	INDICATIONS & DOSAGES	NURSING CONSIDERATIONS
ceftizoxime sodium *(continued)*	fections: up to 200 mg/kg/day in divided doses. Don't exceed 12 g/day. ***Adjust-a-dose:*** Adjust dosage in patients with CrCl < 80 ml/min.	▪ For I.M. use, inject deeply into large muscle. Divide larger doses (2 g) and inject at two separate sites. ▪ Monitor for superinfection.
ceftriaxone sodium Rocephin *Antibiotic* Pregnancy Risk Category: B	*Most infections from susceptible organisms* — **Adults:** 1 to 2 g I.M. or I.V. once daily or b.i.d., depending on severity of infection. *Serious lower respiratory and urinary tract, gynecologic, bone, joint, intra-abdominal, and skin infections; bacteremia; septicemia; Lyme disease from susceptible organisms* — **Adults and children > 12 yr:** 1 to 2 g I.M. or I.V. q.d. or divided b.i.d. Maximum 4 g q.d. **Children 12 yr:** 50 to 75 mg/kg I.M. or I.V., maximum 2 g q.d., divided q 12 hr. *Meningitis* — **Adults and children:** initially, 100 mg/kg I.M. or I.V. (maximum 4 g); then 100 mg/kg I.M. or I.V. q.d. or divided q 12 hr, maximum 4 g, for 1 to 2 wk. *Acute bacterial otitis media* — **Children**: 50 mg/kg (maximum 1 g) I.M. as single dose. *Uncomplicated gonococcal infections* — **Adults:** single dose of 125 mg to 250 mg I.M.	▪ Obtain specimen for culture and sensitivity tests before 1st dose. ▪ For I.M. use, inject deeply into large muscle. ▪ Monitor for superinfection. ▪ Commonly used in home antibiotic programs for outpatient treatment of serious infections such as osteomyelitis.
cefuroxime axetil Ceftin **cefuroxime sodium** Kefurox, Zinacef	*Injectable form for serious infections and for perioperative prophylaxis. Oral form used for otitis media, pharyngitis, tonsillitis, infections of urinary and lower respiratory tracts, and*	▪ Obtain specimen for culture and sensitivity tests before 1st dose. ▪ ***I.V. use:*** For direct injection, inject into large vein or into tubing of free-flowing

Antibiotic
Pregnancy Risk Category: B

skin and skin-structure infections from susceptible organisms — **Adults and children ≥ 12 yr:** 750 mg to 1.5 g of cefuroxime sodium I.M. or I.V. q 8 hr for 5 to 10 days. For life-threatening infections and less-susceptible organisms, 1.5 g I.M. or I.V. q 6 hr; for bacterial meningitis, up to 3 g I.V. q 8 hr. Or, 250 to 500 mg of cefuroxime axetil P.O. q 12 hr. **Children and infants > 3 mo:** 50 to 100 mg/kg/day of cefuroxime sodium I.M. or I.V. in divided doses q 6 to 8 hr (higher doses for meningitis). Or, 125 mg of cefuroxime axetil P.O. q 12 hr; for bacterial meningitis, 200 to 240 mg/kg I.V. in divided doses q 6 to 8 hr.

Otitis media — **Children 3 mo to 12 yr:** 15 mg/kg (suspension) P.O. b.i.d. for 10 days, up to 1,000 mg/day or 250 mg (tablet) P.O. b.i.d. for 10 days.

Pharyngitis and tonsillitis from S. pyogenes — **Adults and children ≥ 12:** 125 to 500 mg P.O. b.i.d. for 10 days. **Children 3 mo to 12 yr:** 10 mg/kg (suspension) P.O. b.i.d. for 10 days (up to 500 mg/day). Or, 125 to 250 mg (tablet) P.O. b.i.d. for 10 days.

Impetigo — **Children 3 mo to 12 yr:** 15 to 30 mg/kg (suspension) P.O. b.i.d. for 10 days, up to 1,000 mg/day. Or, 250 mg P.O. b.i.d. for 10 days (tablets).

Early Lyme disease from B. burgdorferi — **Adults and children ≥ 13 yr:** 500 mg P.O.

I.V. solution over 3 to 5 min.

- For I.M. doses, inject deeply into large muscle.
- Food enhances absorption of cefuroxime axetil.
- With large doses or prolonged therapy, monitor for superinfection, especially in high-risk patients.
- Advise patient to report pain at I.V. site.
- Tell patient to report adverse reactions promptly.
- ***ALERT*** Cefuroxime tablets and oral suspensions aren't bioequivalent and can't be substituted on a mg-to-mg basis.

(continued)

DRUG & CLASS	INDICATIONS & DOSAGES	NURSING CONSIDERATIONS
cefuroxime axetil *(continued)*	b.i.d. for 20 days. *Acute bacterial maxillary sinusitis from susceptible organisms* — **Adults and adolescents ≥ 13 yr:** 250 mg (tablet) P.O. b.i.d. for 10 days. **Infants and children 3 mo to 12 yr:** 30 mg/kg (suspension) P.O. in 2 divided doses for 10 days (up to 1,000 mg/day). Or, 250 mg (tablet) P.O. b.i.d. for 10 days. ***Adjust-a-dose:*** When giving parenterally, adjust dosage in patients with CrCl < 20 ml/min.	
celecoxib Celebrex *NSAID* Pregnancy Risk Category: C	*Relief from signs and symptoms of osteoarthritis* — **Adults:** 200 mg P.O. q.d. as single dose or divided b.i.d. *Relief from signs and symptoms of rheumatoid arthritis* — **Adults:** 100 to 200 mg P.O. b.i.d. *Adjunct to familial adenomatous polyposis to reduce number of adenomatous colorectal polyps* — **Adults:** 400 mg b.i.d. with food for up to 6 mo. ***Adjust-a-dose:*** In patients < 50 kg (110 lb), start at lowest dosage. In patients with moderate hepatic impairment (Child-Pugh class II), start therapy with reduced dosage.	▪ Patients with history of ulcers or GI bleeding are at higher risk for GI bleeding while taking NSAIDs. Other risk factors for GI bleeding include treatment with corticosteroids or anticoagulants, longer NSAID treatment, smoking, alcoholism, older age, and poor overall health. ▪ NSAIDs may be hepatotoxic. Monitor patient for nausea, fatigue, lethargy, and jaundice.
cephalexin hydrochloride Keftab **cephalexin**	*Respiratory and GI tract, skin, soft tissue, bone, and joint infections and otitis media from* E. coli *and other coliform bacteria, group A beta-hemolytic streptococci,* Kleb-	▪ Ask about previous allergic reactions to cephalosporins or penicillin before giving 1st dose. ▪ Obtain specimen for culture and sensitivi-

monohydrate Apo-Cephalex†, Biocef, Cefanex, Keflex *Antibiotic* Pregnancy Risk Category: B	siella, P. mirabilis, S. pneumoniae, *and staphylococci* — **Adults:** 250 mg to 1 g P.O. q 6 hr. **Children:** 6 to 12 mg/kg P.O. q 6 hr (monohydrate only). Maximum 25 mg/kg q 6 hr.	ty tests before 1st dose. ▪ With large doses or prolonged therapy, monitor patient for superinfection. ▪ ***ALERT*** Treat group A beta-hemolytic streptococcal infections for ≥ 10 days.
cephradine Velosef *Antibiotic* Pregnancy Risk Category: B	*Serious respiratory, GI, or GU tract, skin and soft tissue, and bone and joint infections; septicemia; endocarditis; otitis media from susceptible organisms; perioperative prophylaxis* — **Adults:** 250 to 500 mg P.O. q 6 hr. **Children > 9 mo:** 25 to 50 mg/kg P.O. q.d. in divided doses q 6 or 12 hr. ***Adjust-a-dose:*** Patients with a CrCl < 20 ml/min require a dosage reduction. *Otitis media* — **Children:** 75 to 100 mg/kg P.O. q.d. Don't exceed 4 g q.d. Any patient, regardless of age or weight, may receive up to 1 g q.i.d. for severe or chronic infections.	▪ Obtain specimen for culture and sensitivity tests before 1st dose. ▪ ***ALERT*** Treat group A beta-hemolytic streptococcal infections for ≥ 10 days. ▪ With large doses or prolonged therapy, monitor for superinfection, especially in high-risk patients. ▪ Tell patient to take with food or milk. ▪ Instruct patient to shake oral suspension well before measuring dose. ▪ Advise patient to report rash immediately.
cetirizine hydrochloride Zyrtec *Antihistamine* Pregnancy Risk Category: B	*Seasonal allergic rhinitis; perennial allergic rhinitis; chronic urticaria* — **Adults and children ≥ 12 yr:** 5 or 10 mg P.O. q.d. depending on symptom severity; 5 mg P.O. q.d. in renal or hepatic impairment. **Children 6 to 11 yr**: 5 or 10 mg (1 or 2 tsp) P.O. q.d. depending on symptom severity. ***Adjust-a-dose:*** In renally impaired patients with CrCl of 11 to 31 ml/min, those on dialysis (CrCl < 7 ml/min), or those with hepatic impairment, give 5 mg P.O. q.d.	▪ Don't give to breast-feeding patients. ▪ Warn patient to avoid hazardous activities until CNS effects known. ▪ Advise patient to avoid alcohol and other CNS depressants.

†Canadian ‡Australian

DRUG & CLASS	INDICATIONS & DOSAGES	NURSING CONSIDERATIONS
cevimeline hydrochloride Evoxac *Prosecretory drug* Pregnancy Risk Category: C	*Dry mouth in patients with Sjögren's syndrome* — **Adults:** 30 mg P.O. t.i.d.	▪ Don't use in patients with uncontrolled asthma, or when miosis is undesirable, such as in acute iritis or narrow-angle glaucoma. ▪ Monitor patients with history of asthma, COPD, or chronic bronchitis for increased wheezing, sputum production, or cough. ▪ Monitor patients with history of cardiac disease for increased frequency, severity, or duration of angina or heart rate change. ▪ Drug may cause visual disturbances, especially at night, that can impair the patient's ability to drive. ▪ Monitor elderly patients closely because of likelihood of other disease; decreased renal, hepatic, and cardiac function; and drug interactions.
chloral hydrate Aquachloral Supprettes, Noctec, Novo-Chlorhydrate† *Sedative-hypnotic* Pregnancy Risk Category: C Controlled Substance Schedule: IV	*Sedation* — **Adults:** 250 mg P.O. or P.R. t.i.d. after meals. **Children:** 8.3 mg/kg or 250 mg/m² P.O. or P.R. t.i.d. Maximum 500 mg t.i.d. *Insomnia* — **Adults:** 500 mg to 1 g P.O. or P.R. 15 to 30 min before h.s. **Children:** 50 mg/kg or 1.5 g/m² P.O. or P.R. 15 to 30 min before h.s. Maximum single dose 1 g. *Preoperative* — **Adults:** 500 mg to 1 g P.O. or P.R. 30 min before surgery. *Premedication for EEG* — **Children:** 20 to	▪ ***ALERT*** Note 2 strengths of oral liquid form. Double-check dose, especially when giving to children. Fatal overdoses have occurred. ▪ To minimize unpleasant taste and stomach irritation, dilute or give with liquid and after meals. ▪ Take steps to prevent hoarding or self-overdosing by depressed, suicidal, or drug-dependent patients or those with history of drug abuse.

	25 mg/kg P.O. or P.R.	▪ Don't give for 48 hr before fluorometric test. ▪ Monitor BUN; large dosage may raise BUN.
chlorambucil Leukeran *Antineoplastic* Pregnancy Risk Category: D	*Chronic lymphocytic leukemia; malignant lymphomas, including lymphosarcoma, giant follicular lymphoma, and Hodgkin's disease* — **Adults:** 0.1 to 0.2 mg/kg P.O. q.d. for 3 to 6 wk; then adjusted for maintenance (usually 4 to 10 mg q.d.).	▪ Monitor CBC and serum uric acid level. ▪ If WBC count $< 2,000/mm^3$ or granulocyte count $< 1,000/mm^3$, follow infection control policy in immunocompromised patients. ▪ Don't give I.M. when platelet count $< 100,000/mm^3$.
chloramphenicol (ophthalmic) AK-Chlor, Chloromycetin Ophthalmic, Chloroptic, Chloroptic S.O.P. *Antibiotic* Pregnancy Risk Category: C	*Surface bacterial infection involving conjunctiva or cornea* — **Adults and children:** 1 or 2 drops of solution in eye q 3 to 6 hr or more often, p.r.n. Or, small amount of ointment to lower conjunctival sac q 3 to 6 hr or more often, p.r.n. Continue for ≥ 48 hr after eye appears normal.	▪ If drops are given q hr and then dosage is tapered, follow order closely to ensure adequate anterior chamber levels. ▪ Teach patient how to instill drops or apply ointment. ▪ Tell patient to apply light pressure on lacrimal sac for 1 min after drops are instilled.
chlordiazepoxide Libritabs **chlordiazepoxide hydrochloride** Librium, Novo-Poxide† *Anxiolytic, anticonvulsant, sedative-hypnotic* Pregnancy Risk Category: D Controlled Substance Schedule: IV	*Mild to moderate anxiety* — **Adults:** 5 to 10 mg P.O. t.i.d. or q.i.d. **Children > 6 yr:** 5 mg P.O. b.i.d. to q.i.d. Maximum 10 mg P.O. b.i.d. or t.i.d. *Severe anxiety* — **Adults:** 20 to 25 mg P.O. t.i.d. or q.i.d. **Elderly:** 5 mg P.O. b.i.d. to q.i.d. *Withdrawal symptoms of acute alcoholism* — **Adults:** 50 to 100 mg P.O., I.M., or I.V.; repeat in 2 to 4 hr, p.r.n. Maximum 300 mg q.d. *Note:* Don't give parenteral form to children < 12 yr. ***Adjust-a-dose:*** Give debilitated patients 5 mg P.O. b.i.d. to q.i.d.	▪ ***I.V. use:*** Use 5 ml 0.9% NaCl or sterile water for injection as diluent; don't give packaged diluent. Give over 1 min. ▪ When giving I.V., be sure equipment for emergency airway management is available. Monitor respirations every 5 to 15 min and before each repeated I.V. dose. ▪ Injectable form comes in two types of ampules. Read directions carefully. ▪ Don't withdraw abruptly.

†Canadian ‡Australian

DRUG & CLASS	INDICATIONS & DOSAGES	NURSING CONSIDERATIONS
chloroquine hydrochloride Aralen HCl, Chlorquin‡ **chloroquine phosphate** Aralen Phosphate, Chlorquin‡ *Antimalarial, amebicide, anti-inflammatory* Pregnancy Risk Category: C	*Acute malarial attacks* — **Adults:** 1 g (600 mg base) P.O.; then 500 mg (300 mg base) at 6, 24, and 48 hr. Or, 160 to 200 mg (base) I.M. initially; repeat in 6 hr, p.r.n. Switch to P.O. as soon as possible. **Children:** 10 mg (base)/kg P.O.; then 5 mg (base)/kg at 6, 24, and 48 hr (maximum < adult dose). Or 5 mg (base)/kg I.M. initially; repeated in 6 hr, p.r.n. Maximum 10 mg (base)/kg/24 hr. Switch to P.O. as soon as possible. *Malaria prophylaxis* — **Adults and children:** 5 mg (base)/kg P.O. (maximum 300 mg) weekly (begun 2 wk before exposure and continued for 4 to 6 wk after). If treatment begins after exposure, double initial dose in 2 divided doses P.O. q 6 hr.	▪ ***ALERT*** Monitor patient for overdose, which can quickly lead to toxic symptoms. Children are extremely susceptible to toxicity. ▪ Obtain baseline and periodic ophthalmic and autometric exams. ▪ Monitor CBC and LFT results. ▪ Advise patient to take immediately before or after meals on same day each wk. ▪ Tell patient to report adverse reactions promptly. ▪ Instruct patient to avoid exposure to sunlight.
chlorpheniramine maleate Aller-Chlor L, Chlor-Trimeton, Teldrin *Antihistamine (H_1-receptor antagonist)* Pregnancy Risk Category: B	*Rhinitis; allergy symptoms* — **Adults:** 4 mg P.O. q 4 to 6 hr, up to 24 mg/day; or 8 to 12 mg timed-release capsule P.O. q 8 to 12 hr, up to 24 mg q.d. Or, 5 to 20 mg I.M., I.V., or S.C. as single dose. Maximum 40 mg/24 hr. **Children 6 to 12 yr:** 2 mg P.O. q 4 to 6 hr, up to 12 mg/day. Or, may give 8 mg timed-release capsule P.O. h.s. **Children 2 to 6 yr:** 1 mg P.O. q 4 to 6 hr, maximum 4 mg q.d.	▪ ***I.V. use:*** Available in 10-mg/ml ampules. Don't give 100-mg/ml strength I.V. Drug compatible with most I.V. solutions, but check with pharmacist before mixing to verify specific compatibilities. Give over 1 min. ▪ If symptoms occur during or after injection, stop drug.

chlorpromazine hydrochloride Chlorpromanyl-5†, Chlorpromanyl-20†, Chlorpromanyl-40†, Ormazine, Thorazine *Antipsychotic, antiemetic* Pregnancy Risk Category: C	*Psychosis* — **Adults:** 25 to 75 mg P.O. q.d. in 2 to 4 divided doses. Increase by 20 to 50 mg twice weekly until symptoms controlled. May need up to 800 mg q.d. Or, 25 to 50 mg I.M. q 1 to 4 hr, p.r.n. I.M. doses gradually increased over several days to maximum 400 mg q 4 to 6 hr. Switch to P.O. as soon as possible. **Children ≥ 6 mo:** 0.55 mg/kg P.O. q 4 to 6 hr or I.M. q 6 to 8 hr; or 1.1 mg/kg P.R. q 6 to 8 hr. Maximum I.M. dose in children < 5 yr or < 22.7 kg (50 lb): 40 mg. Maximum I.M. dose in children 5 to 12 yr or 22.7 to 45.5 kg (100 lb): 75 mg. *Nausea and vomiting* — **Adults:** 10 to 25 mg P.O. q 4 to 6 hr, p.r.n.; or 50 to 100 mg P.R. q 6 to 8 hr, p.r.n.; or 25 to 50 mg I.M. q 3 to 4 hr, p.r.n. **Children ≥ 6 mo:** 0.55 mg/kg q 4 to 6 hr; or I.M. q 6 to 8 hr; or 1.1 mg/kg P.R. q 6 to 8 hr. Maximum I.M. dose in children < 5 yr (< 22.7 kg): 40 mg. Maximum I.M. dose in children 5 to 12 yr (22.7 to 45.5 kg): 75 mg.	▪ Obtain baseline BP before therapy and monitor BP regularly. Watch for orthostatic hypotension, especially with parenteral use. Monitor BP before and after giving I.M.; keep patient supine 1 hr afterward and instruct to get up slowly. ▪ Monitor patient for tardive dyskinesia, which may occur mo or yr after prolonged use and may disappear spontaneously or persist for life despite stopping drug. ▪ Watch for signs of neuroleptic malignant syndrome. ▪ Treat acute dystonic reactions with diphenhydramine.
chlorthalidone Apo-Chlorthalidone†, Hygroton, Novo-Thalidone†, Thalitone, Uridon† *Diuretic, antihypertensive* Pregnancy Risk Category: D	*Edema* — **Adults:** initially, 50 to 100 mg P.O. q.d., or up to 200 mg P.O. every other day. **Children:** 2 mg/kg or 60 mg/m^2 P.O. 3 times q wk. *Hypertension* — **Adults:** 12.5 to 50 mg P.O. q.d.	▪ To prevent nocturia, give in morning. ▪ Monitor I&O, weight, BP, electrolytes, glucose, creatinine, BUN, and uric acid. ▪ Watch for signs of hypokalemia. ▪ Don't confuse various brands.

†Canadian ‡Australian

DRUG & CLASS	INDICATIONS & DOSAGES	NURSING CONSIDERATIONS
cholestyramine LoCholest, Prevalite, Questran, Questran Light *Antilipemic, bile acid sequestrant* Pregnancy Risk Category: B	*Primary hyperlipidemia or pruritus from partial bile obstruction; adjunct for reduction of elevated serum cholesterol in primary hypercholesterolemia* — **Adults:** 4 g once daily or b.i.d. Maintenance: 8 to 16 g q.d. into 2 divided doses. Maximum 24 g q.d.	▪ Monitor cholesterol and triglycerides regularly. ▪ If patient also receiving cardiac glycoside, monitor serum levels of this drug. ▪ Don't give in dry form. ▪ Monitor bowel habits. Encourage high-fiber diet and fluids.
choline magnesium trisalicylate (choline salicylate and magnesium salicylate) Tricosal, Trilisate *Nonnarcotic analgesic, antipyretic, anti-inflammatory* Pregnancy Risk Category: C	*Rheumatoid arthritis (RA) and other inflammatory conditions* — **Adults:** initially, 1.5 to 2.5 g P.O. q.d. as single dose or in 2 or 3 divided doses. Adjust dosage according to response. Maintenance: 1 to 4.5 g q.d. *Juvenile RA* — **Children:** 60 to 110 mg/kg/day P.O. in divided doses (q 6 to 8 hr). *Mild to moderate pain and fever* — **Adults:** 2 to 3 g P.O. q.d. in divided doses q 4 to 6 hr. **Children $\leq$ 37 kg (81.5 lb):** 25 mg/kg P.O. b.i.d. **Children > 37 kg:** 2,250 mg/day.	▪ Monitor Hgb and PT in long-term or high-dose therapy. ▪ ***ALERT*** Monitor serum salicylate in long-term therapy. In arthritis, therapeutic level is 10 to 30 mg/100 ml.
cidofovir Vistide *Antiviral* Pregnancy Risk Category: C	*CMV retinitis in patients with AIDS* — **Adults:** initially, 5 mg/kg I.V. infused over 1 hr once weekly for 2 consecutive wk; then maintenance dose of 5 mg/kg I.V. infused over 1 hr once q 2 wk. Must give probenecid and prehydration with 0.9% NaCl I.V. together (may lower nephrotoxicity potential). ***Adjust-a-dose:*** In patients with renal failure, if serum creatinine increases 0.3 to 0.4 mg/dl above baseline, reduce dose to 3 mg/kg at	▪ Give 1 L 0.9% NaCl, usually over 1 to 2 hr, immediately before each infusion. ▪ Monitor eye exam results periodically. ▪ To prepare for infusion, transfer dose to bag containing 100 ml 0.9% NaCl. ▪ Mutagenic; prepare drug by facility protocols. ▪ If drug contacts skin, wash mucous membranes and flush thoroughly with water. ▪ Don't give by intraocular injection.

	same rate and frequency. If serum creatinine ≥ 0.5 mg/dl above baseline, stop drug.	▪ ***ALERT*** Don't give to patients with a serum creatinine concentration > 1.5 mg/dl, a calculated CrCl ≤ 55 ml/min, or a urine protein ≥ 100 mg/dl (or ≥ +2 protein).
cilostazol Pletal *Platelet aggregation inhibitor, vasodilator* Pregnancy Risk Category: C	*Reduction of symptoms of intermittent claudication* — **Adults:** 100 mg P.O. b.i.d., taken at least 30 min before or 2 hr after breakfast and dinner. Decrease dose to 50 mg P.O. b.i.d. when giving with drugs that may increase cilostazol levels.	▪ Give at least ½ hr before or 2 hr after breakfast and dinner. ▪ Beneficial effect may not occur for up to 12 wk after starting therapy. ▪ ***ALERT*** Use cautiously with other drugs metabolized by the cytochrome P-450 enzyme system. May need to start therapy at a lower dose in patients taking other drugs metabolized by the cytochrome P-450 enzyme system. ▪ Grapefruit juice inhibits cytochrome P-450A4 enzyme and increases drug levels; tell patient to avoid grapefruit juice while taking drug. ▪ Several drugs that inhibit the enzyme phosphodiesterase have caused lower survival rates than placebo in patients with class III-IV heart failure.
cimetidine Tagamet, Tagamet HB *Antiulcer agent* Pregnancy Risk Category: B	*Duodenal ulcer (short-term treatment and maintenance)* — **Adults and children ≥ 16 yr:** 800 mg P.O. h.s. Or, 400 mg P.O. b.i.d. or 300 mg q.i.d. with meals and h.s. Maintenance therapy: 400 mg h.s. Parenteral therapy: 300 mg diluted to 20 ml by I.V. push over ≥ 5 min q 6 hr; or 300 mg diluted in 50	▪ ***I.V. use:*** Dilute I.V. solutions with 0.9% NaCl, D_5W, and $D_{10}W$ (and combinations of these), lactated Ringer's, or 5% sodium bicarbonate injection. Don't dilute with sterile water. ▪ Don't infuse I.V. too rapidly; bradycardia may occur. May infuse *(continued)*

†Canadian ‡Australian

DRUG & CLASS	INDICATIONS & DOSAGES	NURSING CONSIDERATIONS
cimetidine *(continued)*	ml D_5W or other compatible I.V. solution by I.V. infusion over 15 to 20 min q 6 hr; or 300 mg I.M. q 6 hr (no dilution necessary). Maximum 2,400 mg q.d., p.r.n. Or, 900 mg/day (37.5 mg/hr) I.V. diluted in 100 to 1,000 ml by continuous I.V. infusion. *Active benign gastric ulceration* — **Adults:** 800 mg P.O. h.s., or 300 mg P.O. q.i.d. (with meals and h.s.) for up to 6 wk. *Gastroesophageal reflux disease* — **Adults:** 800 mg P.O. b.i.d. or 400 mg q.i.d. before meals and h.s. for up to 12 wk.	over ≥ 30 min to reduce risk of adverse cardiac effects. May give as continuous I.V. infusion. Use infusion pump if given in total volume of 250 ml over ≤ 24 hr. ▪ Identify tablet strength when obtaining drug history. ▪ Schedule dose at end of hemodialysis. ▪ Up to 10-g overdose can occur without adverse reactions.
ciprofloxacin Cipro, Cipro I.V., Ciproxin‡ *Antibiotic* Pregnancy Risk Category: C	*Mild to moderate UTI from susceptible organisms* — **Adults:** 250 mg P.O. or 200 mg I.V. q 12 hr. *Severe or complicated UTI or mild to moderate bone, joint, skin, or skin-structure infections from susceptible organisms* — **Adults:** 500 mg P.O. or 400 mg I.V. q 12 hr. If severe infection, 400 mg I.V. q 8 hr. *Mild to moderate acute sinusitis from* Haemophilus influenzae, Streptococcus pneumoniae, *or* Moraxella catarrhalis; *mild to moderate chronic bacterial prostatitis from* Escherichia coli *or* Proteus mirabilis — **Adults:** 400 mg I.V. infusion given over 60 min q 12 hr. *To reduce the incidence of progression of*	▪ Obtain specimen for culture and sensitivity tests before 1st dose. ▪ Give oral form 2 hr after meal or 2 hr before or after taking antacids, sucralfate, or products that contain iron. ▪ ***I.V. use:*** Infuse slowly over 1 hr into large vein. ▪ Preferable to give I.V. dose 2 hr after meal. ▪ Don't give antacids, magnesium, aluminum, or iron products within 4 hr before or 2 hr after I.V. dose. ▪ Instruct patient to avoid excessive artificial ultraviolet light and to stop drug and call doctor if phototoxicity occurs. ▪ Encourage high fluid intake to avoid crystalluria.

	disease following exposure to aerosolized Bacillus anthracis *(anthrax)* — **Adults:** 500 mg P.O. q 12 hr for 60 days, beginning as soon as possible after exposure. **Children:** 15 mg/kg/dose P.O. q 12 hr for 60 days, beginning as soon as possible after exposure. Maximum dose 500 mg. *Chronic bacterial prostatitis from* E. coli *or* P. mirabilis — **Adults:** 500 mg P.O. q 12 hr for 28 days. ***Adjust-a-dose:*** In patients with renal failure, if CrCl < 50 ml/min, reduce dose or frequency.	
ciprofloxacin hydrochloride Ciloxan *Antibiotic* Pregnancy Risk Category: C	*Corneal ulcers caused by susceptible organisms* — **Adults and children > 12 yr:** 2 drops in affected eye q 15 min for first 6 hr; then 2 drops q 30 min for remainder of day 1. On day 2, 2 drops q hr. On days 3 to 14, 2 drops q 4 hr. *Bacterial conjunctivitis caused by susceptible organisms* — **Adults and children > 12 yr:** 1 or 2 drops in affected eye q 2 hr *while awake* for first 2 days. Then 1 or 2 drops q 4 hr *while awake* for next 5 days.	▪ Teach patient how to instill drops. ▪ Instruct patient to apply light pressure on lacrimal sac for 1 min after drops instilled. ▪ Stop drug at signs of hypersensitivity and notify doctor. ▪ Prolonged use may cause superinfection.
cisplatin (cis-platinum, CDDP) Platamine‡, Platinol, Platinol AQ *Antineoplastic* Pregnancy Risk Category: D	*Adjunct therapy in metastatic testicular cancer* — **Adults:** 20 mg/m^2 I.V. q.d. for 5 days. Repeated q 3 wk for 3 or more cycles. *Adjunct therapy in metastatic ovarian cancer* — **Adults:** 100 mg/m^2 I.V.; repeated q 4 wk. Or 75 to 100 mg/m^2 I.V. once q 4 wk	▪ Monitor CBC, electrolyte levels, platelet count, and renal function studies. ▪ Hydrate patient with 0.9% NaCl before therapy. Maintain urine output of ≥ 100 ml/hr for 4 hr before therapy and for 24 hr after therapy. *(continued)*

†Canadian ‡Australian

DRUG & CLASS	INDICATIONS & DOSAGES	NURSING CONSIDERATIONS
cisplatin *(continued)*	combined with cyclophosphamide. *Advanced bladder cancer* — **Adults:** 50 to 70 mg/m^2 I.V. q 3 to 4 wk. Patients who have received other antineoplastics or radiation therapy should receive 50 mg/m^2 q 4 wk.	▪ Monitor for tinnitus. ▪ Have anaphylactic medications readily available when giving drugs. ▪ Parenteral form carries carcinogenic, mutagenic, and teratogenic risks for personnel. ▪ ***ALERT*** Don't use needles or I.V. sets that contain aluminum. ▪ Give antiemetics.
citalopram hydrobromide Celexa *Antidepressant* Pregnancy Risk Category: C	*Depression* — **Adults:** initially, 20 mg P.O. q.d., increasing to 40 mg q.d. after ≥ 1 wk. Maximum dose 40 mg q.d. **Elderly:** 20 mg q.d. P.O. with titration to 40 mg q.d. only for nonresponding patients. ***Adjust-a-dose:*** For patients with hepatic impairment, give 20 mg q.d. P.O. with titration to 40 mg q.d. only for nonresponding patients.	▪ Use cautiously in patients with history of mania, seizures, suicidal ideation, or hepatic or renal impairment. ▪ Risk of suicide is inherent in depression and may persist until significant remission occurs. Closely supervise high-risk patients at the start of therapy. Reduce risk of overdose by limiting amount of drug available per refill. ▪ Allow ≥ 2 wk between MAO inhibitor and citalopram treatment.
cladribine (2-chlorodeoxy-adenosine, CdA) Leustatin *Antineoplastic* Pregnancy Risk Category: D	*Active hairy cell leukemia* — **Adults:** 0.09 mg/kg/day by continuous I.V. infusion for 7 consecutive days.	▪ ***I.V. use:*** For 24-hr infusion, add calculated dose to 500-ml infusion bag of 0.9% NaCl for injection. Don't use dextrose solutions. ▪ ***ALERT*** Because of risk of hyperuricemia from tumor lysis, give allopurinol during therapy. ▪ Monitor hematologic function closely. ▪ Fever is common during 1st mo of therapy.

Drug	Indications and dosages	Nursing considerations
clarithromycin Biaxin *Antibiotic* Pregnancy Risk Category: C	*Pharyngitis or tonsillitis from* S. pyogenes — **Adults:** 250 mg P.O. q 12 hr for 10 days. **Children:** 15 mg/kg/day P.O. in divided doses q 12 hr for 10 days. *Acute maxillary sinusitis from* S. pneumoniae, H. influenzae, *or* M. (Branhamella) catarrhalis — **Adults:** 500 mg P.O. q 12 hr for 14 days. **Children:** 15 mg/kg/day P.O. in divided doses q 12 hr for 10 days. *MAC disease in HIV infection* — **Adults:** 500 mg P.O. q 12 hr, with other antimycobacterial drugs, for life. **Children:** 7.5 mg/kg P.O. (maximum 500 mg) q 12 hr, with other antimycobacterial drugs, for life. H. pylori *infection* — **Adults:** 500 mg P.O. q 8 hr for 2 wk with omeprazole 40 mg P.O. q morning. Continue omeprazole (20 mg P.O. q morning) for 4 wk.	▪ Obtain specimen for culture and sensitivity tests before 1st dose. ▪ May cause overgrowth of nonsusceptible bacteria or fungi. Monitor for superinfection. ▪ May give with or without food. Instruct patient not to refrigerate suspension. ▪ Tell patient to report persistent adverse reactions. ▪ Don't give to patients if CrCl < 25 ml/min. ▪ May give without dosage adjustment in patients with hepatic impairment but normal renal function.
clemastine fumarate Antihist-1,Tavist, Tavist-1 *Antihistamine* Pregnancy Risk Category: B	*Rhinitis, allergy symptoms* — **Adults and children ≥ 12 yr:** 1.34 mg P.O. q 12 hr, or 2.68 mg P.O. once daily to t.i.d., p.r.n. Maximum 8.04 mg/day. **Children 6 to 11 yr:** 0.67 to 1.34 mg (syrup only) P.O. b.i.d. Maximum 4.02 mg/day. *Urticaria, angioedema* — **Adults and children ≥ 12 yr:** 2.68 mg P.O. once daily to t.i.d. Maximum dose 8.04 mg/day. **Children 6 to 11 yr:** 1.34 mg (syrup only) P.O. b.i.d. Maximum 4.02 mg/day.	▪ Monitor blood counts during long-term therapy, as ordered; observe for blood dyscrasia. ▪ Instruct patient not to drink alcohol and to avoid activities that require alertness until CNS effects are known. ▪ Tell patient to report tolerance to drug.

DRUG & CLASS	INDICATIONS & DOSAGES	NURSING CONSIDERATIONS
clindamycin hydrochloride Cleocin HCl, Dalacin C†‡ **clindamycin palmitate hydrochloride** Cleocin Pediatric, Dalacin C **clindamycin phosphate** Cleocin Phosphate, Cleocin T, Dalacin C†‡ *Antibiotic* Pregnancy Risk Category: B	*Infections from sensitive aerobic and anaerobic organisms* — **Adults:** 150 to 450 mg P.O. q 6 hr; or, 300 to 600 mg I.M. or I.V. q 6, 8, or 12 hr. **Children >1 mo:** 8 to 20 mg/kg P.O. q.d. in divided doses q 6 to 8 hr; or, 20 to 40 mg/kg I.M. or I.V. q.d. in divided doses q 6 or 8 hr. *Endocarditis prophylaxis for dental procedures in patients allergic to penicillin* — **Adults:** initially, 600 mg P.O. 1 hr before procedure. **Children:** initially, 10 mg/kg P.O. 1 hr before procedure. *Pelvic inflammatory disease* — **Adults:** 900 mg I.V. q 8 hr with gentamicin. Continue ≥ 48 hr after symptoms improve; then switch to oral clindamycin 450 mg 5 times daily for total of 10 to 14 days.	▪ Obtain specimen for culture and sensitivity tests before 1st dose. ▪ ***I.V. use:*** Check I.V. site daily for phlebitis and irritation. For infusion, dilute each 300 mg in 50 ml solution, and give no faster than 30 mg/min (over 10 to 60 min). Never give undiluted as bolus. ▪ ***ALERT*** For I.M. use, inject deeply. Rotate sites. Give ≤ 600 mg per injection. ▪ Observe for signs of superinfection. ▪ Don't give opioid antidiarrheals to treat drug-induced diarrhea; may prolong and worsen diarrhea.
clindamycin phosphate Cleocin T Gel, Lotion, Solution; Cleocin Vaginal Cream *Antibiotic* Pregnancy Risk Category: B	*Inflammatory acne vulgaris* — **Adults and adolescents:** Apply to skin b.i.d., morning and evening. *Bacterial vaginosis* — **Adults:** 1 applicatorful intravaginally h.s. for 7 consecutive days.	▪ Drug can cause excessive dryness. ▪ Tell patient to avoid too-frequent washing of area and to cover entire affected area but avoid contact with eyes, nose, mouth, and other mucous membranes. ▪ ***ALERT*** Warn patient not to smoke while applying topical solution.
clomipramine hydrochloride Anafranil	*Obsessive-compulsive disorder* — **Adults:** initially, 25 mg P.O. q.d. with meals, gradually increased to 100 mg q.d. in divided doses	▪ Gradually stop drug several days before surgery. ▪ Adverse anticholinergic effects can occur

Antiobsessional agent Pregnancy Risk Category: C	during first 2 wk. Thereafter, increase to maximum 250 mg q.d. in divided doses with meals, p.r.n. After adjustment, total daily dose may be given h.s. **Children and adolescents:** initially, 25 mg P.O. q.d. with meals, gradually increased over first 2 wk to daily maximum 3 mg/kg or 100 mg P.O. in divided doses, whichever smaller. Maximum daily dose 3 mg/kg or 200 mg, whichever smaller; may be given h.s. after adjustment. Periodic reassessment and adjustment necessary.	rapidly. ▪ Advise patient to use sunblock, wear protective clothing, and avoid prolonged exposure to strong sunlight. ▪ Don't withdraw abruptly.
clonazepam Klonopin *Anticonvulsant* Pregnancy Risk Category: C Controlled Substance Schedule: IV	*Lennox-Gastaut syndrome; atypical absence seizures; akinetic and myoclonic seizures* — **Adults:** initially, not to exceed 1.5 mg P.O. q.d. in 3 divided doses. May increase by 0.5 to 1 mg q 3 days until seizures controlled. If given in unequal doses, give largest dose h.s. Maximum daily dose 20 mg. **Children ≤ 10 yr or 30 kg (66 lb):** initially, 0.01 to 0.03 mg/kg P.O. q.d. (maximum 0.05 mg/kg q.d.), in 2 or 3 divided doses. Increase by 0.25 to 0.5 mg q 3rd day to maximum maintenance of 0.1 to 0.2 mg/kg q.d., p.r.n.	▪ Don't withdraw suddenly because seizures may worsen. Monitor patient for oversedation. Call doctor if adverse reactions occur. ▪ ***ALERT*** Monitor blood drug levels. Therapeutic level is 20 to 80 ng/ml. ▪ Withdrawal symptoms resemble those of barbiturate withdrawal.
clonidine Catapres-TTS **clonidine hydrochloride** Catapres, Dixarit†‡ *Antihypertensive*	*Essential and renal hypertension* — **Adults:** initially, 0.1 mg P.O. b.i.d.; then increase by 0.1 to 0.2 mg q.d. on weekly basis. Range 0.2 to 0.8 mg q.d. in divided doses. Infrequently, doses up to 2.4 mg q.d. used. Or, as transdermal patch applied to nonhairy	▪ May give to lower BP rapidly in some hypertensive emergencies. ▪ Monitor BP and HR frequently. ▪ Remove transdermal patch before defibrillation to prevent arcing.

(continued)

†Canadian ‡Australian

DRUG & CLASS	INDICATIONS & DOSAGES	NURSING CONSIDERATIONS
clonidine *(continued)* Pregnancy Risk Category: C	area of intact skin on upper arm or torso q 7 days, starting with 0.1-mg system and adjusted with another 0.1-mg or larger system.	▪ Observe for tolerance to therapeutic effects; may need to increased dosage. ▪ ***ALERT*** Transdermal effects may take 2 to 3 days. Oral therapy may have to continue in interim.
clopidogrel bisulfate Plavix *Antiplatelet agent* Pregnancy Risk Category: B	*To reduce atherosclerotic events in patients with atherosclerosis documented by recent CVA, MI, or peripheral arterial disease* — **Adults:** 75 mg P.O. q.d.	▪ Use with caution in patients at risk for increased bleeding from trauma, surgery, or other pathologic conditions, and in patients with hepatic impairment. ▪ Platelet aggregation won't return to normal for at least 5 days after stopping drug. ▪ Use in patients who are hypersensitive or intolerant to aspirin or after stent placement. ▪ Use of NSAIDs may increase risk of GI bleeding. ▪ ***ALERT*** Safety of use with heparin or warfarin has not been established.
clorazepate dipotassium Apo-Clorazepate†, Gen-XENE, Novoclopate†, Tranxene, Tranxene-SD, Tranxene-T-Tab *Anxiolytic, anticonvulsant, sedative-hypnotic* Pregnancy Risk Category: D	*Acute alcohol withdrawal* — **Adults:** day 1: 30 mg P.O. initially, then 30 to 60 mg P.O. in divided doses; day 2: 45 to 90 mg P.O. in divided doses; day 3: 22.5 to 45 mg P.O. in divided doses; day 4: 15 to 30 mg P.O. in divided doses; then gradually reduce dose to 7.5 to 15 mg P.O. q.d. Maximum 90 mg/day. *Adjunct in partial seizure disorder* — **Adults and children > 12 yr:** Maximum initial dose	▪ Reduce dosage in elderly or debilitated patients. ▪ Monitor liver, renal, and hematopoietic function studies periodically, as ordered, with repeated or prolonged therapy. ▪ Abuse and addiction possible. Don't withdraw abruptly after prolonged use; withdrawal symptoms may occur. ▪ Don't give to children < 9 yr.

Controlled Substance Schedule: IV	7.5 mg P.O. t.i.d. Increase $\leq$ 7.5 mg/wk, up to 90 mg q.d. **Children 9 to 12 yr:** maximum initial dose 7.5 mg P.O. b.i.d. Increase $\leq$ 7.5 mg/wk, up to 60 mg q.d. *Anxiety* — **Adults:** 30 mg P.O. q.d., divided; adjust gradually to 15 to 60 mg P.O. q.d.	▪ Instruct patient to avoid alcohol. ▪ Tell patient to avoid activities requiring alertness until CNS effects are known.
clotrimazole Canesten†, Gyne-Lotrimin, Lotrimin, Mycelex, Mycelex-7, Mycelex-G, Mycelex OTC *Antifungal* Pregnancy Risk Category: B	*Superficial fungal infections* — **Adults and children:** Apply thinly and massage into affected and surrounding area, morning and evening, for 2 to 4 wk. If no improvement after 4 wk, reevaluate patient. *Vulvovaginal candidiasis* — **Adults:** two 100-mg vaginal tablets inserted q.d. h.s. for 1 wk, or one 500-mg vaginal tablet q.d. h.s. for 1 day; or 1 applicatorful vaginal cream q.d. h.s. for 1 wk. *Oropharyngeal candidiasis* — **Adults and children $\geq$ 3 yr:** Dissolve lozenge over 15 to 30 min in mouth 5 times q.d. for 2 wk. *Prevention of oropharyngeal candidiasis in immunocompromised patients* — **Adults and children:** Dissolve lozenge over 15 to 30 min in mouth t.i.d. during chemotherapy or until steroid reduced to maintenance levels.	▪ Report irritation or sensitivity; stop using if irritation occurs, and notify doctor. ▪ Warn patient not to use occlusive wrappings or dressings. ▪ Tell patient that frequent or persistent yeast infections may indicate a more serious medical problem.
clozapine Clozaril *Antipsychotic* Pregnancy Risk Category: B	*Schizophrenia in severely ill patients unresponsive to other therapies* — **Adults:** initially, 12.5 mg P.O. once daily or b.i.d., increased after 25 to 50 mg q.d. (if tolerated) to 300 to 450 mg q.d. by end of 2 wk. Indi-	▪ Poses significant risk of agranulocytosis. ▪ Perform WBC counts and blood tests. ▪ Monitor closely for signs of infection. Protective isolation may be needed. *(continued)*

DRUG & CLASS	INDICATIONS & DOSAGES	NURSING CONSIDERATIONS
clozapine *(continued)*	vidual dosage based on response, patient tolerance, and adverse reactions. Don't increase dose more than once or twice weekly, and don't exceed 100-mg q.d. increases. Usual dose is 300 to 600 mg q.d., maximum is 900 mg daily.	▪ Withdraw gradually over 1 to 2 wk. Monitor closely for recurrence of psychotic symptoms. ▪ Don't dispense more than 1-wk supply of drug. ▪ May cause seizures or transient fevers.
codeine phosphate Paveral† **codeine sulfate** *Analgesic, antitussive* Pregnancy Risk Category: C Controlled Substance Schedule: II	*Mild to moderate pain* — **Adults:** 15 to 60 mg P.O. or 15 to 60 mg (phosphate) S.C., I.M., or I.V. q 4 to 6 hr, p.r.n. **Children > 1 yr:** 0.5 mg/kg P.O., S.C., or I.M. q 4 hr, p.r.n. *Nonproductive cough* — **Adults:** 10 to 20 mg P.O. q 4 to 6 hr. Maximum 120 mg daily. **Children 6 to 12 yr:** 5 to 10 mg P.O. q 4 to 6 hr. Maximum 60 mg daily. **Children 2 to 6 yr:** 2.5 to 5 mg P.O. q 4 to 6 hr. Maximum 30 mg daily.	▪ ***I.V. use:*** Give by very slow direct injection into large vein. ▪ Don't mix with other solutions. ▪ For full analgesic effect, give before patient has intense pain. ▪ ***ALERT*** Don't use as antitussive when cough is crucial diagnostic sign or is beneficial (as after thoracic surgery). ▪ Monitor respiratory and circulatory status.
colchicine Colgout‡, Colsalide, Novocolchicine† *Antigout agent* Pregnancy Risk Category: C (P.O.), D (I.V.)	*Prevention or maintenance of acute gout* — **Adults:** 0.5 or 0.6 mg P.O. q.d. Dosage varies with severity and frequency of attacks. *Prevention of acute gout in patients undergoing surgery* — **Adults:** 0.5 or 0.6 mg P.O. t.i.d. 3 days before and 3 days after surgery. *Acute gout; acute gouty arthritis* — **Adults:** 0.5 to 1.3 mg P.O.; then 0.5 or 0.6 mg q 1 to 2 hr until relief, nausea, vomiting, or diarrhea ensues or maximum dose of 8 mg reached. Or, 2 mg I.V.; then 0.5 mg I.V. q 6 hr, p.r.n. Maximum 4 mg daily.	▪ Obtain lab studies before and during therapy. ▪ ***I.V. use:*** Give by slow I.V. push over 2 to 5 min. ▪ Don't give I.M. or S.C. ▪ Give with meals to reduce GI effects. ▪ Monitor I&O; keep output at 2,000 ml/24 hr. ▪ ***ALERT*** First sign of acute overdose may be GI symptoms.

colestipol hydrochloride Colestid *Antilipemic* Pregnancy Risk Category: B	*Primary hypercholesterolemia* — **Adults:** granules: 5 to 30 g P.O. once daily or in divided doses; tablets: 2 to 16 g P.O. once daily or in divided doses.	▪ Monitor cholesterol and triglyceride levels regularly. ▪ Monitor bowel habits. ▪ ***ALERT*** Don't give in dry form. Encourage diet high in fiber and fluids. ▪ In patient also receiving cardiac glycoside, monitor levels of that drug.
co-trimoxazole (trimethoprim-sulfamethoxazole) Apo-Sulfatrim†, Bactrim DS, Cotrim, Septra, Sulfatrim, TMP-SMZ *Antibiotic* Pregnancy Risk Category: C (contraindicated at term)	*Shigellosis or UTI from susceptible* E. coli, Proteus *(indole positive or negative),* Klebsiella, *or* Enterobacter — **Adults:** 160 mg trimethoprim/800 mg sulfamethoxazole (double-strength tablets) P.O. q 12 hr for 10 to 14 days in UTI and for 5 days in shigellosis. For uncomplicated cystitis or acute urethral syndrome, 1 double-strength tablet q 12 hr for 3 days. If indicated, I.V. infusion given: 8 to 10 mg/kg/day in 2 to 4 divided doses q 6, 8, or 12 hr for up to 14 days for severe UTI. Maximum 960 mg trimethoprim. **Children ≥ 2 mo:** 8 mg/kg/day P.O., in 2 divided doses q 12 hr (10 days for UTI; 5 days for shigellosis). If indicated, I.V. infusion given: 8 to 10 mg/kg/day in 2 to 4 divided doses q 6, 8, or 12 hr. Don't exceed adult dose. *Chronic bronchitis; upper respiratory tract infections* — **Adults:** 160 mg trimethoprim/800 mg sulfamethoxazole P.O. q 12 hr for 10 to 14 days.	▪ Dosage for mg/kg/day based on trimethoprim component. ▪ Obtain specimen for culture and sensitivity tests before 1st dose. ▪ ***I.V. use:*** Dilute infusion in D_5W. Don't mix with other drugs or solutions. Infuse slowly over 60 to 90 min. Don't give by rapid infusion or bolus injection. Don't refrigerate. Use within 6 hr. ▪ Adverse reactions, especially hypersensitivity reactions, rash, and fever, are more common in AIDS patients. ▪ Promptly report rash, sore throat, fever, or mouth sores (early signs of blood dyscrasia). ▪ ***ALERT*** Never give I.M.

(continued)

†Canadian ‡Australian

DRUG & CLASS	INDICATIONS & DOSAGES	NURSING CONSIDERATIONS
co-trimoxazole *(continued)*	Pneumocystis carinii — **Adults and children > 2 mo:** 15 to 20 mg/kg/day (as trimethoprim) P.O. or I.V. in equally divided doses q 6 hr for 14 to 21 days. *Prevention of* Pneumocystis carinii—**Adults:** 1 Bactrim DS tablet P.O. q.d. **Children:** 150 mg/m^2/day trimethoprim with 750 mg/m^2/day. Sulfamethoxazole P.O. in divided doses b.i.d. on 3 consecutive days per week. Maximum daily dose is 320 mg trimethoprim/1,600 mg sulfamethoxazole. *UTI in men with prostatitis* — **Adults:** 160 mg trimethoprim/800 mg sulfamethoxazole P.O. b.i.d. for 3 to 6 mo. ***Adjust-a-dose:*** In patients with renal impairment, if CrCl 15 to 30 ml/min, reduce daily dose by 50%. Don't give to patients if CrCl < 15 ml/min.	
cromolyn sodium (sodium cromoglycate) Crolom, Intal, Intal Aerosol Spray, Intal Nebulizer Solution, Nasalcrom *Mast cell stabilizer, antiasthmatic* Pregnancy Risk Category: B	*Mild to moderate persistent asthma* — **Adults and children $\geq$ 5 yr:** 2 metered sprays using inhaler q.i.d. at regular intervals. Or, 20 mg via nebulization q.i.d. at regular intervals. *Prevention and treatment of seasonal and perennial allergic rhinitis* — **Adults and children > 5 yr:** 1 spray in each nostril t.i.d. or q.i.d., up to 6 times daily. *Prevention of exercise-induced bronchospasm* — **Adults and children $\geq$ 5 yr:** 2 me-	▪ ***ALERT*** Except for ophthalmic solution, use only when acute asthma episode has been controlled, airway is clear, and patient can breathe independently. ▪ Dissolve powder in capsules for oral dose in hot water and further dilute with cold water before ingestion. Don't mix with fruit juice, milk, or food. ▪ Watch for recurrence of asthmatic symptoms when dosage decreased.

	tered sprays inhaled < 1 hr before anticipated exercise. *Conjunctivitis* — **Adults and children ≥ 4 yr:** 1 to 2 drops in each eye 4 to 6 times q.d. at regular intervals.	
cyanocobalamin (vitamin B_{12}) Anacobin†, Bedoz†, Crystamine, Crysti-12, Cyanoject, Cyomin, Rubesol-1000 **hydroxocobalamin (vitamin B_{12})** Codroxomin, Hydrobexan, Hydro-Cobex, Hydro-Crysti-12, LA-12 *Vitamin, nutritional supplement* Pregnancy Risk Category: NR	*Vitamin B_{12} deficiency* — **Adults:** 30 mcg hydroxocobalamin I.M. q.d. for 5 to 10 days, depending on severity. Maintenance: 100 to 200 mcg I.M. q mo. **Children:** 1 to 5 mg hydroxocobalamin spread over ≥ 2 wk in doses of 100 mcg I.M., depending on severity. Maintenance: 30 to 50 mcg I.M. q mo. *Pernicious anemia; vitamin B_{12} malabsorption* — **Adults:** 100 mcg cyanocobalamin I.M. or S.C. q.d. for 6 to 7 days; then 100 mcg I.M. or S.C. q mo. **Children:** 30 to 50 mcg I.M. or S.C. q.d. over ≥ 2 wk; then 100 mcg I.M. or S.C. q mo for life. *Methylmalonic aciduria* — **Neonates:** 1,000 mcg cyanocobalamin I.M. q.d.	▪ Use cautiously in anemic patients with coexisting cardiac, pulmonary, or hypertensive disease, and in those with severe vitamin B_{12}–dependent deficiencies. ▪ Use cautiously in premature infants. ▪ Determine reticulocyte count, Hct, B_{12}, iron, and folate levels before therapy. ▪ Don't mix in same syringe with other drugs. ▪ Incompatible with many drugs and solutions. ▪ Closely monitor potassium levels for first 48 hr. ▪ Protect vitamin B_{12} from light. Don't refrigerate or freeze. ▪ ***ALERT*** In pernicious anemia, stress need for monthly injections; anemia will recur if not treated monthly.
cyclobenzaprine hydrochloride Flexeril *Skeletal muscle relaxant* Pregnancy Risk Category: B	*Short-term treatment of muscle spasm* — **Adults:** 10 mg P.O. t.i.d. Maximum 60 mg q.d.; maximum duration of treatment 2 to 3 wk.	▪ Be alert for nausea, headache, and malaise, which may occur with abrupt withdrawal after long-term use. ▪ ***ALERT*** Watch for symptoms of overdose, including cardiac toxicity. Notify doctor immediately and have physostigmine available.

DRUG & CLASS	INDICATIONS & DOSAGES	NURSING CONSIDERATIONS
cyclophosphamide Cycloblastin‡, Cytoxan, Cytoxan Lyophilized, Endoxan-Asta‡, Neosar, Procytox† *Antineoplastic* Pregnancy Risk Category: D	*Breast and ovarian cancers; Hodgkin's disease; chronic lymphocytic leukemia; chronic myelocytic leukemia; acute lymphoblastic leukemia; acute myelocytic and monocytic leukemia; neuroblastoma; retinoblastoma; malignant lymphoma; multiple myeloma; mycosis fungoides; sarcoma* — **Adults and children:** initially, 40 to 50 mg/kg I.V. in divided doses over 2 to 5 days. Or, 10 to 15 mg/kg I.V. q 7 to 10 days, 3 to 5 mg/kg I.V. twice weekly, or 1 to 5 mg/kg P.O. q.d., depending on patient tolerance. Subsequent dosages adjusted according to response. *Minimal change nephrotic syndrome in children* — **Children:** 2.5 to 3 mg/kg P.O. q.d. for 60 to 90 days.	▪ Parenteral form carries carcinogenic, mutagenic, and teratogenic risks for personnel. ▪ After reconstitution, give by direct I.V. injection or infusion. For I.V. infusion, dilute with compatible solution such as D_5W. ▪ ***ALERT*** Don't give drug h.s.; may increase the possibility of cystitis. If cystitis occurs, stop drug and notify doctor. Mesna may be given to lower the incidence and severity of bladder toxicity. ▪ Monitor serum uric acid level. ▪ Encourage voiding q 1 to 2 hr while awake and drinking $\geq$ 3 L fluid q.d.
cyclosporine (cyclosporin) Neoral, Sandimmun‡, Sandimmune *Immunosuppressant* Pregnancy Risk Category: C	*Prevention of organ rejection in kidney, liver, or heart transplant* — **Adults and children:** 15 mg/kg P.O. 4 to 12 hr before transplant and continued q.d. postoperatively for 1 to 2 wk. Then reduce dose 5% each wk to maintenance level of 5 to 10 mg/kg/day. Or, 5 to 6 mg/kg I.V. concentrate 4 to 12 hr before transplant. Postoperatively, repeat dose q.d. until patient can tolerate oral form. *Rheumatoid arthritis; psoriasis* — **Adults:** 1.25 mg/kg (Neoral) P.O. q 12 hr initially. Maximum of 4 mg/kg/day.	▪ To increase palatability of oral solutions, mix with whole milk or fruit juice. Use glass container. ▪ ***ALERT*** Neoral and Sandimmune aren't bioequivalent. Less Neoral may be needed to yield the same blood level derived from Sandimmune. ▪ ***I.V. use:*** Give I.V. concentrate at ⅓ oral dose and dilute before use. Dilute each ml of concentrate in 20 to 100 ml of D_5W or 0.9% NaCl for injection immediately before giving; infuse over 2 to 6 hr.

	Adjust-a-dose: In patients with adverse reactions such as hypertension, elevated serum creatinine (30% above pretreatment level), or abnormal CBC and LFT results, decrease dose by 25% to 50%.	▪ Monitor cyclosporine blood levels, BUN, LFTs, and creatinine levels.
cytarabine (ara-C, cytosine arabinoside) Alexan†, Cytosar†, Cytosar-U *Antineoplastic* Pregnancy Risk Category: D	*Acute nonlymphocytic leukemia; acute lymphocytic leukemia; blast phase of chronic myelocytic leukemia* — **Adults and children:** 100 mg/m² q.d. by continuous I.V. infusion or 100 mg/m² I.V. q 12 hr. Give for 7 days and repeat q 2 wk. Maintenance: 1 mg/kg S.C. once or twice a wk. *Meningeal leukemia* — **Adults and children:** highly variable from 5 mg/m² to 75 mg/m² intrathecally. Frequency also varies from once a day for 4 days to once q 4 days.	▪ Give antiemetic before giving drugs. ▪ Parenteral form has carcinogenic, mutagenic, and teratogenic risks for personnel. ▪ For I.V. infusion, dilute using 0.9% NaCl for injection or D_5W. ▪ ***ALERT*** When given intrathetically, use preservative-free 0.9% NaCl. ▪ Maintain high fluid intake and give allopurinol to avoid urate nephropathy. ▪ Monitor uric acid level, LFTs, renal function studies, and CBC. ▪ Assess patient for neurotoxicity.
cytomegalovirus immune globulin (human), intravenous (CMV-IGIV) CytoGam *Immune globulin* Pregnancy Risk Category: C	*To attenuate primary CMV in seronegative patients who received a kidney from CMV-seropositive donor* — **Adults:** give I.V. based on time after transplant: within 72 hr, 150 mg/kg; 2 wk after, 100 mg/kg; 4 wk after, 100 mg/kg; 6 wk after, 100 mg/kg; 8 wk after, 100 mg/kg; 12 wk after, 50 mg/kg; 16 wk after, 50 mg/kg. *Prevention of CMV from lung, liver, pancreas, and heart transplants* — **Adults:** used with ganciclovir in organ transplants from CMV-seropositive donors into seronegative recipi-	▪ ***I.V. use:*** Give through separate I.V. line with constant infusion pump. If unable to give through separate line, piggyback into preexisting line. Don't dilute more than 1:2 with diluent. ▪ Begin infusion within 6 hr of entering vial; finish within 12 hr. ▪ Monitor vital signs closely. ▪ Give 1st dose at 15 mg/kg/hr. Increase to 30 mg/kg/hr after 30 min if no adverse reactions, then to 60 mg/kg/hr after another 30 min if no reactions. *(continued)*

†Canadian ‡Australian

DRUG & CLASS	INDICATIONS & DOSAGES	NURSING CONSIDERATIONS
cytomegalovirus immune globulin *(continued)*	ents. Maximum total dosage per infusion is 150 mg/kg given I.V. as follows, based on time after transplant: within 72 hr: 50 mg/kg; 2 wk after: 150 mg/kg; 4 wk after: 50 mg/kg; 6 wk after: 150 mg/kg; 8 wk after: 50 mg/kg; 12 wk after: 100 mg/kg; 16 wk after: 100 mg/kg.	Volume maximum 75 ml/hr. Subsequent doses may be given at 15 mg/kg/hr for 15 min, increasing q 15 min in steps to 60 mg/kg/hr. Volume maximum 75 ml/hr. ▪ For anaphylaxis or drop in BP, stop infusion, notify doctor, and be prepared to perform cardiac resuscitation and give diphenhydramine and epinephrine. ▪ Refrigerate at 36° to 46° F (2° to 8° C). ▪ Monitor patient closely during and after each rate change.
dacarbazine (DTIC) DTIC†, DTIC-Dome *Antineoplastic* Pregnancy Risk Category: C	*Metastatic malignant melanoma* — **Adults:** 2 to 4.5 mg/kg I.V. q.d. for 10 days; repeated q 4 wk as tolerated. Or 250 mg/m^2 I.V. q.d. for 5 days, repeated q 3 wk. *Hodgkin's disease* — **Adults:** 150 mg/m^2 I.V. q.d. (in combination with other agents) for 5 days, repeated q 4 wk; or 375 mg/m^2 on 1st day of combination, repeated q 15 days.	▪ ***ALERT*** Avoid extravasation during infusion. If I.V. solution infiltrates, stop immediately, apply ice to area for 24 to 48 hr, and notify doctor. ▪ To prevent bleeding, avoid all I.M. injections when platelet count < 100,000/mm^3. ▪ Toxicity often accompanies therapeutic effects. Monitor CBC and platelet count.
daclizumab Zenapax *Immunosuppressant* Pregnancy Risk Category: C	*Prevention of acute organ rejection in patients receiving renal transplants combined with immunosuppressive regimen that includes cyclosporine and corticosteroids* — **Adults:** 1 mg/kg I.V. Standard course of therapy is 5 doses. Give 1st dose no more than 24 hr before transplant; give remaining 4 doses q 14 days.	▪ Use only under supervision of doctor experienced in immunosuppressive therapy and management of organ transplant. ▪ Monitor for lipoproliferative disorders and opportunistic infections. ▪ Keep drugs used for anaphylactic reactions immediately available. ▪ ***I.V. use:*** Don't use as direct I.V. injection.

Dilute in 50 ml sterile 0.9% NaCl before giving. Don't shake. Inspect for particulate matter or discoloration before use.

- Patient and family members shouldn't receive vaccinations during daclizumab therapy unless approved by doctor.

---

dactinomycin (actinomycin D)
Cosmegen
Antineoplastic
Pregnancy Risk Category: C

Dosage and indications vary. Check treatment protocol with doctor.

Sarcoma; trophoblastic tumors in women; testicular cancer — **Adults:** 500 mcg (0.5 mg) I.V. q.d. for 5 days. Maximum 15 mcg/kg/day, or 400 to 600 mcg/m^2/day for 5 days. After bone marrow recovery, may repeat course.

Wilms' tumor; rhabdomyosarcoma; Ewing's sarcoma — **Children:** 10 to 15 mcg/kg or 450 mcg/m^2/day I.V. for 5 days. Maximum 500 mcg/day. Or, 2.5 mg/m^2 I.V. in equally divided daily doses over 7 days. After bone marrow recovery, may repeat course.

- ***I.V. use:*** Give by direct injection into vein or through tubing of free-flowing I.V. solution of 0.9% NaCl for injection or D_5W.
- For I.V. infusion, dilute with up to 50 ml D_5W or 0.9% NaCl for injection; infuse over 15 min.
- ***ALERT*** If extravasation occurs, severe tissue necrosis may result. If infiltration occurs, apply cold compresses and notify doctor.
- If skin contact occurs, irrigate with water for $\geq$ 15 min.
- Monitor CBC, platelet counts, and renal and hepatic functions, as ordered. Observe for stomatitis, diarrhea, and leukopenia.

---

dalteparin sodium
Fragmin
Anticoagulant
Pregnancy Risk Category: B

Prevention of deep vein thrombosis (DVT) in patients undergoing abdominal surgery who are at risk for thromboembolic complications — **Adults:** 2,500 IU S.C. q.d., starting 1 to 2 hr before surgery and repeated q.d. for 5 to 10 days postoperatively.

Prevention of DVT in patients undergoing hip replacement surgery — **Adults:** 1st

- Have patient sit or lie supine when giving. Give S.C. injection deeply. Rotate sites daily.
- ***ALERT*** Not interchangeable unit for unit with unfractionated heparin or other low-molecular-weight heparin.
- ***ALERT*** Patients receiving dalteparin who require neuraxial *(continued)*

DRUG & CLASS	INDICATIONS & DOSAGES	NURSING CONSIDERATIONS
dalteparin sodium *(continued)*	dose, 2,500 IU S.C. ≤ 2 hr before surgery and 2nd dose 2,500 IU S.C. the evening of surgery (≥ 6 hr after 1st dose). If surgery is performed in evening, omit 2nd dose on day of surgery. Starting on 1st postoperative day, give 5,000 IU S.C. q.d. for 5 to 10 days. Or, 5,000 IU S.C. evening before surgery, then 5,000 IU S.C. q.d. starting evening of surgery for 5 to 10 days postoperatively. *Unstable angina; non–Q-wave MI* — **Adults:** 120 IU/kg (maximum 10,000 IU/dose) S.C. q 12 hr with aspirin therapy. Usual duration of treatment is 5 to 8 days.	anesthesia or spinal puncture may be at increased risk for developing an epidural or spinal hematoma, which can cause long-term or permanent paralysis. ▪ Periodic, routine CBC and fecal occult blood tests recommended. Regular monitoring of PT or activated PTT not required. ▪ Monitor closely for thrombocytopenia. ▪ Discontinue if thromboembolic event occurs despite dalteparin prophylaxis.
danaparoid sodium Orgaran *Anticoagulant, antithrombotic* Pregnancy Risk Category: B	*Prevention of postoperative deep vein thrombisis (DVT) in patients undergoing elective hip replacement surgery* — **Adults:** 750 anti-Xa units S.C. b.i.d. starting 1 to 4 hr preoperatively, and then ≥ 2 hr after surgery. Treat for 1 to 2 wk postoperatively or until risk of DVT diminished.	▪ To give, have patient lie down. Give S.C. injection deeply. Never give I.M. Don't rub afterward. ▪ ***ALERT*** Not interchangeable (unit for unit) with heparin or low–molecular-weight heparin. ▪ Perform routine CBC and fecal occult blood tests during therapy. ▪ Has little effect on PT, PTT, fibrinolytic activity, or bleeding time. ▪ Monitor Hct and BP closely; decrease in either may signal hemorrhage. ▪ If serious bleeding occurs, stop drug and transfuse blood products.

danazol
Cycloment†, Danocrine
Antiestrogen, androgen
Pregnancy Risk Category: X

Mild endometriosis — **Women:** initially, 100 to 200 mg P.O. b.i.d. uninterrupted for 3 to 6 mo; may continue for 9 mo. Subsequent dosage based on patient response.
Moderate to severe endometriosis — **Women:** 400 mg P.O. b.i.d. uninterrupted for 3 to 6 mo; may continue for 9 mo.
Fibrocystic breast disease — **Women:** 100 to 400 mg P.O. q.d. in 2 divided doses uninterrupted for 2 to 6 mo.

- Unless contraindicated, instruct patient to use with diet high in calories and protein.
- Monitor closely for virilization signs. Some androgenic effects, such as voice deepening, may be irreversible.
- Periodic dosage decreases or gradual drug withdrawal preferred.
- Instruct patient to use nonhormonal contraceptive measures during therapy. Stop drug if pregnancy suspected.

dantrolene sodium
Dantrium
Skeletal muscle relaxant
Pregnancy Risk Category: C

Spasticity and sequelae from severe chronic disorders (such as multiple sclerosis, cerebral palsy, spinal cord injury, CVA) — **Adults:** 25 mg P.O. q.d. Increase gradually in 25-mg increments, up to 100 mg b.i.d. to q.i.d. **Children:** initially, 0.5 mg/kg P.O. b.i.d.; increase to t.i.d., then q.i.d. Increase, p.r.n., by 0.5 mg/kg q.d. to 3 mg/kg b.i.d. to q.i.d., to maximum 100 mg q.i.d.

- Watch for hepatitis (fever and jaundice), severe diarrhea, severe weakness, or sensitivity reactions (fever and skin eruptions). Withhold dose and notify doctor if these occur.
- Prepare oral suspension for single dose by dissolving capsule contents in juice or other liquid.
- Obtain LFT results at start of therapy.
- Caution patient about exposure to sunlight; photosensitivity may occur.

dapsone
Avlosulfon†, Dapsone 100‡
Antileprotic, antimalarial
Pregnancy Risk Category: C

All forms of leprosy (Hansen's disease) — **Adults:** 100 mg P.O. q.d., indefinitely; give with rifampin 600 mg P.O. q.d. for 6 mo. **Children:** 1.4 mg/kg P.O. q.d. for ≥ 3 yr.
Dermatitis herpetiformis — **Adults:** 50 mg P.O. q.d.; increase to 300 mg q.d., p.r.n.

- ***ALERT*** Monitor for signs and symptoms of erythema nodosum reaction (malaise, fever, painful inflammatory induration in skin and mucosa, iritis, neuritis).
- Be prepared to reduce dose or stop drug with decreased Hgb or RBC or WBC count.
- If generalized,

(continued)

†Canadian ‡Australian

DRUG & CLASS	INDICATIONS & DOSAGES	NURSING CONSIDERATIONS
dapsone *(continued)*		diffuse dermatitis occurs, notify doctor. ▪ Give antihistamine to combat allergic dermatitis.
daunorubicin hydrochloride Cerubidine†, Cerubidine *Antineoplastic* Pregnancy Risk Category: D	Dosage and indications vary. *Remission induction in acute nonlymphocytic (myelogenous, monocytic, erythroid) leukemia* — **Adults:** in combination, 30 to 45 mg/m²/day I.V. on days 1, 2, and 3 of 1st course and on days 1 and 2 of subsequent courses with cytarabine infusions. *Remission induction in acute lymphocytic leukemia* — **Adults:** in combination, 45 mg/m²/day I.V. on days 1, 2, and 3 of 1st course. **Children ≥ 2 yr:** 25 mg/m² I.V. on day 1 q wk, for up to 6 wk, p.r.n. **Children < 2 yr or body surface area < 0.5 m²:** dose calculated based on body weight (1 mg/kg). ***Adjust-a-dose:*** May reduce dosage in patients with impaired renal or hepatic function.	▪ Take preventive measures (including adequate hydration) before treatment starts. ▪ ***I.V. use:*** Withdraw into syringe containing 10 to 15 ml 0.9% NaCl for injection. Inject into tubing of free-flowing I.V. solution of D_5W or 0.9% NaCl for injection over 2 to 3 min. Or, dilute in 50 ml 0.9% NaCl for injection, and infuse over 10 to 15 min, or dilute in 100 ml and infuse over 30 to 45 min. If extravasation occurs, stop infusion immediately, apply ice for 24 to 48 hr, and notify doctor. ▪ Monitor CBC, LFTs, and pulse, as ordered; monitor ECG q mo during therapy. Monitor for nausea and vomiting, which may last 24 to 48 hr. ▪ Stop drug and notify doctor if signs of heart failure or cardiomyopathy develop.
delavirdine mesylate Rescriptor *Antiretroviral* Pregnancy Risk Category: C	*HIV-1 infection when therapy is warranted* — **Adults:** 400 mg P.O. t.i.d. with other appropriate antiretroviral agents.	▪ Drug-induced rash is more common in patients with lower CD4+ cell counts and usually occurs within first 3 wk of treatment. ▪ Monitor LFTs and renal function tests; effects in patients with hepatic or renal impairment unknown.

demeclocycline hydrochloride Declomycin, Ledermycin‡ *Antibiotic* Pregnancy Risk Category: D	*Infections from susceptible gram-positive and -negative organisms,* Rickettsia, M. pneumoniae, C. trachomatis; *psittacosis; granuloma inguinale* — **Adults:** 150 mg P.O. q 6 hr or 300 mg P.O. q 12 hr. **Children > 8 yr:** 6 to 12 mg/kg P.O. q.d. in divided doses q 6 to 12 hr. *Gonorrhea* — **Adults:** initially, 600 mg P.O.; then 300 mg P.O. q 12 hr for 4 days (total 3 g).	▪ Obtain specimen for culture and sensitivity tests before 1st dose. ▪ Don't expose to light or heat; store in tightly capped container. ▪ Monitor for superinfection. ▪ Check tongue for signs of candidal infection. Stress good oral hygiene.
desipramine hydrochloride Norpramin, Pertofran‡, Pertofrane *Antidepressant* Pregnancy Risk Category: C	*Depression* — **Adults:** 100 to 200 mg P.O. q.d. in divided doses, increased to maximum 300 mg q.d. Or give entire dose h.s. **Elderly and adolescents:** 25 to 100 mg P.O. q.d. in divided doses, increased gradually to maximum 150 mg q.d., if needed.	▪ Record mood changes. Monitor for suicidal tendencies, and allow only minimum drug supply. ▪ Produces fewer anticholinergic effects than other TCAs. Such effects can occur rapidly. ▪ Stop gradually several days before surgery.
desmopressin acetate DDAVP, Minirin‡, Stimate *Antidiuretic agent, hemostatic* Pregnancy Risk Category: B	*Nonnephrogenic diabetes insipidus; temporary polyuria and polydipsia with pituitary trauma* — **Adults:** 0.1 to 0.4 ml intranasally q.d. in 1 to 3 doses. Adjust morning and evening doses separately for adequate diurnal rhythm of water turnover. Or, give injectable form 0.5 to 1 ml I.V. or S.C. q.d., usually in 2 divided doses. **Children 3 mo to 12 yr:** 0.05 to 0.3 ml intranasally q.d. in 1 or 2 doses. *Management of primary nocturnal enuresis* — **Children ≥ 6 yr:** 20 mcg (0.2 ml) intranasally h.s, ½ the dose given per nostril. Or, initially, 0.2 mg P.O. h.s. May increase to 0.6 mg for	▪ ***ALERT*** Overdose may cause oxytocic or vasopressor activity. Withhold drug and notify doctor. ▪ Intranasal use can cause changes in nasal mucosa resulting in erratic, unreliable absorption. Report worsening condition to doctor; may prescribe injectable DDAVP. ▪ Adjust fluid intake to reduce risk of water intoxication and sodium depletion, especially in children and elderly patients.

(continued)

†Canadian ‡Australian

DRUG & CLASS	INDICATIONS & DOSAGES	NURSING CONSIDERATIONS
desmopressin acetate *(continued)*	desired response. For patients previously on intranasal DDAVP therapy, start tablet at night 24 hr after last intranasal dose. *Hemophilia A and von Willebrand's disease (Type I)* — **Adults and children > 3 mo:** 0.3 mcg/kg I.V. slowly over 15 to 30 min. Or, 1 spray (1.5 mg/ml solution) per nostril for total dose of 300 mcg. In patients < 50 kg, 150 mcg given as single spray.	
dexamethasone (injectable) Decadron, Hexadrol **dexamethasone acetate** Dalalone D.P., Decadron-LA, Dexasone-L.A. **dexamethasone sodium phosphate** Dalalone, Decadron Phosphate, Dexasone *Anti-inflammatory, immunosuppressant* Pregnancy Risk Category: C	*Cerebral edema* — **Adults:** initially, 10 mg (phosphate) I.V.; then 4 to 6 mg I.M. q 6 hr until symptoms subside (usually 2 to 4 days); then taper over 5 to 7 days. *Inflammatory conditions; allergic reactions; neoplasias* — **Adults:** 0.75 to 9 mg/day P.O. or 0.5 to 9 mg/day (phosphate) I.M.; or 4 to 16 mg (acetate) I.M. into joint or soft tissue q 1 to 3 wk; or 0.8 to 1.6 mg (acetate) into lesions q 1 to 3 wk. *Shock* — **Adults:** 1 to 6 mg/kg (phosphate) I.V. as single dose; or 40 mg I.V. q 2 to 6 hr, p.r.n.; continue only until patient stabilized.	▪ For better results and less toxicity, give once-daily dose in morning with food. ▪ Inspect skin for petechiae. ▪ Monitor weight, BP, serum electrolytes, and blood glucose. ▪ Watch for depression or psychotic episodes, especially with high-dose therapy. ▪ ***I.V. use:*** When giving as direct injection, inject undiluted over ≥ 1 min.
dexamethasone (ophthalmic) Maxidex Ophthalmic Suspension	*Uveitis; iridocyclitis; inflammatory conditions of eyelids, conjunctiva, cornea, anterior segment of globe; corneal injury from chemical or thermal burns or penetration of*	▪ Use cautiously in patients with corneal abrasions that may be infected (especially with herpes). ▪ Increase glaucoma medications.

dexamethasone sodium phosphate Ak-Dex, Decadron Phosphate Ophthalmic, Maxidex Ophthalmic *Ophthalmic anti-inflammatory* Pregnancy Risk Category: C	*foreign bodies; allergic conjunctivitis; suppression of graft rejection after keratoplasty* — **Adults and children:** 1 to 2 drops suspension or solution or 1.25 to 2.5 cm ointment into conjunctival sac. In severe disease, use drops q hr, tapering off as condition improves. In mild conditions, use drops ≤ 6 times daily or ointment t.i.d. or q.i.d.; taper to b.i.d., then once daily.	▪ Monitor for corneal ulceration. ▪ Tell patient to shake suspension well before use. ▪ Teach patient how to use drug. ▪ Warn patient to stop drug and call doctor if visual acuity changes or visual field diminishes. ▪ Treatment may extend from days to weeks.
dexamethasone (topical) Aeroseb-Dex, Decaderm, Decaspray **dexamethasone sodium phosphate** Decadron *Anti-inflammatory* Pregnancy Risk Category: C	*Inflammation from corticosteroid-responsive dermatoses* — **Adults and children:** For ointment, clean area, part hair, and apply sparingly t.i.d. to q.i.d. For aerosol use on scalp, shake can gently and apply to dry scalp after shampooing. Spray (about 2 sec) while moving to all affected areas, keeping spray under hair. Spot-spray inadequately covered areas. Don't massage drug into scalp or spray forehead or near eyes.	▪ Gently wash skin before applying. Rub in gently, leaving thin coat. Don't apply near eyes, on mucous membranes, or in ear canal. ▪ Notify doctor if skin infection, striae, atrophy, or fever develops. ▪ When using aerosol around face, cover patient's eyes and warn against inhaling spray. To avoid freezing tissues, don't spray > 1 to 2 sec or closer than 6" (15 cm). ▪ Continue treatment for several days after lesions clear, as ordered.
dextroamphetamine sulfate Dexedrine, Dexedrine Spansule, Spancap #1 *CNS stimulant, short-term adjunctive anorexigenic* Pregnancy Risk Category: C	*Narcolepsy* — **Adults:** 5 to 60 mg P.O. q.d. in divided doses. **Children ≥ 12 yr:** 10 mg P.O. q.d., increase by 10-mg increments q wk, p.r.n. Give 1st dose on awakening, then 1 or 2 more doses, q 4 to 6 hr. **Children 6 to 11 yr:** 5 mg P.O. q.d., with 5-mg increments q wk, p.r.n. *Short-term adjunct in exogenous obesity* — **Adults and children ≥ 12 yr:** 5 to 30 mg P.O.	▪ Don't use to prevent fatigue. ▪ Make sure obese patient is on weight-reduction program. ▪ If tolerance to anorexigenic effect develops, stop drug and notify doctor. ▪ Advise patient to avoid activities requiring alertness until CNS effects are known. *(continued)*

DRUG & CLASS	INDICATIONS & DOSAGES	NURSING CONSIDERATIONS
dextroamphetamine sulfate *(continued)* Controlled Substance Schedule: II	q.d. 30 to 60 min before meals in divided doses of 5 to 10 mg. Or, one 10- or 15-mg sustained-release capsule q.d. in morning. *Attention deficit disorder with hyperactivity* — **Children ≥ 6 yr:** 5 mg P.O. daily or b.i.d. Add 5-mg increments weekly, p.r.n. **Children 3 to 5 yr:** 2.5 mg P.O. daily. Add 2.5-mg increments weekly, p.r.n.	▪ Tell patient to report excessive stimulation. ▪ Fatigue may occur as drug wears off.
dextrose (d-glucose) *TPN component, caloric supplement, fluid volume replacement* Pregnancy Risk Category: C	*Fluid replacement and caloric supplementation* — **Adults and children:** Dosage varies. Peripheral I.V. infusion of 2.5% to 10% solution or central I.V. infusion of 20% solution for minimal fluid needs. 25% solution for acute hypoglycemia in neonates or infants. 50% solution for insulin-induced hypoglycemia. Solution of 10% to 70% diluted in admixtures, for TPN given through central vein.	▪ ***I.V. use:*** Control infusion rate carefully; maximum rate 0.5 g/kg/hr. Use infusion pump when infusing with amino acids for TPN. ▪ Use central veins to infuse dextrose solutions with concentration > 10%. ▪ Monitor serum glucose carefully. ▪ Never stop hypertonic solutions abruptly. ▪ Monitor I&O and weight carefully. ▪ Check vital signs frequently.
diazepam Apo-Diazepam†, Diazepam Intensol, Valium *Anxiolytic, skeletal muscle relaxant, amnesic agent, anticonvulsant, sedative-hypnotic* Pregnancy Risk Category: D Controlled Substance	*Anxiety* — **Adults:** 2 to 10 mg P.O. b.i.d. to q.i.d., or 15 to 30 mg extended-release capsules P.O. q.d. Or, 2 to 10 mg I.M. or I.V. q 3 to 4 hr, p.r.n. **Elderly:** 2 to 2.5 mg once daily to b.i.d.; increased gradually. **Children ≥ 6 mo:** 1 to 2.5 mg P.O. t.i.d. to q.i.d., increased gradually, p.r.n. *Muscle spasm* — **Adults:** 2 to 10 mg P.O. b.i.d. to q.i.d., or 15 to 30 mg extended-	▪ ***ALERT*** Have emergency resuscitation equipment and oxygen at bedside. Monitor respirations q 5 to 15 min and before each I.V. dose. ▪ Don't mix injectable form with other drugs. ▪ Don't store parenteral solution in plastic syringes. ▪ ***I.V. use:*** Give no faster than 5 mg/min.

Schedule: IV	release capsules q.d. Or, 5 to 10 mg I.M. or I.V. initially; then 5 to 10 mg I.M. or I.V. q 3 to 4 hr, p.r.n. **Children $\geq$ 5 yr:** 5 to 10 mg I.M. or I.V. q 3 to 4 hr, p.r.n. **Children > 30 days to 4 yr:** 1 to 2 mg I.M. or I.V. slowly, repeated q 3 to 4 hr, p.r.n. *Status epilepticus and severe recurrent seizures* — **Adults:** 5 to 10 mg I.V. (preferred) or I.M. Repeat q 10 to 15 min, p.r.n., to maximum 30 mg. Repeat q 2 to 4 hr. **Children $\geq$ 5 yr:** 1 mg I.V. q 2 to 5 min to maximum 10 mg. Repeat q 2 to 4 hr, p.r.n. **Children > 30 days to 4 yr:** 0.2 to 0.5 mg I.V. slowly q 2 to 5 min to maximum 5 mg. Repeat q 2 to 4 hr, p.r.n.	Check daily for phlebitis at injection site. ▪ I.V. route most reliable parenteral route; don't give I.M. because absorption is variable and injection painful. ▪ Avoid extravasation. Don't inject into small veins.
diazoxide Hyperstat IV *Antihypertensive* Pregnancy Risk Category: C	*Hypertensive crisis* — **Adults and children:** 1 to 3 mg/kg by I.V. bolus undiluted (to maximum 150 mg) q 5 to 15 min until adequate response occurs. Repeat at 4- to 24-hr intervals, p.r.n.	▪ ***I.V. use:*** Monitor BP and ECG continuously. Keep patient supine during and 1 hr after infusion. Protect I.V. solutions from light. ▪ Avoid extravasation. ▪ Monitor fluid balance and glucose level.
diclofenac potassium Cataflam **diclofenac sodium** Fenac‡, Voltaren, Voltaren SR† *Antarthritic, anti-inflammatory* Pregnancy Risk Category: B	*Ankylosing spondylitis* — **Adults:** 25 mg P.O. q.i.d. (and h.s., p.r.n.). *Osteoarthritis* — **Adults:** 50 mg P.O. b.i.d. or t.i.d., or 75 mg P.O. b.i.d. (sodium form only). *Rheumatoid arthritis* — **Adults:** 50 mg P.O. t.i.d. or q.i.d. Or, 75 mg P.O. b.i.d. (sodium form only) or 50 to 100 mg P.R. h.s. as substitute for last P.O. dose of day. Maximum 225 mg/day.	▪ Can decrease renal blood flow and lead to reversible renal impairment. Monitor patient closely. ▪ Monitor serum transaminase periodically during therapy. ▪ May mask symptoms of infection. ▪ To minimize GI distress, instruct patient to take with milk or meals.

(continued)

†Canadian ‡Australian

DRUG & CLASS	INDICATIONS & DOSAGES	NURSING CONSIDERATIONS
diclofenac potassium *(continued)*	*Analgesia and primary dysmenorrhea* — **Adults:** 50 mg P.O. t.i.d. (potassium form only).	▪ Tell patient not to crush, chew, or break enteric-coated tablets.
dicyclomine hydrochloride Antispas, Bentyl, Dibent, Di-Spaz, Spasmoban† *Antimuscarinic, GI antispasmodic* Pregnancy Risk Category: B	*Irritable bowel syndrome; other functional GI disorders* — **Adults:** initially, 20 mg P.O. q.i.d., increased to 40 mg q.i.d., or 20 mg I.M. q 4 to 6 hr.	▪ Don't give S.C. or I.V. ▪ Give 30 min to 1 hr before meals and h.s. Bedtime dose can be larger; give ≥ 2 hr after last meal. ▪ Monitor vital signs and urine output. ▪ Prepare to adjust dosage according to patient's needs and response, as ordered.
didanosine (ddI) Videx *Antiviral* Pregnancy Risk Category: B	*HIV infection requiring antiretroviral therapy* — **Adults ≥ 60 kg (132 lb):** 200 mg (tablets) P.O. q 12 hr; or 250 mg buffered powder P.O. q 12 hr. **Adults < 60 kg:** 125 mg (tablets) P.O. q 12 hr; or 167 mg buffered powder P.O. q 12 hr. **Children:** 120 mg/m^2 P.O. q 12 hr. ***Adjust-a-dose:*** Adjust dosage in patients with reduced renal function or on dialysis.	▪ Give on empty stomach. ▪ ***ALERT*** Pediatric powder for oral solution must be prepared by pharmacist before dispensing. ▪ Drug causes diarrhea. ▪ Don't use fruit juice or other acidic beverages to dissolve powder.
diflunisal Dolobid *Nonnarcotic analgesic, antipyretic, anti-inflammatory* Pregnancy Risk Category: C	*Mild to moderate pain; osteoarthritis; rheumatoid arthritis* — **Adults > 65 yr:** half of usual adult dose. **Adults:** 500 to 1,000 mg P.O. q.d. in 2 divided doses, usually q 12 hr. Maximum 1,500 mg q.d.	▪ ***ALERT*** Don't give to children or teenagers with chickenpox or flulike illness because of risk of Reye's syndrome. ▪ Tell patient to take with water, milk, or meals.
digoxin Digoxin, Lanoxicaps, Lanoxin, Novodigoxin†	*Heart failure; PSVT; atrial fibrillation and flutter* — **Adults > 65 yr:** 0.125 mg P.O. q.d. as maintenance dose. **Adults ≤ 65 yr:** loading	▪ Before therapy, obtain baseline data (apical pulse, HR, BP, and electrolytes) and ask about use of cardiac glycosides within

Antiarrhythmic, inotropic
Pregnancy Risk Category: C

dose 0.5 to 1 mg I.V. or P.O. in divided doses over 24 hr; maintenance: 0.125 to 0.5 mg I.V. or P.O. q.d. (average: 0.25 mg). **Children > 2 yr:** loading dose 0.02 to 0.04 mg/kg P.O. q.d., divided q 8 hr over 24 hr. I.V. loading dose, 0.015 to 0.035 mg/kg; maintenance dose, 0.012 mg/kg P.O. q.d., divided q 12 hr. **Children 1 mo to 2 yr:** loading dose 0.035 to 0.06 mg/kg P.O. in 3 divided doses over 24 hr; I.V. loading dose 0.03 to 0.05 mg/kg; maintenance: 0.01 to 0.02 mg/kg P.O. q.d., divided q 12 hr.

Neonates: loading dose 0.025 to 0.035 mg/kg P.O., divided q 8 hr over 24 hr; I.V. loading dose 0.02 to 0.03 mg/kg; maintenance: 0.01 mg/kg P.O. q.d., divided q 12 hr. **Premature neonates:** loading dose 0.015 to 0.025 mg/kg I.V. in 3 divided doses over 24 hr; maintenance: 0.01 mg/kg q.d., divided q 12 hr.

Adjust-a-dose: Reduce loading and maintenance doses if renal function impaired.

previous 2 to 3 wk.

- Before therapy, take apical-radial pulse for 1 min. Record and report significant changes. If changes occur, check BP and obtain ECG.
- Therapeutic level ranges from 0.8 to 2 ng/ml. However, patient should be evaluated based on clinical response.
- ***ALERT*** Slowing of pulse (≤ 60 beats/min) may signal digitalis toxicity. Withhold drug and notify doctor.
- ***I.V. use:*** Infuse slowly over ≥ 5 min.
- Encourage consumption of potassium-rich foods.
- Smaller doses given in patients with impaired renal function or who are frail.

---

digoxin immune Fab (ovine)

Digibind
Cardiac glycoside antidote
Pregnancy Risk Category: C

Potentially life-threatening digoxin or digitoxin intoxication — **Adults and children:** I.V. dosage varies according to amount of digoxin or digitoxin to be neutralized. Each vial binds about 0.5 mg of digoxin or digitoxin. Average dosage, 6 vials (228 mg). However, if toxicity is from acute digoxin ingestion and if digoxin and estimated ingestion amount unknown, 20 vials (760 mg)

- ***ALERT*** Use only for life-threatening overdose in shock or cardiac arrest or with ventricular arrhythmias, progressive bradycardia, or 2nd- or 3rd-degree AV block not responsive to atropine.
- ***I.V. use:*** Reconstitute 38-mg vial with 4 ml sterile water for injection. Gently roll vial to dissolve powder. Reconstituted solution contains 9.5 mg/ml.

(continued)

DRUG & CLASS	INDICATIONS & DOSAGES	NURSING CONSIDERATIONS
digoxin immune Fab *(continued)*	may be needed. See package insert for complete, specific dosage instructions.	May give by direct injection if cardiac arrest seems imminent. Or, dilute with 0.9% NaCl for injection to appropriate volume and give by intermittent infusion over 30 min through 0.22-micron membrane filter. ▪ Monitor serum potassium closely. ▪ Interferes with digitalis immunoassay measurements; standard serum digoxin levels misleading until drug cleared from body (about 2 days).
dihydroergotamine mesylate D.H.E. 45, Dihydergot‡, Migranal *Vasoconstrictor* Pregnancy Risk Category: X	*To prevent or abort vascular or migraine headache* — **Adults:** 1 mg I.M. or I.V. Repeat q 1 to 2 hr, p.r.n., to total of 2 mg I.V. or 3 mg I.M. per attack. Maximum weekly dose 6 mg. Or, 1 spray (0.5 mg), into each nostril. Repeat dose in 15 min.	▪ Most effective when used at first sign of migraine or soon after onset. ▪ ***I.V. use:*** Directly inject solution into vein over 3 min. ▪ Be alert for ergotamine rebound. ▪ Protect ampules from heat and light.
diltiazem hydrochloride Apo-Diltiaz†, Cardizem, Cardizem CD, Cardizem SR, Dilacor-XR, Tiamate, Tiazac *Antianginal* Pregnancy Risk Category: C	*Vasospastic angina (Prinzmetal's [variant] angina); classic chronic stable angina pectoris* — **Adults:** 30 mg P.O. t.i.d. or q.i.d. before meals and h.s. Increase gradually up to 360 mg/day in divided doses. Or, 120 or 180 mg (extended-release capsules). Adjust dose, p.r.n. up to 480 mg q.d. *Hypertension* — **Adults:** 60 to 120 mg P.O. b.i.d. (sustained-release). Adjust dose to effect. Maximum 360 mg/day. Or, 180 to 240 mg q.d. (extended-release) initially. Adjust	▪ ***I.V. use:*** Don't infuse > 24 hr. ▪ Monitor BP and HR during initiation of therapy and dosage adjustments. ▪ ***ALERT*** If systolic BP < 90 or HR < 60, withhold dose and notify doctor. ▪ Tell patient to avoid hazardous activities during initiation of therapy. ▪ Advise patient that drug may be taken with S.L. nitroglycerin p.r.n., if angina acute.

dose, p.r.n.
Atrial fibrillation or flutter; PSVT — **Adults:** 0.25 mg/kg as I.V. bolus injection over 2 min. If response inadequate, 0.35 mg/kg I.V. after 15 min, then continuous infusion of 10 mg/hr. Some patients respond well to 5 mg/hr; maximum 15 mg/hr.

---

dimenhydrinate
Calm-X, Dimetabs, Dinate, Dramamine, Dymenate, Triptone
Antihistamine, antiemetic, antivertigo agent
Pregnancy Risk Category: B

Prevention and treatment of motion sickness — **Adults and children ≥ 12 yr:** 50 to 100 mg P.O. q 4 to 6 hr; 50 mg I.M., p.r.n.; or 50 mg I.V. diluted in 10 ml NaCl for injection, injected over 2 min. Maximum 400 mg q.d. **Children 6 to 11 yr:** 25 to 50 mg P.O. q 6 to 8 hr, not to exceed 150 mg in 24 hr. **Children 2 to 5 yr:** 12.5 to 25 mg P.O. q 6 to 8 hr, not to exceed 75 mg in 24 hr. **Children < 2 yr:** 1.25 mg/kg or 37.5 mg/m^2 I.M. q.i.d. Maximum 300 mg q.d.

- ***ALERT*** Most I.V. products contain benzyl alcohol, associated with fatal "gasping syndrome" in premature and low-birth-weight infants.
- May mask symptoms of ototoxicity, brain tumor, or intestinal obstruction.
- ***I.V. use:*** Before giving, dilute each ml of drug with 10 ml sterile water for injection, D_5W, or 0.9% NaCl for injection. Give by direct injection over ≥ 2 min.
- ***ALERT*** Don't mix parenteral preparation with other drugs.

---

diphenhydramine hydrochloride
Allerdryl†, Benadryl, Hydramine, Nytol Maximum Strength, Sominex
Antihistamine, antiemetic, antivertigo agent, antitussive, sedative-hypnotic, antidyskinetic
Pregnancy Risk Category: B

Rhinitis, allergy symptoms, motion sickness, Parkinson's disease — **Adults and children ≥ 12 yr:** 25 to 50 mg P.O. t.i.d. or q.i.d.; or, 10 to 50 mg deep I.M. or I.V. Maximum I.M. or I.V. dose 400 mg q.d. **Children < 12 yr:** 5 mg/kg q.d. P.O., deep I.M., or I.V. in divided doses q.i.d. Maximum 300 mg q.d.
Sedation — **Adults:** 25 to 50 mg P.O., or deep I.M., p.r.n.
Nonproductive cough — **Adults:** 25 mg P.O. q 4 to 6 hr (maximum 150 mg q.d.). **Children 6**

- Children < 12 yr should use only as directed by doctor.
- Alternate injection sites to prevent irritation. Give I.M. injection deeply into large muscle.
- Tell patient to take 30 min before travel to prevent motion sickness.
- Instruct patient to take with food or milk to reduce GI distress.
- Tell patient to use sunscreen and to avoid overexposure to sunlight.

(continued)

†Canadian ‡Australian

DRUG & CLASS	INDICATIONS & DOSAGES	NURSING CONSIDERATIONS
diphenhydramine hydrochloride *(continued)*	**to 12 yr:** 12.5 mg P.O. q 4 to 6 hr (maximum 75 mg q.d.). **Children 2 to 6 yr:** 6.25 mg P.O. q 4 to 6 hr (maximum 25 mg/day). *Insomnia* — **Adults and children ≥ 12 yr:** 50 mg P.O. h.s. p.r.n.	
diphenoxylate hydrochloride and atropine sulfate Lomocot, Lomotil, Lonox *Antidiarrheal* Pregnancy Risk Category: C Controlled Substance Schedule: V	*Acute, nonspecific diarrhea* — **Adults:** initially, 5 mg P.O. q.i.d.; then adjusted, p.r.n. **Children 2 to 12 yr:** 0.3 to 0.4 mg/kg liquid form P.O. q.d. in 4 divided doses. For maintenance, initial dose reduced, p.r.n., up to 75%.	▪ Use cautiously in children ≥ 2 yr; patients with hepatic disease, narcotic dependence, or acute ulcerative colitis; and pregnant patients. Stop therapy immediately and notify doctor if abdominal distention or other signs of toxic megacolon develop. ▪ Correct fluid and electrolyte disturbances before starting drug. Monitor fluid and electrolyte balance. Dehydration, especially in young children, may increase risk of delayed toxicity. ▪ Don't use to treat antibiotic-induced diarrhea. ▪ Drug unlikely to be effective if no response occurs within 48 hr. ▪ Risk of physical dependence increases with high dosage and long-term use. Atropine sulfate helps discourage abuse.
diphtheria and tetanus toxoids and acellular pertussis vaccine	*Primary immunization* — **Children 6 wk to 6 yr:** 0.5 ml I.M. 4 to 8 wk apart for 3 doses and 4th dose 1 yr later. Booster, 0.5 ml I.M. when starting school, unless 4th dose in se-	▪ Obtain history of allergies and reaction to immunization. ▪ Keep epinephrine 1:1,000 available to treat anaphylaxis.

Acel-Imune, DTaP, Tripedia **diphtheria and tetanus toxoids and whole-cell pertussis vaccine (DTP, DPT)** DTwP, Tri-Immunol *Diphtheria, tetanus, and pertussis prophylaxis agent* Pregnancy Risk Category: C	ries given after 4th birthday; then, booster not needed at time of school entrance. Not recommended for adults or children > 6 yr. Products containing acellular pertussis vaccine may now be used for any dose in DTP immunization.	▪ Shake before using. Store refrigerated. ▪ Give only by deep I.M. injection, preferably in thigh or deltoid muscle. Don't give S.C. ▪ Acellular vaccine may be associated with lower incidence of local pain and fever.
dipivefrin Propine *Antiglaucoma agent* Pregnancy Risk Category: B	*IOP reduction in chronic open-angle glaucoma* — **Adults:** for initial glaucoma therapy, 1 drop of 0.1% solution q 12 hr. Adjust dosage based on patient response, as determined by tonometric readings.	▪ Often used with other antiglaucoma drugs. ▪ May cause fewer adverse reactions than conventional epinephrine therapy.
dipyridamole I.V. Persantine, Persantin‡, Persantine *Coronary vasodilator, platelet aggregation inhibitor* Pregnancy Risk Category: B	*Inhibition of platelet adhesion in prosthetic heart valves* — **Adults:** 75 to 100 mg P.O. q.i.d. with coumarin anticoagulant. *Alternative to exercise in CAD evaluation during thallium (^{201}Tl) myocardial perfusion scintigraphy* — **Adults:** 0.57 mg/kg as I.V. infusion at constant rate over 4 min (0.142 mg/kg/min).	▪ If patient develops GI distress, give ≤ 1 hr before meals. ▪ ***I.V. use:*** If using as diagnostic agent, dilute in 0.45% or 0.9% NaCl or D_5W in ≥ 1:2 ratio for total volume of 20 to 50 ml. Inject ^{201}Tl within 5 min after completing dipyridamole infusion. ▪ Observe for signs of bleeding or other adverse reactions. ▪ Adverse effects are usually dose-related and transient.

†Canadian ‡Australian

DRUG & CLASS	INDICATIONS & DOSAGES	NURSING CONSIDERATIONS
dirithromycin Dynabac *Antibiotic* Pregnancy Risk Category: C	*Acute bacterial exacerbations of chronic bronchitis from* M. catarrhalis, S. pneumoniae, *or* H. influenzae; *secondary bacterial infections of acute bronchitis from* M. catarrhalis *or* S. pneumoniae; *uncomplicated skin or skin-structure infections from* S. aureus *(methicillin-susceptible strains) or* S. pyogenes — **Adults and children ≥ 12 yr:** 500 mg P.O. q.d. with food (or within 1 hr of a meal) for 5 to 7 days. *Community-acquired pneumonia due to* L. pneumophila, M. pneumoniae, *or* S. pneumoniae — **Adults and children ≥ 12 yr:** 500 mg P.O. q.d. for 14 days.	▪ Obtain culture and sensitivity results to ensure organism is sensitive to drug. Not for empiric use. ▪ Don't use in patients who may have bacteremia. ▪ Give ≤ 1 hr before meals. ▪ Monitor for superinfection. ▪ Safety in children < 12 yr not established. ▪ Use with caution in patients with moderate to severe hepatic disease.
disopyramide Rythmodan† **disopyramide phosphate** Norpace, Norpace CR, Rythmodan-LA† *Antiarrhythmic* Pregnancy Risk Category: C	*Ventricular tachycardia and life-threatening ventricular arrhythmias* — **Adults > 50 kg (110 lb):** 150 mg q 6 hr with conventional capsules or 300 mg q 12 hr with extended-release preparation. **Adults ≤ 50 kg:** 100 mg P.O. q 6 hr or 200 mg q 12 hr as extended-release capsules. **Children 12 to 18 yr:** 6 to 15 mg/kg P.O. q.d. **Children 4 to 12 yr:** 10 to 15 mg/kg P.O. q.d. **Children 1 to 4 yr:** 10 to 20 mg/kg P.O. q.d. **Children < 1 yr:** 10 to 30 mg/kg P.O. q.d. *Note:* For pediatric dosages, divide into equal amounts and give q 6 hr. ***Adjust-a-dose:*** In patients with advanced renal insufficiency, if CrCl is 30 to 40 ml/min,	▪ Check apical pulse before giving. Notify doctor if < 60 or > 120 beats/min. ▪ ***ALERT*** Stop drug and notify doctor if heart block develops, QRS complex widens by more than 25%, or QT interval lengthens by more than 25% above baseline. ▪ Watch for recurrence of arrhythmias and check for adverse reactions; notify doctor if any occur. ▪ Correct electrolyte abnormalities before therapy begins, as ordered. ▪ Don't give extended-release capsules if CrCl ≤ 40 ml/min.

give 100 mg q 8 hr; 15 to 30 ml/min, 100 mg q 12 hr; < 15 ml/min, 100 mg q 24 hr.

disulfiram Antabuse *Alcoholic deterrent* Pregnancy Risk Category: NR	*Adjunct in management of chronic alcoholism* — **Adults:** 250 to 500 mg P.O. as single dose in morning for 1 to 2 wk or in evening if drowsiness occurs. Maintenance, 125 to 500 mg P.O. q.d. (average dose 250 mg) until permanent self-control established. Treatment may be required for months to years.	▪ Use only under close medical and nursing supervision. Never give until patient has abstained from alcohol for ≥ 12 hr. Patient should clearly understand consequences of drug and give permission for its use. Use only in patients who are cooperative, well motivated, and receiving supportive psychiatric therapy. ▪ Complete physical exam and lab studies, including CBC, SMA-12, and transaminase level, should precede therapy and be repeated regularly, as ordered. ▪ ***ALERT*** The disulfiram–alcohol reaction includes headache, nausea, vomiting, angina, anxiety, hypotension, vertigo, weakness, syncope, confusion, and palpitations.
dobutamine hydrochloride Dobutrex *Inotropic* Pregnancy Risk Category: B	*To increase cardiac output in short-term treatment of cardiac decompensation caused by depressed contractility, such as during refractory heart failure; adjunct in cardiac surgery* — **Adults:** 0.5 to 2.0 mcg/kg/min I.V. infusion. Rates up to 40 mcg/kg/min may be needed (rare).	▪ Before starting therapy, correct hypovolemia with plasma volume expanders. ▪ Give after cardiac glycoside in patients with atrial fibrillation. ▪ Continuously monitor ECG, BP, PAWP, cardiac condition, and urine output. ▪ ***I.V. use:*** Give through large vein. Use infusion pump. Avoid extravasation. ▪ Dilute concentrate for injection before giving. Don't exceed 5 mg/ml concentration.

DRUG & CLASS	INDICATIONS & DOSAGES	NURSING CONSIDERATIONS
docetaxel Taxotere *Antineoplastic* Pregnancy Risk Category: D	*Patients with locally advanced or metastatic breast cancer who have progressed during anthracycline-based therapy or have relapsed during anthracycline-based adjuvant therapy* — **Adults:** 60 to 100 mg/m^2 I.V. over 1 hr q 3 wk. *Locally advanced or metastatic non–small-cell lung cancer after failure of platinum-based chemotherapy* — **Adults:** 75 mg/m^2 I.V. over 1 hr q 3 wk. Premedicate with dexamethasone 8 mg b.i.d. for 3 days, starting 1 day before docetaxel therapy.	▪ Monitor LFT results. ▪ Wear gloves when preparing and giving. If solution contacts skin, wash immediately and thoroughly with soap and water. Mark all waste materials with CHEMOTHERAPY HAZARD labels. ▪ ***ALERT*** Bone marrow toxicity most frequent and dose-limiting toxic effect. Monitor blood count frequently during therapy. ▪ Monitor for hypersensitivity reactions.
docusate calcium Dioctocal, Kasof, Surfak **docusate sodium** Colace, Genasoft *Emollient laxative* Pregnancy Risk Category: C	*Stool softener* — **Adults and children > 12 yr:** 50 to 500 mg P.O. q.d. until bowel movements normal. **Children 6 to 12 yr:** 40 to 120 mg docusate sodium P.O. q.d. **Children 3 to 5 yr:** 20 to 60 mg docusate sodium P.O. q.d. **Children < 3 yr:** 10 to 40 mg docusate sodium P.O. q.d.	▪ Give liquid in milk, fruit juice, or infant formula to mask bitter taste. ▪ Before giving, determine if patient has adequate fluid intake, exercise routine, and diet. ▪ Teach patient about dietary sources of bulk fiber. ▪ Instruct patient to use only occasionally and not for > 1 wk without doctor's knowledge.
dofetilide Tikosyn *Class III antiarrhythmic* Pregnancy Risk Category: C	*Maintenance of normal sinus rhythm in patients with symptomatic atrial fibrillation or atrial flutter of > 1 wk's duration who have been converted to normal sinus rhythm; con*	▪ Continuous ECG monitoring is required for 3 ≥ days. ▪ Patients shouldn't be discharged within 12 hr of conversion to

(continued)

version of atrial fibrillation and atrial flutter to normal sinus rhythm — **Adult:** 500 mcg P.O. b.i.d. if CrCl > 60 ml/min. Obtain QT interval before 1st dose and q 2 to 3 hr after each dose in hospital. If QT interval increases by > 15% or is > 500 msec (550 msec in ventricular conduction abnormalities) 2 to 3 hr after 1st dose, adjust as follows: If 1st dose was 500 mcg P.O. b.i.d., give 250 mcg P.O. b.i.d. If 1st dose was 250 mcg P.O. b.i.d., give 125 mcg P.O. b.i.d. If 1st dose was 125 mcg P.O. b.i.d., give 125 mcg P.O. q.i.d. If QT interval > 500 msec (550 msec in ventricular conduction abnormalities) any time after 2nd dose, stop drug.
Adjust-a-dose: If CrCl is 40 to 60 ml/min, starting dose is 250 mcg b.i.d.; if 20 to 40 ml/min, starting dose is 125 mcg b.i.d. If CrCl is < 20 ml/min, drug is contraindicated.

normal sinus rhythm.

- Monitor the patient for prolonged diarrhea, sweating, and vomiting and report to prescriber because electrolyte imbalance may increase the potential for arrhythmia development.
- Hypokalemia and hypomagnesemia, conditions associated with potassium-depleting diuretic therapy, increase the potential for developing torsades de pointes. Potassium levels should be normal before dofetilide is given and maintained at a normal range.
- If patient doesn't convert to normal sinus rhythm within 24 hr of receiving dofetilide, electrical conversion should be considered.
- If dofetilide needs to be stopped to allow dosing of other interacting drugs, ≥ 2 days should be allowed before other drug therapy is started.

---

dolasetron mesylate
Anzemet
Antinauseant, antiemetic
Pregnancy Risk Category: B

Prevention of nausea and vomiting from cancer chemotherapy — **Adults:** 100 mg P.O. given as single dose 1 hr before chemotherapy; or 1.8 mg/kg (or a fixed dose of 100 mg) as single I.V. dose 30 min before chemotherapy. **Children 2 to 16 yr:** 1.8 mg/kg P.O. 1 hr before chemotherapy; or 1.8 mg/kg as single I.V. dose 30 min before chemotherapy. Injection can be mixed with apple juice and given P.O. Maximum 100 mg.

- Give with caution in patients who have or may develop prolonged cardiac conduction intervals, such as those with electrolyte abnormalities, history of arrhythmias, or cumulative high-dose anthracycline therapy.
- Don't give to children < 2 yr.
- Injection for P.O. use is stable in apple or apple-grape juice for 2 hr at room temperature.

(continued)

DRUG & CLASS	INDICATIONS & DOSAGES	NURSING CONSIDERATIONS
dolasetron mesylate *(continued)*	*Prevention of postoperative nausea and vomiting* — **Adults:** 100 mg P.O. ≤ 2 hr before surgery; 12.5 mg as single I.V. dose 15 min before stopping anesthesia. **Children 2 to 16 years:** 1.2 mg/kg P.O. ≤ 2 hr before surgery, up to 100 mg; or 0.35 mg/kg (up to 12.5 mg) as single I.V. dose 15 min before stopping anesthesia. Injection can be mixed with apple juice and given P.O. *Postoperative nausea and vomiting* — **Adults:** 12.5 mg as single I.V. dose when nausea or vomiting occurs. **Children 2 to 16 years:** 0.35 mg/kg, up to 12.5 mg, as single I.V. dose when nausea or vomiting occurs.	▪ ***I.V. use:*** Injection can be infused as rapidly as 100 mg/30 sec or diluted in 50 ml compatible solution and infused over 15 min. ▪ Report nausea and vomiting to doctor.
donepezil hydrochloride Aricept *CNS agent for Alzheimer's disease* Pregnancy Risk Category: C	*Mild to moderate dementia of Alzheimer's type* — **Adults:** initially, 5 mg P.O. q.d. h.s. After 4 to 6 wk, may increase to 10 mg q.d.	▪ Monitor for symptoms of active or occult GI bleeding.
dopamine hydrochloride Intropin, Revimine† *Inotropic, vasopressor* Pregnancy Risk Category: C	*To treat shock and correct hemodynamic imbalances; to improve perfusion to vital organs; to increase cardiac output; to correct hypotension* — **Adults:** initially, 1 to 5 mcg/kg/min by I.V. infusion. Titrate dose to desired hemodynamic or renal response; may increase infusion by 1 to 4 mcg/kg/min	▪ If volume deficit exists, replace fluid before giving drug. ▪ ***I.V. use:*** Don't mix with alkaline solutions. Use central line or large vein to minimize risk of extravasation. ▪ Frequently monitor ECG, BP, cardiac output, CVP, PAWP, pulse rate, urine output,

	at 10- to 30-min intervals.	and color and temperature of hands and feet.
dorzolamide hydrochloride Trusopt *Antiglaucoma agent* Pregnancy Risk Category: C	*Increased IOP in patients with ocular hypertension or open-angle glaucoma* — **Adults:** 1 drop in conjunctival sac of affected eye t.i.d. ***Adjust-a-dose:*** Adjust dosage in patients with renal failure.	▪ If patient receiving > 1 topical ophthalmic drug, give drugs ≥ 10 min apart.
doxazosin mesylate Cardura *Antihypertensive* Pregnancy Risk Category: C	*Essential hypertension* — **Adults:** 1 mg P.O. q.d.; determine effect on standing and supine BP at 2 to 6 hr and 24 hr after dosing. Increase to 2 mg q.d. p.r.n. Adjust dosage slowly. May increase to 4 mg q.d., then 8 mg. Maximum, 16 mg/day. *Benign prostatic hyperplasia* — **Adults:** initially, 1 mg P.O. q.d. in morning or evening; may increase to 2 mg and, thereafter, 4 mg and 8 mg q.d., p.r.n. Adjustment interval 1 to 2 wk.	▪ Monitor BP closely. ▪ If syncope occurs, place patient in recumbent position and treat supportively. Transient hypotensive response doesn't contraindicate continued therapy. ▪ ***ALERT*** Orthostatic hypotension most common after 1st dose but also can occur during dosage adjustment or interruption.
doxepin hydrochloride Adapin, Deptran‡, Novo-Doxepin†, Sinequan, Triadapin† *Antidepressant* Pregnancy Risk Category: NR	*Depression or anxiety* — **Adults:** initially, 25 to 75 mg P.O. q.d. in divided doses to maximum 300 mg q.d. Or, give entire maintenance dose q.d. with maximum 150 mg P.O.	▪ Record mood changes. Monitor patient for suicidal tendencies, and allow only minimal drug supply. ▪ Stop gradually several days before surgery. ▪ ***ALERT*** Dilute oral concentrate with 120 ml (4 oz) of water, milk, or juice (not grape juice).
doxorubicin hydrochloride Adriamycin‡, Adriamycin PFS, Adriamycin RDF,	Dosage and indications vary. Check treatment protocol with doctor. *Bladder, breast, lung, ovarian, stomach, and thyroid cancers; osteogenic and soft tissue*	▪ Never give I.M. or S.C. ▪ Perform cardiac function studies (including ECG) before treatment and periodically throughout. *(continued)*

†Canadian ‡Australian

DRUG & CLASS	INDICATIONS & DOSAGES	NURSING CONSIDERATIONS
doxorubicin hydrochloride *(continued)* Rubex *Antineoplastic* Pregnancy Risk Category: D	*sarcoma; non-Hodgkin's lymphoma; Hodgkin's disease; acute lymphoblastic and myeloblastic leukemia; Wilms' tumor; neuroblastoma; lymphoma; sarcoma* — **Adults:** 60 to 75 mg/m^2 I.V. as single dose q 3 wk; or 30 mg/m^2 I.V. as single daily dose, days 1 to 3 of 4-wk cycle. Or, 20 mg/m^2 I.V. once weekly. Maximum cumulative dose 550 mg/m^2. ***Adjust-a-dose:*** Reduce dosage in patients with myelosuppression or impaired cardiac or hepatic function or if serum bilirubin level rises. Give 50% of dosage when bilirubin 1.2 to 3 mg/100 ml; give 25% of dosage when bilirubin > 3 mg/100 ml.	▪ May be given with dexrazoxane if accumulated doxorubicin dose is 300 mg/m^2. ▪ ***ALERT*** Don't place I.V. line over joints or in extremities with poor venous or lymphatic drainage. If extravasation occurs, stop immediately, apply ice for 24 to 48 hr, and notify doctor. Monitor area closely. May consult plastic surgeon. ▪ If vein streaking occurs, slow infusion rate. If welts occur, stop infusion and report to doctor. ▪ Monitor CBC and hepatic function tests, as ordered; monitor ECG monthly. If tachycardia develops, be prepared to stop drug or slow infusion rate and notify doctor. ▪ ***ALERT*** For signs of heart failure, stop drug and notify doctor. Heart failure can be prevented by limiting cumulative dose to 550 mg/m^2 (400 mg/m^2 when patient receives cyclophosphamide or radiation therapy to cardiac area). ▪ Monitor patient for hematologic toxicity.
doxycycline calcium Vibramycin **doxycycline hyclate**	*Infections caused by susceptible gram-positive and -negative organisms* Rickettsia, M. pneumoniae, C. trachomatis, *and* B. burgdorferi (*Lyme disease); psittacosis; granuloma inguinale* — **Adults and children**	▪ Obtain specimen for culture and sensitivity tests before 1st dose. ▪ ***ALERT*** Check expiration date. Outdated or deteriorated tetracyclines have been associated with reversible nephrotoxicity (Fan-

Doryx, Doxy-Caps, Doxycin†, Monodox, Vibramycin, Vibra-tabs
doxycycline hydrochloride
Cyclidox†, Doryx‡, Doxylin‡, Vibramycin‡, Vibra-Tabs 50‡
doxycycline monohydrate
Monodox, Vibramycin
Antibiotic
Pregnancy Risk Category: D

> 8 yr weighing ≥ 45 kg (99 lb): 100 mg P.O. q 12 hr on 1st day; then 100 mg P.O. q.d.; or 200 mg I.V. on 1st day in 1 or 2 infusions; then 100 to 200 mg I.V. q.d. **Children > 8 yr weighing < 45 kg:** 4.4 mg/kg P.O. or I.V. q.d., in divided doses q 12 hr on 1st day; then 2.2 to 4.4 mg/kg q.d. in 1 or 2 divided doses. Give I.V. infusion slowly (≥ 1 hr). Infusion must be completed within 12 hr (within 6 hr in lactated Ringer's solution or dextrose 5% in lactated Ringer's solution).
Uncomplicated urethral, endocervical, or rectal infections caused by C. trachomatis *or* U. urealyticum — **Adults:** 100 mg P.O. b.i.d. for ≥ 7 days (10 days for epididymitis).
Pelvic inflammatory disease — **Adults:** 100 mg I.V. q 12 hr and continued for ≥ 2 days after symptomatic improvement; then, 100 mg P.O. q 12 hr for total course of 2 wk.

coni's syndrome).
- Give with milk or food if adverse GI reactions develop.
- Don't expose to light or heat. Protect from sunlight during infusion.
- Check tongue for signs of fungal infection. Stress good oral hygiene.
- Don't give to children ≤ 8 yr; drug can permanently discolor tooth enamel.

---

dronabinol
Marinol
Antiemetic, appetite stimulant
Pregnancy Risk Category: C
Controlled Substance Schedule: II

Nausea and vomiting from cancer chemotherapy — **Adults:** 5 mg/m^2 P.O. 1 to 3 hr before chemotherapy. Then same dose q 2 to 4 hr after chemotherapy for total of 4 to 6 doses per day. Increase in 2.5-mg/m^2 increments p.r.n., up to 15 mg/m^2 per dose.
Anorexia and weight loss from AIDS — **Adults:** 2.5 mg P.O. b.i.d. before lunch and dinner. If unable to tolerate, decrease dose to 2.5 mg P.O., q.d. in evening or h.s. May gradually increase to 20 mg/day.

- ***ALERT*** Principal active substance in *Cannabis sativa* (marijuana); can produce physical and psychological dependence and has high abuse potential.
- CNS effects intensify at higher dosages.
- Effects may persist for days after treatment.

†Canadian ‡Australian

DRUG & CLASS	INDICATIONS & DOSAGES	NURSING CONSIDERATIONS
droperidol Inapsine *Sedative-hypnotic* Pregnancy Risk Category: C	*Premedication* — **Adults and children > 12 yr:** 2.5 to 10 mg I.M. 30 to 60 min preoperatively. **Children 2 to 12 yr:** 1 to 1.5 mg per 9 to 11 kg (20 to 25 lb) of body weight I.M. ***Adjust-a-dose:*** Reduce dose in debilitated or elderly patients, and those who receive other depressant drugs. *For induction as adjunct to general anesthesia* — **Adults and children > 12 yr:** 2.5 mg per 9 to 11 kg of body weight I.V. For maintenance, 1.25 to 2.5 mg, usually I.V. **Children 2 to 12 yr:** 1 to 1.5 mg per 9 to 11 kg of body weight I.V. *Use without general anesthetic in diagnostic procedures* — **Adults and children > 12 yr:** 2.5 to 10 mg I.M. 30 to 60 min before procedure. May give additional doses of 1.25 to 2.5 mg, usually I.V. *Adjunct to regional anesthesia when additional sedation required* — **Adults:** 2.5 to 5 mg I.M. or slow I.V.	▪ Use cautiously in patients with hepatic or renal dysfunction and in breast-feeding patients. ▪ Use cautiously in patients with pheochromocytoma; severe hypertension and tachycardia can occur. ▪ Have fluids and other measures to manage hypotension readily available. ▪ ***ALERT*** Monitor for signs and symptoms of neuroleptic malignant syndrome (fever, altered consciousness, extrapyramidal symptoms, tachycardia). ▪ Give I.V. doses slowly.

efavirenz Sustiva *Antiretroviral* Pregnancy Risk Category: C	*HIV-1 infection* — **Adults:** 600 mg P.O. q.d. **Children ≥ 3 yr weighing ≥ 40 kg (88 lb):** 600 mg P.O. q.d. **Children ≥ 3 yr weighing 10 to < 40 kg (22 to < 88 lb):** *10 to 15 kg (22 to 33 lb),* 200 mg P.O. q.d.; *15 to 20 kg (33 to 44 lb),* 250 mg P.O. q.d.; *20 to 25 kg (44 to 55 lb),* 300 mg P.O. q.d.; *25 to 32.5 kg (55 to 72 lb),* 350 mg P.O. q.d.; *32.5 to 40 kg (72 to 88 lb),* 400 mg P.O. q.d.	▪ Use cautiously in patients with hepatic impairment or in those also receiving hepatotoxic drugs. Monitor liver function tests in patients with history of hepatitis B or C and in those also taking ritonavir. ▪ Rule out pregnancy before starting therapy. ▪ ***ALERT*** Use with protease inhibitors or nucleoside reverse transcriptase inhibitors; resistant viruses emerge when used alone. ▪ Give h.s. to decrease CNS adverse effects. ▪ Give with water, juice, milk, or soda and without regard to meals. ▪ Report rash immediately.
enalaprilat Vasotec I.V. **enalapril maleate** Amprace‡, Renitec‡, Vasotec *Antihypertensive* Pregnancy Risk Category: C (D in 2nd and 3rd trimesters)	*Hypertension* — **Adult:** patient not on diuretics: initially 2.5 to 5 mg P.O. q.d., then adjust according to response. Dosage range 10 to 40 mg q.d. as single dose or 2 divided doses. Or, 1.25 mg I.V. infusion q 6 hr over 5 min. Patient on diuretics: initially 2.5 mg P.O. q.d. Or, 0.625 mg I.V. over 5 min; repeat in 1 hr, p.r.n., then 1.25 mg I.V. q 6 hr. *To switch from I.V. to P.O. therapy* — **Adults:** initially, 5 mg P.O. q.d.; if patient was receiving 0.625 mg I.V. q 6 hr, then 2.5 mg P.O. q.d. Adjust dosage to response. *To switch from P.O. to I.V. therapy* — **Adults:** 1.25 mg I.V. over 5 min q 6 hr.	▪ Monitor potassium intake and serum potassium level. ▪ Monitor CBC with differential. ▪ ***I.V. use:*** Inject slowly over ≥ 5 min, or dilute in 50 ml compatible solution and infuse over 15 min. ▪ Monitor BP. ▪ Advise patient to report adverse reactions, such as cough. ▪ Advise caution in hot weather and during repositioning or exercise to avoid lightheadedness and syncope. ▪ Don't give to patients with renal artery stenosis.

(continued)

†Canadian ‡Australian.

DRUG & CLASS	INDICATIONS & DOSAGES	NURSING CONSIDERATIONS
enalaprilat *(continued)*	***Adjust-a-dose:*** In hypertensive patients with CrCl $\leq$ 30 ml/min, initiate therapy at 2.5 mg P.O. q.d. and gradually adjust.	
enoxaparin sodium Lovenox *Anticoagulant* Pregnancy Risk Category: B	*To prevent pulmonary embolism (PE) and DVT after hip or knee replacement surgery* — **Adults:** 30 mg S.C. q 12 hr for 7 to 10 days. Give 1st dose between 12 and 24 hr postoperatively if hemostasis established. *To prevent PE and DVT after abdominal surgery* — **Adults:** 40 mg S.C. daily with 1st dose 2 hr before surgery. Give next dose, if hemostasis established, 24 hr after 1st preoperative dose and continue q.d. for 7 to 10 days. Continue treatment during postoperative period until risk of DVT diminished. *To prevent ischemic complications of unstable angina and non–Q-wave MI* — **Adults:** 1 mg/kg S.C. q 12 hr until stabilized ($\geq$ 2 days) with aspirin 100 to 325 mg P.O. once daily. *Inpatient treatment of acute DVT with and without PE when administered with warfarin sodium* — **Adults:** 1 mg/kg S.C. q 12 hr; or, 1.5 mg/kg S.C. q.d. (at same time daily) for 5 to 7 days until INR 2 to 3. Start warfarin sodium within 72 hr of injection.	▪ Don't expel gas bubble from syringe before injection. ▪ Never give I.M. Don't massage after S.C. injection. Watch for signs of bleeding. Rotate sites and keep record.

	Outpatient treatment of acute DVT without PE — **Adults:** 1 mg/kg S.C. q 12 hr for 5 to 7 days until INR 2 to 3. Start warfarin sodium within 72 hr of injection. ***Adjust-a-dose:*** If patient weighs < 45 kg or has a CrCl < 30 ml/min, decrease dose.	
entacapone Comtan *Antiparkinsonian* Pregnancy Risk Category: C	*Adjunct to levodopa-carbidopa to treat patients with Parkinson's disease who experience end-of-dose wearing-off of signs and symptoms* — **Adults:** 200 mg P.O. with each dose of levodopa-carbidopa to maximum of 8 times daily. Maximum daily dose of entacapone is 1,600 mg/day. May need to reduce daily levodopa dose or extend the interval between doses to optimize patient's response.	▪ Antiparkinsonian effects of drug occur only when used with levodopa-carbidopa. ▪ Levodopa-carbidopa dosage requirements are usually lower when given with entacapone; levodopa-carbidopa dose should be lowered or dosing interval increased to avoid adverse effects. ▪ Hallucinations may occur or worsen when this drug is taken. ▪ Monitor BP closely. Watch for orthostatic hypotension. ▪ Rapid withdrawal or abrupt reduction in dose may lead to signs and symptoms of Parkinson's disease and to hyperpyrexia and confusion, a symptom complex resembling neuroleptic malignant syndrome. Gradually stop drug, and monitor patient closely. Adjust other dopaminergic treatments as needed.

DRUG & CLASS

epinephrine (adrenaline)
Adrenalin, Bronkaid Mist, Bronkaid Mistometer†, Primatene Mist

epinephrine bitartrate
AsthmaHaler Mist, Bronitin Mist, Bronkaid Suspension Mist, Medihaler-Epi

epinephrine hydrochloride
Adrenalin Chloride, Asthma-Nefrin†, EpiPen, EpiPen Jr., Racepinephrine, Sus-Phrine, Vaponefrin

Bronchodilator, vasopressor, cardiac stimulant

Pregnancy Risk Category: C

INDICATIONS & DOSAGES

Bronchospasm; hypersensitivity reactions; anaphylaxis — **Adults:** 0.1 to 0.5 ml of 1:1,000 S.C. or I.M. Repeat q 10 to 15 min, p.r.n. Or, 0.1 to 0.25 ml of 1:1,000 I.V. slowly over 5 to 10 min. **Children:** 0.01 ml (10 mcg) of 1:1,000/kg S.C.; repeat q 20 min to 4 hr, p.r.n. Or, 0.004 to 0.005 ml/kg of 1:200 (Sus-Phrine) S.C.; repeat q 8 to 12 hr, p.r.n.

Acute asthmatic attacks — **Adults and children ≥ 4 yr:** 160 to 250 mcg (metered aerosol), equivalent to 1 inhalation, repeated once p.r.n. after 1 min; p.r.n. repeat dose after ≥ 3 hr. Or, 1% (1:100) solution epinephrine or 2.25% solution racepinephrine by hand-bulb nebulizer as 1 to 3 deep inhalations, repeated q 3 hr, p.r.n.

To restore cardiac rhythm in cardiac arrest — **Adults:** 0.5 to 1 mg I.V. May repeat q 3 to 5 min, p.r.n. Higher-dose epinephrine may be used: 3 to 5 mg (about 0.1 mg/kg) repeated q 3 to 5 min. **Children:** 0.01 mg/kg (0.1 ml/kg 1:10,000 injection) I.V. Initial dose through ET tube 0.1 mg/kg (0.1 ml/kg 1:1,000 injection) diluted in 1 to 2 ml 0.45% or 0.9% NaCl. Subsequent I.V. or intratracheal doses 0.1 to 0.2 mg/kg (0.1 to 0.2 ml/kg of 1:1,000 injection). May repeat q 3 to 5 min.

NURSING CONSIDERATIONS

- ***I.V. use:*** Don't mix with alkaline solutions.
- When giving I.V., monitor BP, HR, and ECG at start and during therapy.
- Don't inject parenteral suspension I.M. into buttocks. Gas gangrene may occur.
- Massage site after I.M. injection.
- Observe closely for adverse reactions. Notify doctor if these develop.
- If more than 1 inhalation ordered, tell patient to wait ≥ 2 min before repeating.
- If patient also uses steroid inhaler, tell to use bronchodilator first, then wait 5 min before using steroid.
- Teach patient with acute hypersensitivity reactions (bee stings, food allergies) how to self-inject drug (EpiPen, EpiPen Jr.) at home, p.r.n..

epirubicin hydrochloride
Ellence
Antineoplastic
Pregnancy Risk Category: D

Adjuvant therapy in patients with axillary node tumor involvement following primary breast cancer resection — **Adults:** 100 to 120 mg/m^2 I.V. infusion over 3 to 5 min via free-flowing I.V. solution on day 1 of each cycle q 3 to 4 wk; or divided equally into two doses on days 1 and 8 of each cycle. Maximum cumulative (lifetime) dose is 900 mg/m^2.

Dosage modification after the 1st cycle is based on toxicity. For patients with platelet counts < 50,000/mm^3, absolute neutrophil count (ANC) < 250/mm^3, neutropenic fever, or grade 3 or 4 nonhematologic toxicity, the day 1 dose in subsequent cycles should be reduced to 75% of the day 1 dose given in the current cycle. Day 1 therapy in subsequent cycles should be delayed until platelets are ≥ 100,000/mm^3, ANC ≥ 1,500/mm^3, and nonhematologic toxicity recovers to grade 1.

For patients receiving divided doses (days 1 and 8), the day 8 dose should be 75% of the day 1 dose if platelet counts are 75,000 to 100,000/mm^3 and ANC is 1,000 to 1,499/mm^3. If day 8 platelet counts are < 75,000/mm^3, ANC < 1,000/mm^3, or grade 3 or 4 nonhematologic toxicity has occurred, the day 8 dose should be omitted.

Adjust-a-dose: In patients with bone mar-

- Patients receiving 120 mg/m^2 of epirubicin should also receive prophylactic antibiotic therapy with trimethoprim-sulfamethoxazole or a fluoroquinolone.
- Monitor left ventricular ejection fraction (LVEF) regularly during therapy; drug should be stopped at the first sign of impaired cardiac function. Early signs of cardiac toxicity may include sinus tachycardia, ECG abnormalities, tachyarrhythmias, bradycardia, AV block, and bundle branch block.
- Get total and differential WBC, RBC, and platelet counts before and during each cycle of therapy.
- Epirubicin should be given under the supervision of a physician who is experienced in the use of cancer chemotherapy. Pregnant nurses shouldn't handle drug.
- ***ALERT*** Drug is a vesicant. Never give I.M. or S.C. Always give through free-flowing I.V. solution of 0.9 % NaCl or D_5W over 3 to 5 min.
- Avoid veins over joints or in extremities with compromised venous or lymphatic drainage.
- Plasma clearance is decreased in elderly women. Monitor closely for toxicity in elderly patients, especially women over age 70.

(continued)

DRUG & CLASS	INDICATIONS & DOSAGES	NURSING CONSIDERATIONS
epirubicin hydrochloride *(continued)*	row dysfunction (heavily pretreated patients, patients with bone marrow depression, or those with neoplastic bone marrow infiltration), start at lower doses of 75 to 90 mg/m^2. In hepatic dysfunction, if bilirubin is 1.2 to 3 mg/dl or AST is 2 to 4 times the upper limit of normal, give ½ the starting dose. If bilirubin is > 3 mg/dl or AST is more than 4 times the upper limit of normal, give ¼ the starting dose. In patients with severe renal dysfunction (serum creatinine > 5 mg/dl), consider lower dosages.	
epoetin alfa (erythropoietin) Epogen, Procrit *Antianemic* Pregnancy Risk Category: C	*Anemia from reduced production of endogenous erythropoietin caused by end-stage renal disease* — **Adults:** dosage individualized. Initially, 50 to 100 U/kg I.V. 3 times/wk. (Can give S.C. or I.V. in nondialysis patients with chronic renal failure or patients receiving continuous peritoneal dialysis.) Reduce dosage when target Hct reached or if Hct rises > 4 points in 2 wk. Increase dosage if Hct doesn't increase by 5 to 6 points after 8 wk of therapy. Maintenance dosage highly individualized. *Anemia from cancer chemotherapy* — **Adults:** 150 U/kg S.C. 3 times q wk for 8 wk or until target Hgb level reached. If target not reached after 8 wk, can increase to 300/kg 3 times q wk.	▪ Monitor BP before therapy. BP may rise, especially when Hct increases in early therapy. Monitor blood count. Elevated Hct may cause excessive clotting. ▪ ***I.V. use:*** Give undiluted by direct injection. Solution contains no preservatives. Discard unused portion. Don't mix with other drugs. ▪ Give iron supplement when treatment starts and throughout therapy. ▪ Response depends on amount of endogenous erythropoietin in plasma. Patients with ≥ 500 U/L usually have transfusion-dependent anemia and probably won't respond. Those with levels < 500 U/L usually respond well.

	Anemia in pediatric patients with chronic renal failure who are undergoing dialysis—**Infants and children ages 1 mo to 16 yr:** 50 units/kg I.V. or S.C. 3 times q wk. Reduce dosage when target Hct level reached or if level rises > 4 points within 2 wk. Increase dosage if Hct level doesn't rise by 5 to 6 points after 8 wk of therapy and is below target range. Maintenance dose is highly individualized to maintain Hct level within target range.	
eprosartan mesylate Teveten *Antihypertensive* Pregnancy Risk Category: C (D in 2nd and 3rd trimesters)	*Hypertension, alone or with other antihypertensives* — **Adults:** initially, 600 mg P.O. daily. Daily dose ranges from 400 to 800 mg given as single daily dose or 2 divided doses.	▪ Contraindicated in patients who are hypersensitive to drug or its components. Use cautiously in patients with an activated renin-angiotensin system, such as volume- or salt-depleted patients, and in patients whose renal function may depend on the activity of the renin-angiotensin-aldosterone system, such as patients with severe heart failure. Also use cautiously in patients with renal artery stenosis. ▪ Monitor blood pressure closely when starting treatment. If hypotension occurs, place patient in supine position and, if necessary, give I.V. infusion of normal saline. ▪ A transient episode of hypotension isn't a contraindication to continued treatment. Drug may be restarted when BP is stable.

(continued)

†Canadian ‡Australian.

DRUG & CLASS	INDICATIONS & DOSAGES	NURSING CONSIDERATIONS
eprosartan mesylate *(continued)*		▪ Drug may be used alone or with other antihypertensives, such as diuretics and calcium channel blockers. Maximal BP response may take 2 to 3 wk. ▪ Monitor patient for facial or lip swelling because angioedema has occurred with other angiotensin II antagonists. ▪ Expect a slightly decreased response to drug in elderly patients. No initial dose adjustment is necessary.
eptifibatide Integrilin *Platelet aggregation inhibitor* Pregnancy Risk Category: B	*Acute coronary syndrome (unstable angina or non–Q-wave MI), including patients to be managed medically and those undergoing percutaneous coronary intervention* — **Adults:** I.V. bolus of 180 mcg/kg (up to 22.6 mg) immediately after diagnosis, followed by continuous I.V. infusion of 2 mcg/kg/min (up to infusion rate of 15 mg/hr) for up to 72 hr. Infusion rate may be decreased to 0.5 mcg/kg/min during percutaneous coronary intervention. Infusion should then be continued for additional 20 to 24 hr after procedure, for up to 96 hr of therapy. *Patients without acute coronary syndrome who are having percutaneous coronary intervention* — **Adults:** I.V. bolus of 135 mcg/kg given immediately before procedure,	▪ Drug intended for use with heparin and aspirin. ▪ If patient is to undergo CABG surgery, stop infusion before surgery. ▪ Minimize use of arterial and venous punctures, I.M. injections, urinary catheters, nasotracheal tubes, and NG tubes, and avoid use of noncompressible I.V. sites (subclavian or jugular veins). ▪ ***I.V. use:*** May give drug in same I.V. line as alteplase, atropine, dobutamine, heparin, lidocaine, meperidine, metoprolol, midazolam, morphine, nitroglycerin, verapamil, 0.9% NaCl, and D_5W and 0.9% NaCl; line may also contain up to 60 mEq/L of potassium chloride. ▪ If patient's platelet count is < 100,000/

	followed by continuous infusion of 0.5 mcg/kg/min for 20 to 24 hr.	mm³, discontinue eptifibatide and heparin. ▪ Withdraw bolus dose from 10-ml vial into syringe and give by I.V. push over 1 to 2 min. Give I.V. infusion undiluted directly from 100-ml vial using infusion pump. ▪ Monitor patient for bleeding. ▪ Don't give to patients with recent transplant surgery, trauma, or stroke.
ergotamine tartrate Ergodryl Mono‡, Ergomar, Gynergen†, Medihaler Ergotamine *Vasoconstrictor* Pregnancy Risk Category: X	*Vascular or migraine headache* — **Adults:** initially, 2 mg P.O. or S.L., then 1 to 2 mg P.O. q hr or S.L. q ½ hr, to maximum 6 mg q.d. and 10 mg q wk. Or, aerosol inhaler: 1 spray (360 mcg) initially, repeated q 5 min, p.r.n., to maximum of 6 sprays (2.16 mg/24 hr) or 15 sprays (5.4 mg/wk).	▪ Most effective when used in prodromal stage of headache or soon after onset. ▪ Obtain dietary history to determine if condition is caused by certain foods. ▪ Be alert for ergotamine rebound. ▪ With long-term use, check for and report coldness or tingling in hands or feet. ▪ Instruct patient not to exceed recommended dose.
erythromycin (topical) Akne-Mycin, Erycette, EryDerm, Erygel, Ery-Sol **erythromycin** *Topical antibiotic* Pregnancy Risk Category: C	*Inflammatory acne vulgaris* — **Adults and children:** apply in thin film to affected areas b.i.d.	▪ Wash, rinse, and dry affected areas before application. ▪ May require prolonged use when treating acne vulgaris; may cause overgrowth of nonsusceptible organisms.
erythromycin (ophthalmic) Ilotycin Ophthalmic Ointment	*Acute and chronic conjunctivitis, trachoma, other eye infections* — **Adults and children:** 1-cm length applied directly to infected eye up to 6 times daily.	▪ To prevent ophthalmia neonatorum, apply ≤ 1 hr after birth. Use in neonates born either by vaginal delivery or by cesarean section. Gently massage *(continued)*

†Canadian ‡Australian.

DRUG & CLASS	INDICATIONS & DOSAGES	NURSING CONSIDERATIONS
erythromycin *(continued)* *Ophthalmic antibiotic* Pregnancy Risk Category: NR	*Prevention of ophthalmia neonatorum from* N. gonorrhoeae *or* C. trachomatis — **Neonates:** apply ribbon of ointment about 1 cm long in lower conjunctival sac of each eye shortly after birth.	eyelids for 1 min to spread ointment. ▪ Use only when sensitivity studies show drug effective against infecting organisms. ▪ Store at room temperature in tightly closed, light-resistant container.
erythromycin base E-Mycin, Eramycin, Eryc, Eryc333, PCE, Ery-Tab, Robimycin **erythromycin estolate** Ilosone **erythromycin ethylsuccinate** EES, EryPed, EryPed 200 **erythromycin lactobionate** Erythrocin **erythromycin stearate** Erythrocin Stearate, My-E *Antibiotic* Pregnancy Risk Category: B	*Acute pelvic inflammatory disease from* N. gonorrhoeae — **Adults:** 500 mg I.V. (or lactobionate) q 6 hr for 3 days, then 250 mg (base, estolate, stearate) or 400 mg (ethylsuccinate) P.O. q 6 hr for 7 days. *Mild to moderate severe respiratory tract, skin, or soft-tissue infections* — **Adults:** 250 to 500 mg (base, estolate, stearate) P.O. q 6 hr; or 400 to 800 mg (ethylsuccinate) P.O. q 6 hr; or 15 to 20 mg/kg I.V. q.d. (lactobionate) continuous infusion or divided doses q 6 hr for 10 days. **Children:** 30 to 50 mg/kg (oral erythromycin salts) P.O. q.d., divided doses q 6 hr; or 15 to 20 mg/kg I.V. q.d., divided doses q 4 to 6 hr for 10 days.	▪ Obtain urine specimen for culture and sensitivity tests before 1st dose. ▪ Monitor hepatic function, especially with erythromycin estolate. ▪ When giving suspension, note concentration. ▪ ***I.V. use:*** Reconstitute according to directions; dilute each 250 mg in ≥ 100 ml 0.9% NaCl. Infuse over 1 hr. Watch for phlebitis, which is common. ▪ Don't give erythromycin lactobionate with other drugs. ▪ Monitor patient for superinfection. ▪ Tell patient to take oral form with water 1 hr before or 2 hr after meals or with food if GI upset occurs. Coated tablets may be taken with meals. ▪ Caution patient not to drink juice with drug, not to swallow chewable tablets whole, and not to crush or chew delayed-release or coated tablets.

esmolol hydrochloride Brevibloc *Antiarrhythmic, antihypertensive* Pregnancy Risk Category: C	*Supraventricular tachycardia; to control ventricular rate in atrial fibrillation or flutter in perioperative, postoperative, or other emergent circumstances; noncompensatory sinus tachycardia when HR requires specific interventions* — **Adults:** loading dose: 500 mcg/kg/min by I.V. infusion over 1 min, then 4-min maintenance infusion of 50 mcg/kg/min. If no adequate response in 5 min, repeat loading dose and follow with maintenance infusion of 100 mcg/kg/min for 4 min. Repeat loading dose and increase maintenance infusion by 50-mcg/kg/min increments. Maximum maintenance infusion for tachycardia 200 mcg/kg/min. *Perioperative, postoperative tachycardia or hypertension* — **Adults:** perioperative treatment of tachycardia or hypertension: 80 mg (about 1 mg/kg) I.V. bolus over 30 sec; then 150 mcg/kg/min I.V. infusion, p.r.n. Adjust rate, p.r.n., to maximum 300 mcg/kg/min.	▪ ***I.V. use:*** Don't give by I.V. push; use infusion control device. May use 10-mg/ml single-dose vials without diluting, but always dilute injection concentrate (250 mg/ml) to maximum concentration of 10 mg/ml before infusion. Remove 20 ml from 500 ml of D_5W, lactated Ringer's, or 0.45% or 0.9% NaCl, and add 2 ampules esmolol (final concentration 10 mg/ml). ▪ Esmolol solutions are incompatible with diazepam, furosemide, sodium bicarbonate, and thiopental sodium. ▪ Monitor ECG and BP continuously during infusion; hypotension possible. ▪ Hypotension usually can be reversed within 30 min by decreasing dose or, if necessary, stopping infusion. Notify doctor. ▪ Instruct patient to report adverse reactions promptly. ▪ Use with caution in patients with hyperthyroidism, diabetes, or asthma.
estazolam ProSom *Hypnotic* Pregnancy Risk Category: X Controlled Substance Schedule: IV	*Insomnia* — **Adults:** 1 to 2 mg P.O. h.s. **Elderly:** 1 mg P.O. h.s. Use higher doses with extreme care.	▪ Avoid prolonged use. ▪ Monitor liver and renal functions and CBC. ▪ Patient should avoid activities that require mental alertness or physical coordination. ▪ Warn patient that alcohol can cause additive depressant effects.

†Canadian ‡Australian.

DRUG & CLASS	INDICATIONS & DOSAGES	NURSING CONSIDERATIONS
esterified estrogens Estratab, Menest, Neo-Estrone† *Estrogen replacement, antineoplastic* Pregnancy Risk Category: X	*Inoperable prostate cancer* — **Men:** 1.25 to 2.5 mg P.O. t.i.d. *Osteoporosis prevention*—**Adults:** initially, 0.3 mg P.O. q.d.; may be increased to 1.25 mg q.d. *Breast cancer* — **Men and postmenopausal women:** 10 mg P.O. t.i.d. for ≥ 3 mo. *Female hypogonadism* — **Women:** 2.5 to 7.5 mg q.d. in divided doses in cycles of 20 days on, 10 days off. *Female castration; primary ovarian failure* — **Women:** 1.25 mg q.d. in cycles of 3 wk on, 1 wk off. Adjust for symptoms.	▪ ***ALERT*** Stop ≥ 1 mo before procedures featuring prolonged immobilization or thromboembolism. ▪ Warn patient to immediately report adverse reactions. ▪ Tell diabetic patient to report elevated blood glucose. ▪ Teach patient how to perform routine breast self-exam. ▪ Don't give to patients in liver failure.
estradiol Climara, Estrace, Estraderm, Vivelle **estradiol cypionate** depGynogen, Depo-Estradiol, E-Cypionate **estradiol valerate (oestradiol valerate)** Delestrogen, Estra-L 40, Gynogen L.A., Menaval-20, Valergen *Estrogen replacement, antineoplastic* Pregnancy Risk Category: X	*Vasomotor menopausal symptoms; female hypogonadism; female castration; primary ovarian failure* — **Adults:** 1 to 2 mg P.O. (estradiol) q.d. in cycles of 3 wk on and 1 wk off, or cycles of 5 days on and 2 days off; or 1 transdermal system (Estraderm) delivering 0.05 mg/24 hr, or (Climara) delivering 0.05 mg/ 24 hr or 0.1 mg/24 hr and applied q wk in cycles of 3 wk on and 1 wk off. Or, 1 to 5 mg (cypionate) I.M. q 3 to 4 wk, or 10 to 20 mg (valerate) I.M. q 4 wk, p.r.n. *Palliative treatment of advanced, inoperable breast cancer*— **Men and postmenopausal women:** 10 mg P.O. (estradiol) t.i.d. for 3 mo.	▪ Ensure that patient undergoes physical exam before and during therapy. ▪ Ask patient about allergies, especially to foods or plants. ▪ Never give I.V. ▪ Apply transdermal patch to clean, dry, hairless, intact skin on abdomen or buttocks. Don't apply to areas where clothing can loosen patch. ▪ Rotate application sites. ▪ Warn patient to immediately report adverse reactions. ▪ Tell diabetic patient to report elevated blood glucose levels. ▪ Don't apply patch to breasts.

Palliative treatment of advanced inoperable prostate cancer — **Men:** 30 mg I.M. (valerate) q 1 to 2 wk, or 1 to 2 mg P.O. (estradiol) t.i.d.

Prevention of postmenopausal osteoporosis — **Women:** 0.5 mg P.O. (estadiol) q.d. in cycles of 3 wk on, 1 wk off; or transdermal patch (Climara) 0.025 mg q.d. or (Estraderm) 0.05 mg q.d.

---

estradiol/norethindrone acetate transdermal system

Activella, CombiPatch

Estrogen replacement, antineoplastic

Pregnancy Risk Category: X

Moderate-to-severe vasomotor menopausal symptoms, vulvar and vaginal atrophy, hypoestrogenemia from hypogonadism, castration, or primary ovarian failure in women with intact uterus — **Women:** *Continuous combined regimen:* 9-cm^2 patch worn on lower abdomen. Remove old system and apply new system twice weekly during 28-day cycle. May increase to 16-cm^2 patch. *Continuous sequential regimen:* apply as sequential regimen in combination with 0.05-mg estradiol transdermal patch worn for first 2 wk of 28-day cycle; replace system twice weekly. For rest of 28-day cycle, apply 9-cm^2 patch system to lower abdomen. May increase to 16-cm^2 patch, p.r.n.

Prevention of postmenopausal osteoporosis — **Women:** 1 tablet Activella P.O. q.d.

- Use cautiously in patients with impaired liver function, asthma, epilepsy, migraine, and cardiac or renal dysfunction, and in breast-feeding patients.
- Women not currently receiving continuous estrogen or estrogen/progestin therapy may start therapy at any time.
- Women receiving continuous hormone replacement therapy should complete current cycle of therapy before beginning estradiol therapy. Start therapy on 1st day of withdrawal bleeding.
- Apply patch system to smooth (fold-free), clean, dry, nonirritated area of skin on lower abdomen, avoiding the waistline. Rotate application sites waiting ≥ 1 wk between applications to same site.
- Monitor patient's BP.
- Don't apply patch to breasts.

†Canadian ‡Australian.

DRUG & CLASS	INDICATIONS & DOSAGES	NURSING CONSIDERATIONS
estrogens, conjugated (estrogenic substances, conjugated; oestrogens, conjugated) C.E.S.†, Premarin, Premarin Intravenous *Estrogen replacement, antineoplastic, antiosteoporotic* Pregnancy Risk Category: X	*Abnormal uterine bleeding (hormonal imbalance)* — **Women:** 25 mg I.V. or I.M., repeated in 6 to 12 hr, p.r.n. *Female castration; primary ovarian failure* — **Women:** 1.25 mg P.O. q.d. in cycles of 3 wk on, 1 wk off. *Osteoporosis* — **Postmenopausal women:** 0.625 mg P.O. q.d. in cycles of 3 wk on, 1 wk off.	▪ ***I.V. use:*** When giving by direct injection, give slowly to avoid flushing reaction. ▪ When giving I.M., inject deeply into large muscle. Rotate injection sites to prevent muscle atrophy. ▪ Warn patient to immediately report adverse reactions. ▪ Tell diabetic patient to report elevated blood glucose levels so that antidiabetic dosage can be adjusted.
estropipate (piperazine estrone sulfate) Ogen, OrthoEST *Estrogen replacement* Pregnancy Risk Category: X	*Primary ovarian failure; female castration; female hypogonadism* — **Women:** 1.25 to 7.5 mg P.O. q.d. for first 3 wk, then rest period of 8 to 10 days. If bleeding doesn't occur by end of rest period, repeat cycle. *Vasomotor menopausal symptoms* — **Women:** 0.625 mg to 5 mg P.O. q.d. in cycles of 3 wk on, 1 wk off. *Prevention of osteoporosis* — **Women:** 0.625 mg P.O. q.d. for 25 days of 31-day cycle.	▪ Ensure that patient undergoes thorough physical exam before therapy starts and yearly thereafter. Periodically monitor serum lipid levels, BP, weight, and hepatic function. ▪ ***ALERT*** Warn patient to immediately report adverse reactions. ▪ Teach patient how to perform routine breast self-exams.
etanercept Enbrel *Disease-modifying antirheumatic* Pregnancy Risk Category: B	*Moderately to severely active rheumatoid arthritis in patients who don't respond well to one or more antirheumatics plus methotrexate or to methotrexate alone* — **Adults:** 25 mg S.C. twice weekly. *Moderately to severely active polyarticular-course juvenile rheumatoid arthritis* — **Children ages 4 to 17:** 0.4 mg/kg (up to 25 mg/	▪ Don't give live vaccines during therapy. ▪ Reconstitute aseptically with 1 ml of supplied sterile bacteriostatic water for injection, USP (0.9% benzyl alcohol). Inject diluent slowly into vial. Don't filter reconstituted solution. ▪ Injection sites should be ≥ 1 inch apart. Rotate sites regularly.

	dose) S.C. twice weekly, 72 to 96 hr apart. *Moderately to severely active rheumatoid arthritis and delay of structural damage* — **Adults:** 25 mg S.C. twice weekly 72 to 96 hr apart.	▪ Use when patient has no resposne to other antirheumatics. ▪ Most common adverse effect is injection site reaction.
ethacrynate sodium Edecrin Sodium **ethacrynic acid** Edecrin *Diuretic* Pregnancy Risk Category: B	*Acute pulmonary edema* — **Adults:** 50 mg or 0.5 to 1 mg/kg I.V. Usually only 1 dose necessary, though 2nd dose may be required.	▪ ***I.V. use:*** Reconstitute vacuum vial with 50 ml D_5W or 0.9% NaCl. Give slowly through tubing or running infusion over several min. ▪ Don't give S.C. or I.M. ▪ If more than one dose is needed, use new injection site to avoid thrombophlebitis. ▪ Monitor I&O, weight, BP, and electrolyte and uric acid levels. ▪ Watch for signs of hypokalemia.
ethambutol hydrochloride Etibi†, Myambutol *Antituberculotic* Pregnancy Risk Category: C	*Adjunctive treatment in pulmonary TB* — **Adults and children > 13 yr:** initial treatment for patients who haven't received previous antitubercular therapy, 15 mg/kg P.O. as single dose q.d. **Retreatment:** 25 mg/kg P.O. q.d. as single dose for 60 days (or until bacteriologic smears and cultures become negative) with more than one other antitubercular; then decrease to 15 mg/kg/day as single dose.	▪ Obtain AST and ALT levels before therapy and monitor levels q 3 to 4 wk. ▪ Always give with other antituberculotics to prevent development of resistant organisms. ▪ Tell patient to report adverse effects, especially blurred vision, red-green color blindness, or changes in urinary elimination. ▪ Reassure that visual disturbances should disappear few wk to mo after drug stopped. ▪ Monitor uric acid levels in patients with gout.
ethinyl estradiol Estinyl *Estrogen replacement, antineoplastic*	*Palliative treatment of metastatic breast cancer (≥ 5 yr after menopause)* — **Women:** 1 mg P.O. t.i.d. for ≥ 3 mo. *Female hypogonadism* — **Women:** 0.05 mg	▪ Tell patient to immediately report adverse reactions. ▪ Tell diabetic patient to report elevated blood glucose levels. *(continued)*

†Canadian ‡Australian.

DRUG & CLASS	INDICATIONS & DOSAGES	NURSING CONSIDERATIONS
ethinyl estradiol *(continued)* Pregnancy Risk Category: X	P.O. daily to t.i.d. 2 wk each mo, then 2 wk of progesterone therapy; continued for 3 to 6 mo, then 2 mo off. *Vasomotor menopausal symptoms* — **Women:** 0.02 to 0.05 mg P.O. q.d. for cycles of 3 wk on and 1 wk off. *Palliative treatment of metastatic inoperable prostate cancer* — **Men:** 0.15 to 2 mg P.O. q.d.	▪ Explain to patient on cyclic therapy for postmenopausal symptoms that, although withdrawal bleeding may occur during wk off drug, fertility isn't restored. ▪ Teach women how to perform breast self-exams.
ethinyl estradiol *monophasic:* w/desogestrel — Desogen; w/ethynodiol diacetate — Demulen 1/35; w/levonorgestrel — Nordette; w/norethindrone — Genora 1/35; w/norethindrone acetate — Loestrin 21 1/20; w/norgestimate — Ortho-Cyclen; w/norgestrel — Ovral; w/norethindrone acetate and ferrous fumarate — Loestrin Fe 1/20; *biphasic:* w/norethindrone — Jenest-28; *triphasic:* w/levonorgestrel — Triphasil; w/norethindrone — Ortho-Novum 7/7/7; w/norgestimate — Ortho Tri-Cyclen	*Contraception* — **Adults:** *Monophasic oral contraceptives:* 1 tablet P.O. q.d., starting on day 5 of menstrual cycle. With 20- and 21-tablet package, new dosing cycle begins 7 days after last tablet taken. With 28-tablet package, dose is 1 tablet q.d. without interruption. *Biphasic oral contraceptives:* 1 color tablet P.O. q.d. for 10 days; then next color tablet for 11 days. With 21-tablet package, new dosing cycle begins 7 days after last tablet taken. With 28-tablet package, dose is 1 tablet q.d. without interruption. *Triphasic oral contraceptives:* 1 tablet P.O. q.d. in sequence specified by brand. With 21-tablet package, new dosing cycle begins 7 days after last tablet taken. With 28-tablet package, dose is 1 tablet q.d. without interruption. *Acne vulgaris* — **Adults:** 1 tablet P.O. q.d., using the 28-tablet package of Ortho Tri-Cyclen. Dosage schedule for acne should fol-	▪ Triphasic contraceptives may cause fewer adverse reactions, such as breakthrough bleeding and spotting. ▪ Monitor serum lipid levels, BP, weight, and hepatic function. ▪ Oral contraceptives affect many lab tests. ▪ Monitor blood glucose levels. ▪ Warn patient to immediately report adverse reactions. ▪ ***ALERT*** Advise patient of increased risk of thrombosis associated with simultaneous use of cigarettes and oral contraceptives. ▪ Instruct patient to take tablets at same time each day; nighttime dosing may reduce nausea and headaches. ▪ Advise patient to use additional method of birth control, such as condoms or diaphragm with spermicide, for 1st wk of administration in 1st cycle (if used for birth control).

mestranol *monophasic:* w/norethin-drone — Genora 1/50 *Oral contraceptive* Pregnancy Risk Category: X	low same guidelines for Ortho Tri-Cyclen as when used as an oral contraceptive.	▪ Stress importance of Papanicolaou tests and annual gynecologic exams.
etodolac Lodine *Antarthritic* Pregnancy Risk Category: C	*Acute and chronic management of pain* — **Adults:** 200 to 400 mg P.O. q 6 to 8 hr, p.r.n., not to exceed 1,200 mg/24 hr. For patients ≤ 60 kg (132 lb), total daily dose shouldn't exceed 20 mg/kg. *Osteoarthritis, rheumatoid arthritis*—300 mg b.i.d. or t.i.d., or 400 mg b.i.d., or 500 mg b.i.d. Adjust to 600 to 1,200 mg/day in divided doses.	▪ Can lead to reversible renal impairment. ▪ To minimize GI discomfort, instruct patient to take with milk or meals. ▪ ***ALERT*** Teach patient about signs and symptoms of GI bleeding; tell him to contact doctor immediately if any occurs. ▪ Advise patient to avoid alcohol and aspirin.
etoposide (VP-16) VePesid, Toposar **etoposide phosphate** Etopophos *Antineoplastic* Pregnancy Risk Category: D	*Testicular cancer* — **Adults:** 50 to 100 mg/m^2 I.V. on 5 consecutive days q 3 to 4 wk; or 100 mg/m^2 on days 1, 3, and 5 q 3 to 4 wk. *Small-cell carcinoma of lung* — **Adults:** 35 mg/m^2/day I.V. for 4 days; or 50 mg/m^2/day I.V. for 5 days. Oral dose: twice I.V. dose, rounded to nearest 50 mg. ***Adjust-a-dose:*** In patients with CrCl 15 to 50 ml/min, give 75% initial dose; if CrCl is < 15 ml/min, may further reduce dose.	▪ Monitor BP q 15 min. If systolic pressure is < 90 mm Hg, stop infusion and notify doctor. ▪ Have emergency drugs and equipment available in case of anaphylaxis. ▪ ***I.V. use:*** Give etoposide by slow I.V. infusion (over ≥ 30 min) to prevent severe hypotension. May give etoposide phosphate over 5 to 210 min. Don't give etoposide through membrane-type in-line filter. ▪ Dilute etoposide for infusion in D_5W or 0.9% NaCl to concentration of 0.2 or 0.4 mg/ml. May give etoposide phosphate without further dilution, or may dilute to concentration as low as 0.1 mg/ml in D_5W or 0.9% NaCl.

†Canadian ‡Australian.

DRUG & CLASS	INDICATIONS & DOSAGES	NURSING CONSIDERATIONS
exemestane Aromasin *Antineoplastic* Pregnancy Risk Category: D	*Advanced breast cancer in postmenopausal women whose disease has progressed following treatment with tamoxifen* — **Adults:** 25 mg P.O. once daily after a meal.	▪ Drug should be used only in postmenopausal women, never in premenopausal women. ▪ Don't give with estrogen-containing drugs because this could interfere with intended action. ▪ Treatment should continue until tumor progression is apparent. ▪ Patient should take drug after a meal.
famciclovir Famvir *Antiviral* Pregnancy Risk Category: B	*Acute herpes zoster infection (shingles)* — **Adults:** 500 mg P.O. q 8 hr for 7 days. *Recurrent episodes of genital herpes* — **Adults:** 125 mg P.O. b.i.d. for 5 days. Start when symptoms occur. *Recurrent herpes simplex virus infections in HIV-infected patients* — **Adults:** 500 mg P.O. b.i.d. for 7 days. ***Adjust-a-dose:*** Reduce dosage in patients with renal failure.	▪ May take without regard to meals. ▪ Inform patient that drug won't cure genital herpes but can decrease symptom length and severity. ▪ Teach patient how to prevent spread of herpes infection. ▪ Urge patient to report early symptoms.
famotidine Pepcid, Pepcid AC, Pepcidine‡ *Antiulcer agent* Pregnancy Risk Category: B	*Duodenal ulcer (short-term treatment)* — **Adults:** acute therapy: 40 mg P.O. once daily h.s. or 20 mg P.O. b.i.d. Maintenance: 20 mg P.O. once daily h.s. *Benign gastric ulcer (short-term)* — **Adults:** 40 mg P.O. q.d. h.s. for 8 wk. *Gastroesophageal reflux disease (GERD)* — **Adults:** 20 mg P.O. b.i.d. up to 6 wk. For	▪ ***I.V. use:*** To prepare injection, dilute 2 ml (20 mg) with compatible I.V. solution to total volume of 5 or 10 ml; inject over ≥ 2 min. Or, give by intermittent I.V. infusion. Dilute 20 mg (2 ml) in 100 ml compatible solution and infuse over 15 to 30 min. Stable for 48 hr at room temperature after dilution.

	esophagitis caused by GERD, 20 to 40 mg b.i.d. up to 12 wk. *Heartburn* — **Adults:** 10 mg (Pepcid AC only) P.O. 1 hr before meals (prevention) or 10 mg (Pepcid AC only) P.O. with water for symptoms. Maximum 20 mg daily. Don't take daily for > 2 wk. *Hospitalized patients with intractable ulcerations or hypersecretory conditions or those who can't take P.O. medication* — **Adults:** 20 mg I.V. q 12 hr.	▪ Prescription drug most effective when taken h.s. ▪ With doctor's knowledge, let patient take antacids with drug, especially at start of therapy when pain is severe. ▪ Urge patient to avoid cigarette smoking.
felodipine Agon SR‡, Plendil, Plendil ER‡, Renedil† **felodipine** *Antihypertensive* Pregnancy Risk Category: C	*Hypertension* — **Adults:** initially, 5 mg P.O. q.d. Adjust according to patient response, generally at intervals ≥ 2 wk. Usual dose 5 to 10 mg q.d.; maximum, 20 mg q.d. **Elderly > 65 yr:** initially, 2.5 mg P.O. q.d. Maximum, 10 mg q.d. ***Adjust-a-dose:*** In patient with impaired hepatic function, give 2.5 mg P.O. q.d.	▪ Monitor BP and for orthostatic hypotension and peripheral edema. ▪ Tell patient to swallow tablets whole and not to crush or chew them. ▪ Tell patient to continue taking even when he feels better and to check with doctor or pharmacist before taking other drugs, including OTC drugs.
fenofibrate (micronized) Lipidil, Micro†, Tricor *Antihyperlipidemic* Pregnancy Risk Category: C	*Adjunct therapy to diet to reduce LDL cholesterol, total cholesterol, triglycerides, and apolipoprotein B in patients with primary hypercholesterolemia or mixed dyslipidemia (Fredrickson types IIa and IIb)* — **Adults:** 200 mg P.O. daily. In patients with severe renal impairment, initial dose is 67 mg/day. Increase after renal function and triglyceride levels evaluated. Don't modify dosage if renal impairment is moderate.	▪ Obtain baseline lipid levels and LFTs before starting therapy. Monitor liver function periodically during therapy. Stop therapy if enzyme levels persist at more than 3 times normal limit. ▪ ***ALERT*** Monitor for symptoms of pancreatitis, myositis, rhabdomyolysis, cholelithiasis, and renal failure. Watch for myalgia, muscle tenderness, or weakness, especially with malaise or fever. *(continued)*

†Canadian ‡Australian.

DRUG & CLASS	INDICATIONS & DOSAGES	NURSING CONSIDERATIONS
fenofibrate *(continued)*	*Adjunct to diet to treat patients with very high serum triglyceride levels (types IV and V hyperlipidemia) who are at risk for pancreatitis and don't respond adequately to determined dietary effort* — **Adults:** initially, 67 mg P.O. q.d. Dose may be increased after repeat serum triglyceride estimations at 4- to 8-wk intervals to maximum of 3 capsules q.d. (201 mg).	▪ Beta blockers, estrogens, and thiazide diuretics may increase plasma triglyceride levels. ▪ Teach patient about diet and glycemic control in diabetes for management of hypertriglyceridemia. ▪ Urge patient to avoid alcohol.
fenoldopam mesylate Corlopam *Antihypertensive* Pregnancy Risk Category: B	*Short-term (up to 48 hr) hospital management of severe hypertension when rapid but quickly reversible reduction of BP is indicated, including malignant hypertension with deteriorating end-organ function* — **Adults:** start infusion rates at 0.1 to 0.3 mcg/kg/min and titrate up or down for desired BP $\leq$ q 15 min. Increments for titration are 0.05 to 0.1 mcg/kg/min.	▪ Drug causes tachycardia. ▪ Drug contains sodium metabisulfite, which may cause allergic-type reactions. ▪ Monitor serum electrolytes and watch for hypokalemia. ▪ ***I.V. use:*** Give by continuous I.V. infusion using infusion pump. Don't use bolus dose. Check BP and HR q 15 min until patient is stable. ▪ Drug is for short-term use. Patients should be converted to P.O. antihypertensive drugs within 48 hr.
fenoprofen calcium Nalfon, Nalfon 200 *Nonnarcotic analgesic, antipyretic, anti-inflammatory* Pregnancy Risk Category: B	*Rheumatoid arthritis; osteoarthritis* — **Adults:** 300 to 600 mg P.O. t.i.d. to q.i.d. Maximum 3.2 g q.d. *Mild to moderate pain* — **Adults:** 200 mg P.O. q 4 to 6 hr, p.r.n. *Fever* — **Adults:** single P.O. doses up to 400 mg.	▪ May lead to reversible renal impairment. ▪ Inform patient that full therapeutic effect for arthritis may take 2 to 4 wk. ▪ Instruct patient to take 30 min before or 2 hr after meals. If adverse GI reactions occur, may be taken with milk or meals. ▪ Tell patient to contact doctor immediately if

		GI bleeding occurs. ▪ Warn patient to avoid alcohol and aspirin.
fentanyl citrate Sublimaze **fentanyl transdermal system** Duragesic **fentanyl transmucosal** Fentanyl Oralet *Analgesic, adjunct to anesthesia, anesthetic* Pregnancy Risk Category: C Controlled Substance Schedule: II	*Preoperative* — **Adults:** 50 to 100 mcg I.M. 30 to 60 min before surgery. Or, 5 mcg/kg as Oralet unit, 20 to 40 min before need. *Adjunct to general anesthetic* — **Adults:** low-dose therapy, 2 mcg/kg I.V. Moderate-dose therapy, 2 to 20 mcg/kg I.V.; then 25 to 100 mcg I.V., p.r.n. High-dose therapy, 20 to 50 mcg/kg I.V.; then 25 mcg to half of initial loading dose I.V., p.r.n. *Adjunct to regional anesthesia* — **Adults:** 50 to 100 mcg I.M. or I.V. over 1 to 2 min, p.r.n. *Induction and maintenance of anesthesia* — **Children 2 to 12 yr:** 2 to 3 mcg/kg I.V. *Postoperative* — **Adults:** 50 to 100 mcg I.M. q 1 to 2 hr, p.r.n. *Management of chronic pain* — **Adults:** 1 transdermal system applied to upper torso skin area not irritated or irradiated. Start with 25-mcg/hr system; adjust dosage p.r.n. and as tolerated. May wear system for 72 hr; some may need applied q 48 hr.	▪ Monitor circulatory and respiratory status and urinary function carefully. ▪ Keep narcotic antagonist and resuscitation equipment available when giving I.V. ▪ Give before onset of intense pain. ▪ Periodically monitor postoperative vital signs and bladder function. ▪ Remove foil overwrap of Oralet just before giving. Have patient place Oralet in mouth and suck (not chew or swallow) it. ▪ Remove Oralet unit using handle after it's consumed, patient shows adequate effect, or patient shows signs of respiratory depression. Place any remaining portion in plastic overwrap and dispose as appropriate for Schedule II drugs or flush in toilet. ▪ Transdermal form not used for postoperative pain. ▪ Use lower doses in elderly patients. ▪ Less histamine release than with other opioid analgesics.
ferrous fumarate Femiron, Feostat, Fumasorb, Fumerin, Novofumar†, Palafer† *Hematinic* Pregnancy Risk Category: A	*Iron deficiency* — **Adults:** 50 to 100 mg elemental iron P.O. t.i.d. **Children:** 4 to 6 mg/kg/day elemental iron P.O. in 3 divided doses.	▪ GI upset may be related to dose. Between-meal doses preferable but can be given with some foods. ▪ Check for constipation; may turn stools black. ▪ Monitor Hgb, Hct, and *(continued)*

†Canadian ‡Australian

DRUG & CLASS	INDICATIONS & DOSAGES	NURSING CONSIDERATIONS
ferrous fumarate *(continued)*		reticulocyte count. ▪ Mix liquid preparation in juice or water and drink with straw to prevent staining of teeth. ▪ Avoid taking with antacids and milk products. ▪ Taking drug with orange juice increases absorption.
ferrous gluconate Fergon, Noroferroglut†, Simron *Hematinic* Pregnancy Risk Category: A	*Iron deficiency* — **Adults:** 50 to 100 mg elemental iron P.O. t.i.d. **Children:** 4 to 6 mg/kg/day elemental iron P.O. in 3 divided doses.	▪ GI upset may be related to dose. Between-meal doses preferable but can be given with some foods. ▪ Check for constipation; may turn stools black. ▪ Monitor Hgb, Hct, and reticulocyte count. ▪ Avoid taking with antacids and milk products. ▪ Taking drug with orange juice increases absorption.
ferrous sulfate Apo-Ferrous Sulfate†, Feosol, Mol-Iron **ferrous sulfate, dried** Feosol *Hematinic* Pregnancy Risk Category: A	*Iron deficiency* — **Adults:** 50 to 100 mg elemental iron P.O. t.i.d. **Children:** 4 to 6 mg/kg/day elemental iron P.O. in 3 divided doses.	▪ GI upset may be related to dose. Between-meal doses preferable but can be given with some foods. Enteric-coated products reduce GI upset but also decrease amount of iron absorbed. ▪ May turn stools black. ▪ Monitor Hgb, Hct, and reticulocyte count. ▪ Avoid taking with antacids and milk products.

fexofenadine Allegra *Antihistaminic* Pregnancy Risk Category: C	*Seasonal allergic rhinitis* — **Adults and children ≥ 12 yr:** 60 mg P.O. b.i.d., or 180 mg q.d. **Children ages 6 to 11:** 30 mg P.O. b.i.d. *Chronic idiopathic urticaria* — **Children ages 12 and older:** 60 mg P.O. b.i.d. **Children ages 6 to 11:** 30 mg P.O. b.i.d. ***Adjust-a-dose:*** In patients with renal impairment or on dialysis, give 60 mg P.O. q.d.	▪ Tell patient to avoid hazardous activities if drowsy. ▪ Instruct patient not to exceed prescribed dosage and to take only p.r.n.
filgrastim (granulocyte colony-stimulating factor; G-CSF) Neupogen *Colony-stimulating factor* Pregnancy Risk Category: C	*To decrease incidence of infection in patients with nonmyeloid malignant disease receiving myelosuppressive antineoplastic agents* — **Adults and children:** 5 mcg/kg/day I.V. or S.C. as 1 dose given ≥ 24 hr after cytotoxic chemotherapy. May increase by 5 mcg/kg for each chemotherapy cycle depending on duration and severity of nadir of absolute neutrophil count (ANC). *To decrease incidence of infection in patients with nonmyeloid malignant disease receiving myelosuppressive antineoplastic agents followed by bone marrow transplantation* — **Adults and children:** 10 mcg/kg/day I.V. or S.C. ≥ 24 hr after cytotoxic chemotherapy and bone marrow infusion. Adjust dosage according to neutrophil response. *Peripheral blood progenitor cell collection and therapy in cancer patient with severe chronic neutropenia* — 10 mcg/kg/day, starting 4 days before first leukapheresis and continuing until last leukaphoresis.	▪ Obtain baseline CBC and platelet count before therapy, then twice weekly during therapy. ▪ ***I.V. use:*** Dilute in 50 to 100 ml D_5W and give by intermittent infusion over 15 to 60 min or continuous infusion over 24 hr. If final concentration will be 2 to 15 mcg/ml, add albumin at concentration of 2 mg/ml (0.2%). ▪ Vials are for single-dose use. Discard unused portion. ▪ Refrigerate at 36° to 46° F (2° to 8° C). Don't freeze; avoid shaking. Store at room temperature up to 6 hr; discard after 6 hr. ▪ Transiently increased neutrophil count common 1 or 2 days after therapy starts. Give daily for up to 2 wk or until ANC returns to 10,000/mm^3 after expected chemotherapy-induced neutrophil nadir.

DRUG & CLASS	INDICATIONS & DOSAGES	NURSING CONSIDERATIONS
finasteride Propecia, Proscar *Androgen synthesis inhibitor* Pregnancy Risk Category: X	*Symptomatic BPH, reduction of risk of acute urinary retention and reduction of need for prostate surgery* — **Adults:** 5 mg (Proscar) P.O. q.d. *Male pattern hair loss in men* — **Adults:** 1 mg (Propecia) P.O. q.d.	▪ Monitor urine volume or urine flow. ▪ Evaluate sustained increases in serum prostate-specific antigen; could signal noncompliance. ▪ Women who are, or may be, pregnant should not handle crushed or broken tablets; this carries a potential risk to male fetus.
flecainide acetate Tambocor *Ventricular antiarrhythmic* Pregnancy Risk Category: C	*PSVT; paroxysmal atrial fibrillation, flutter in patients without structural heart disease; life-threatening ventricular arrhythmias* — **Adults:** For PSVT, 50 mg P.O. q 12 hr. May increase in increments of 50 mg b.i.d. q 4 days until efficacy achieved. Maximum 300 mg/day. For life-threatening ventricular arrhythmias, 100 mg P.O. q 12 hr. Increase in increments of 50 mg b.i.d. q 4 days until efficacy achieved. Maximum 400 mg q.d. ***Adjust-a-dose:*** In renally impaired patients, CrCl $\leq$ 35 ml/min, give 100 mg P.O. or 50 mg b.i.d.	▪ Monitor renally impaired patients for adverse cardiac effects and toxicity. ▪ Stress importance of taking drug exactly as prescribed. ▪ Instruct patient to report adverse reactions promptly and to limit fluid and sodium intake. ▪ Aggressive cardiac monitoring required when starting therapy. ▪ Drug can cause new or worsened supraventricular or ventricular arrhythmias.
fluconazole Diflucan *Antifungal* Pregnancy Risk Category: C	*Oropharyngeal and esophageal candidiasis* — **Adults:** 200 mg P.O. or I.V. on 1st day, then 100 mg q.d. Continue for $\geq$ 2 wk after symptoms resolve. **Children:** 6 mg/kg on 1st day, then 3 mg/kg for $\geq$ 2 wk. *Vaginal candidiasis* — **Adults:** 150 mg P.O. as single dose.	▪ ***I.V. use:*** Give by continuous infusion no faster than 200 mg/hr. Use infusion pump. To prevent air embolism, don't connect in series with other infusions. Don't add other drugs to solution. ▪ Periodically monitor liver function during prolonged therapy.

	Systemic candidiasis — **Adults:** up to 400 mg P.O. or I.V. q.d. Continue for ≥ 2 wk after symptoms resolve. *Cryptococcal meningitis* — **Adults:** 400 mg P.O. or I.V. on 1st day, then 200 to 400 mg q.d. Continue 10 to 12 wk after CSF cultures negative. ***Adjust-a-dose:*** In patients with CrCl < 50 ml/min, reduce dosage by ≥ 50%.	▪ If mild rash occurs, monitor closely. If lesions progress, stop drug and notify doctor. ▪ Incidence of adverse reactions greater in patients with HIV.
flucytosine (5-FC, 5-fluorocytosine) Ancobon, Ancotil† *Antifungal* Pregnancy Risk Category: C	*Severe fungal infections caused by susceptible strains of* Candida *and* Cryptococcus — **Adults:** 50 to 150 mg/kg q.d. P.O. divided q 6 hr. ***Adjust-a-dose:*** In patients with renal impairment, increase dosing intervals to q 12 to 48 hr, depending on CrCl.	▪ Obtain hematologic tests and renal and liver function studies. ▪ Give capsules over 15 min to reduce adverse GI reactions. ▪ Monitor fluid I&O; report marked change. ▪ Instruct patient to report adverse reactions promptly. ▪ Inform patient that therapeutic response may take weeks or months.
fludrocortisone acetate Florinef *Mineralocorticoid replacement therapy* Pregnancy Risk Category: C	*Adrenal insufficiency (partial replacement); salt-losing adrenogenital syndrome* — **Adults:** 0.1 to 0.2 mg P.O. q.d. Decrease to 0.05 mg q.d. if transient hypertension occurs. **Children:** 0.05 to 0.1 mg P.O. q.d. *Orthostatic hypotension, in diabetic and other patients* — **Adults:** 0.1 to 0.4 mg P.O. q.d.	▪ Use with cortisone or hydrocortisone in adrenal insufficiency. ▪ Monitor BP and serum electrolytes. ▪ Weigh patient daily; report sudden gain. ▪ Unless contraindicated, give low-sodium diet that's high in potassium and protein. ▪ Tell patient to report worsening symptoms, such as hypotension, weakness, cramping, and palpitations.

DRUG & CLASS	INDICATIONS & DOSAGES	NURSING CONSIDERATIONS
flumazenil Romazicon *Antidote* Pregnancy Risk Category: C	*Complete or partial reversal of sedative effects of benzodiazepines after anesthesia or short diagnostic procedures (conscious sedation)* — **Adults:** 0.2 mg I.V. over 15 sec. If desired level of consciousness not reached after 45 sec, repeat q 1 min until total dose of 1 mg given (initial dose plus 4 additional doses), p.r.n. Most patients respond after 0.6 to 1 mg. In case of resecation, may repeat after 20 min, but don't give > 1 mg at once or > 3 mg/hr. *Suspected benzodiazepine overdose* — **Adults:** 0.2 mg I.V. over 30 sec. If desired level of consciousness not reached after 30 sec, give 0.3 mg over 30 sec. If poor response, give 0.5 mg over 30 sec; repeat 0.5-mg doses, p.r.n., q 1 min until total dose of 3 mg given. Most patients respond to total doses of 1 to 3 mg; rarely, patients who respond partially after 3 mg may require additional doses, up to 5 mg total. If no response in 5 min after receiving 5 mg, sedation unlikely to be caused by benzodiazepines. In case of resedation, may repeat dose after 20 min, but don't give > 1 mg at once or > 3 mg/hr.	▪ ***I.V. use:*** Give by direct injection or dilute with compatible solution. Discard unused drug drawn into syringe or diluted within 24 hr. ▪ Give into I.V. line in large vein with free-flowing I.V. solution to minimize pain at injection site. Compatible solutions include D_5W, lactated Ringer's for injection, and 0.9% NaCl. ▪ ***ALERT*** Monitor patient closely for possible resedation after reversal of benzodiazepine effects (flumazenil's duration of action shorter than that of benzodiazepines). Duration of monitoring depends on drug being reversed. Monitor closely after long-acting benzodiazepines or after high doses of short-acting benzodiazepines. Severe resedation unlikely in patients showing no signs of resedation 2 hr after 1 mg flumazenil. ▪ Tell patient to avoid alcohol, CNS depressants, and OTC drugs for 24 hr. ▪ Patient won't recall information given after procedure; drug doesn't reverse amnesic effects of benzodiazepines.
flunisolide AeroBid, AeroBid-M, Nasalide (nasal inhalant)	*Persistent asthma* — **Adults:** 2 inhalations (500 mcg) b.i.d. Maximum total 2,000 mcg q.d. (8 inhalations/day). **Children 6 to 15 yr:**	▪ Warn patient that drug won't relieve emergency asthma attacks. ▪ If patient uses a bronchodilator, teach to

Anti-inflammatory, antiasthmatic Pregnancy Risk Category: C	2 inhalations (500 mcg) b.i.d. Don't exceed 4 inhalations/day. *Seasonal or perennial rhinitis* — **Adults:** 2 sprays (50 mcg) in each nostril b.i.d. Increase to 2 sprays in each nostril t.i.d., p.r.n. **Children 6 to 14 yr:** 1 spray in each nostril t.i.d. or 2 sprays in each nostril b.i.d.	use several min before flunisolide. ▪ Instruct patient to wait 1 min before repeating inhalation and to hold breath several seconds, to enhance drug action. ▪ Withdraw slowly after inhaling in patients who've received long-term P.O. corticosteroids. ▪ Advise patient to rinse mouth after P.O. inhalation to prevent thrush.
fluocinonide Lidex, Lidex-E, Topactin† *Anti-inflammatory* Pregnancy Risk Category: C	*Inflammation from corticosteroid-responsive dermatoses* — **Adults and children:** clean area; apply cream, gel, ointment, or topical solution sparingly b.i.d. to q.i.d.	▪ Gently wash skin before applying. Rub in gently, leaving thin coat. When treating hairy sites, part hair and apply directly to lesion. Don't apply near eyes, mucous membranes, or in ear canal. ▪ Notify doctor if skin infection, striae, atrophy, or fever develops. ▪ Watch for symptoms of systemic absorption with occlusive dressings, prolonged treatment, or extensive body-surface treatment. ▪ Continue treatment for several days after lesions clear.
fluorouracil (5-fluorouracil, 5-FU) Adrucil, Efudex, Fluoroplex *Antineoplastic* Pregnancy Risk Category: D (injection), X (topical)	*Colon, rectal, breast, stomach, pancreatic cancers* — **Adults:** 12 mg/kg I.V. q.d. for 4 days; if no toxicity, 6 mg/kg on days 6, 8, 10, and 12; then single weekly maintenance dose of 10 to 15 mg/kg I.V. begun after toxicity from 1st course subsides. Maximum single dose 800 mg/day. *Palliative treatment of advanced colorectal*	▪ Toxicity may be delayed for 1 to 3 wk. ▪ Use plastic I.V. containers to give continuous infusions. Don't refrigerate. Protect from sunlight. ▪ Monitor CBC and platelet counts. Watch for ecchymoses, petechiae, easy bruising, and anemia. Monitor I&O and renal and hepatic function test results. *(continued)*

†Canadian ‡Australian

DRUG & CLASS	INDICATIONS & DOSAGES	NURSING CONSIDERATIONS
fluorouracil *(continued)*	*cancer* — **Adults:** 425 mg/m² I.V. q.d. for 5 days. Give with 20 mg/m² leucovorin I.V. Repeat q 4 wk for 2 more courses; repeat q 4 to 5 wk if tolerated. *Multiple actinic (solar) keratoses; superficial basal cell carcinoma* — **Adults:** apply cream or topical solution b.i.d., usually for 2 to 6 wk.	▪ ***ALERT*** Ingestion and systemic absorption of topical form may cause serious adverse reactions. Application to large ulcerated areas may cause systemic toxicity. ▪ Watch for stomatitis or diarrhea. Discontinue and notify doctor if diarrhea occurs. ▪ Encourage diligent oral hygiene to prevent superinfection of denuded mucosa. ▪ Dosing varies with type of cancer; check hospital guidelines.
fluoxetine hydrochloride Prozac, Prozac 20‡, Sarafem *Antidepressant* Pregnancy Risk Category: B	*Depression; obsessive-compulsive disorder* — **Adults:** initially, 20 mg P.O. in morning; increase dosage per response. May give b.i.d. morning and noon. Gradually increase, p.r.n. and as tolerated, to 60 to 80 mg q.d. *Moderate to severe bulimia nervosa* — **Adults:** 60 mg/day P.O. in morning. *Premenstrual dysphoric disorder* — **Adults:** 20 mg P.O. q.d.	▪ Warn patient to avoid hazardous activities until CNS effects known. ▪ Tell patient to consult doctor before taking other medications and to avoid alcohol. ▪ Tell patient not to take in afternoon because of possible nervousness and insomnia. ▪ Tell patient to promptly report rash or hives, anxiety or nervousness, anorexia, or suspicion of pregnancy. ▪ Tell patient that nausea and vomiting are common but usually subside after 1st few weeks.
fluoxymesterone Android-F, Halotestin, Hysterone *Androgen replacement, antineoplastic* Pregnancy Risk Category: X	*Hypogonadism caused by testicular deficiency* — **Adults:** 5 to 20 mg P.O. q.d., in single dose or in 3 or 4 divided doses. *Delayed puberty* — **Males:** 2.5 to 20 mg q.d. *Palliation of breast cancer in women* — **Adults:** 10 to 40 mg P.O. q.d. in 3 or 4 divid-	▪ Instruct patient to take with food or meals if GI upset occurs. ▪ Tell women to stop drug and report menstrual irregularities or irregular bleeding. ▪ Urge women to report androgenic effects immediately.

Controlled Substance Schedule: III	ed doses. All dosages individualized and reduced to minimum when effect noted.	▪ Watch for hypoglycemia in diabetic patients; check blood glucose. ▪ If LFT results abnormal, notify doctor and stop drug.
fluphenazine decanoate Modecate†‡, Prolixin Decanoate **fluphenazine enanthate** Moditen Enanthate† Prolixin Enanthate **fluphenazine hydrochloride** Moditen HCl†, Permitil Concentrate, Prolixin, Prolixin Concentrate *Antipsychotic* Pregnancy Risk Category: C	*Psychotic disorders* — **Adults:** initially, 0.5 to 10 mg (hydrochloride) P.O. q.d. in divided doses q 6 to 8 hr; may increase cautiously to 20 mg. Maintenance: 1 to 5 mg P.O. q.d. For I.M. doses, give ⅓ to ½ of P.O. doses. Usual I.M. dose 1.25 mg. Give doses > 10 mg/day with caution. **Elderly:** 1 to 2.5 mg q.d. Or, 12.5 to 25 mg (decanoate or enanthate) I.M. or S.C. q 1 to 6 wk; maintenance: 25 to 100 mg, p.r.n.	▪ ***ALERT*** Watch for neuroleptic malignant syndrome. ▪ Monitor therapy with CBC, LFT, and renal function, bilirubin, and ophthalmic tests. ▪ Dilute liquid concentrate with water, fruit juice, milk, or semisolid food. ▪ Oral liquid and parenteral forms can cause contact dermatitis. ▪ Withhold dose and notify doctor if patient develops blood dyscrasia or persistent extrapyramidal reactions. ▪ Warn patient to avoid hazardous activities until CNS effects known. ▪ Tell patient of possible urine discoloration. ▪ Give maintenance dose h.s.
flurazepam hydrochloride Dalmane, Novoflupam, Somnal† *Sedative-hypnotic* Pregnancy Risk Category: X Controlled Substance Schedule: IV	*Insomnia* — **Adults:** 15 to 30 mg P.O. h.s. **Elderly:** 15 mg P.O. h.s.	▪ Check hepatic and renal function and CBC during long-term therapy. ▪ Assess mental status before initiating. ▪ Encourage patient to keep taking even if insomnia occurs on first night. ▪ Instruct patient to avoid alcohol use. ▪ Caution patient not to perform activities that require alertness or physical coordination. ▪ Prevent hoarding or self-overdosing.

†Canadian ‡Australian

DRUG & CLASS	INDICATIONS & DOSAGES	NURSING CONSIDERATIONS
flurbiprofen Ansaid, Apo-Flurbiprofen†, Froben†, Froben SR† *Antarthritic* Pregnancy Risk Category: B	*Rheumatoid arthritis; osteoarthritis* — **Adults:** 200 to 300 mg P.O. q d., divided b.i.d., t.i.d., or q.i.d. Where available, patients on 200 mg q.d. may take one 200-mg extended-release capsule P.O. q.d., in evening after food. **Elderly:** may need a lower dose.	▪ Tell patient to take with food, milk, or antacid if GI upset occurs. ▪ Teach patient signs and symptoms of GI bleeding and tell him to contact doctor immediately if they occur. ▪ Advise patient to avoid alcohol and aspirin. ▪ Tell patient taking extended-release capsules to swallow them whole. ▪ Monitor patients with end-stage renal disease for CNS adverse effects.
flutamide Euflex†, Eulexin *Antineoplastic* Pregnancy Risk Category: D	*Metastatic prostate cancer (stage B_2, C, D_2) in combination with luteinizing hormone–releasing hormone analogues such as leuprolide acetate* — **Adults:** 250 mg P.O. q 8 hr.	▪ Monitor LFTs and CBC periodically. ▪ Drug should be started 8 weeks before and continued during radiation therapy.
fluticasone propionate (inhalation) Flovent Inhalation Aerosol, Flovent Rotadisk *Anti-inflammatory* Pregnancy Risk Category: C	*Maintenance therapy to prevent asthma; treatment of chronic asthma with oral corticosteroid* — ***Flovent Inhalation Aerosol:*** **Adults and children ≥ 12 yr:** in those previously taking bronchodilators alone, initially, inhaled dose of 88 mcg b.i.d. to maximum of 440 mcg b.i.d. **Patients previously taking inhaled corticosteroids:** initially, inhaled dose of 88 to 220 mcg b.i.d. to maximum of 440 mcg b.i.d. **Patients previously taking oral corticosteroids:** inhaled dose of 880 mcg b.i.d. ***Flovent Rotadisk:*** **Adults and adolescents:** in patients previously taking bronchodilators alone, initially, inhaled dose	▪ ***ALERT*** If bronchospasm occurs after dosing with fluticasone inhalation aerosol, treat immediately with a fast-acting inhaled bronchodilator. ▪ Observe for evidence of systemic corticosteroid effects. ▪ Monitor patient, especially postoperatively or during stress, for inadequate adrenal response. ▪ During withdrawal from P.O. corticosteroids, patients may have symptoms of systemically active corticosteroid withdrawal (joint or muscular pain, lassitude, and depression) despite maintenance or even im-

	of 100 mcg b.i.d. up to 500 mcg b.i.d. **Patients previously taking inhaled corticosteroids:** initially, inhaled dose of 100 to 250 mcg b.i.d., up to 500 mcg b.i.d. **Patients previously taking P.O. corticosteroids:** inhaled dose of 1,000 mcg b.i.d. **Children 4 to 11 yr:** for patients previously on bronchodilators alone or on inhaled corticosteroids, initially, inhaled dose of 50 mcg b.i.d., up to 100 mcg b.i.d.	provement of respiratory function. ▪ For patients starting therapy ,who are also receiving P.O. corticosteroids, reduce dose of prednisone to ≤ 2.5 mg/day on weekly basis, beginning after ≥ 1 wk of therapy with fluticasone. ▪ Not for relief of acute bronchospasm.
fluticasone propionate (nasal) Flonase *Topical anti-inflammatory* Pregnancy Risk Category: C	*Seasonal and perennial allergic rhinitis* — **Adults:** initially, 2 sprays (50 mcg each spray) per nostril q.d. Or, 1 spray per nostril b.i.d. After several days, may reduce dose to 1 spray per nostril q.d. **Children ≥ 12 yr:** initially, 1 spray (50 mcg) per nostril q.d. If no response or symptoms severe, increase to 2 sprays per nostril. Depending on response, may decrease dose to 1 spray per nostril q.d. Maximum daily dose, 2 sprays per nostril.	▪ Don't use after recent nasal septal ulcers, nasal surgery, or nasal trauma until healing occurs. ▪ Monitor for signs of immediate hypersensitivity reactions or contact dermatitis after giving intranasally. ▪ Drug effective only with regular use. ▪ Tell patient to notify doctor if exposed to chickenpox or measles. ▪ Instruct patient in proper use of nasal spray.
fluticasone propionate (topical) Cutivate *Topical anti-inflammatory* Pregnancy Risk Category: C	*Inflammatory and pruritic manifestations from corticosteroid-responsive dermatoses* — **Adults:** apply sparingly to affected area b.i.d.; rub in quickly and completely. **Children ≥ 3 mo:** apply sparingly to affected area once daily to b.i.d.; rub in quickly and completely.	▪ Don't mix with other bases or vehicles; may affect potency. ▪ One-time coverage of adult body requires 12 to 26 g. Don't use > 50 g q wk. ▪ Discontinue if local irritation or systemic infection, absorption, or hypersensitivity occurs. ▪ Don't apply in diaper area. ▪ Don't use with occlusive dressing.

DRUG & CLASS	INDICATIONS & DOSAGES	NURSING CONSIDERATIONS
fluvastatin sodium Lescol *Cholesterol-lowering agent, antilipemic* Pregnancy Risk Category: X	*Reduction of LDL and total cholesterol levels in patients with primary hypercholesterolemia (types IIa and IIb)* — **Adults:** initially, 20 mg P.O. h.s. Increase to 40 mg q.d., p.r.n. *Reduction of triglycerides and apolipoprotein B levels in patients with primary hypercholesterolemia and mixed dyslipidemia with inadequate response to dietary restriction and other nonpharmacologic measures* — **Adults:** initially, 20 to 40 mg P.O. h.s., increased p.r.n. up to 80 mg q.d. in divided doses.	▪ Teach patient about proper dietary management, weight control, and exercise. ▪ Initiate only after diet and other nonpharmacologic measures fail. ▪ Get LFT results when therapy starts and periodically thereafter. ▪ Watch for signs of myositis. ▪ Tell patient to avoid alcohol and to stop drug and notify doctor if pregnancy occurs.
fluvoxamine maleate Luvox *Anticompulsive agent* Pregnancy Risk Category: C	*Obsessive-compulsive disorder* — **Adults:** initially, 50 mg P.O. q.d. h.s., increased in 50-mg increments q 4 to 7 days until maximum benefit achieved. Maximum 300 mg q.d. Give total daily doses of > 100 mg in 2 divided doses.	▪ Record mood changes. Watch for suicidal tendencies; provide minimal drug supply. ▪ Warn patient not to engage in hazardous activities until CNS effects known. ▪ Tell patient to notify doctor if allergic reaction occurs. ▪ Advise patient not to discontinue until directed by doctor.
folic acid Folvite, Novofolacid† *Vitamin supplement* Pregnancy Risk Category: A	*Recommended daily allowance (RDA)* — **Breast-feeding women:** 260 to 280 mcg. **Pregnant women:** 400 mcg. **Adolescent and adult women:** 150 to 180 mcg. **Adolescent and adult men:** 150 to 200 mcg. **Children 7 to 10 yr:** 100 mcg. **Children 4 to 6 yr:** 75 mcg. **Birth to 3 yr:** 25 to 50 mcg.	▪ Don't mix with other medications in same syringe when giving I.M. ▪ May need to give parenterally in patients with small-bowel resections and intestinal malabsorption. ▪ Protect from light and heat; store at room temperature.

Megaloblastic or macrocytic anemia from deficiency of folic acid or other nutrient, hepatic disease, alcoholism, intestinal obstruction, excessive hemolysis — **Adults and children > 4 yr:** 0.4 mg to 1 mg P.O., S.C., or I.M. q.d. **Children < 4 yr:** up to 0.3 mg P.O., S.C., or I.M. q.d. **Pregnant and breast-feeding women:** 0.8 mg P.O., S.C., or I.M. q.d.

Prevention of megaloblastic anemia during pregnancy to prevent fetal damage — **Adults:** ≤ 1 mg P.O., S.C., or I.M. q.d. during pregnancy.

- Monitor CBC to measure drug effectiveness.
- Patients undergoing renal dialysis are at risk for folate deficiency.
- Many drugs, such as P.O. contraceptives and alcohol, can cause folic acid deficiencies.
- Teach patient about dietary sources of folic acid, such as yeast, whole grains, leafy vegetables, beans, nuts, and fruit.
- Inform patient that overcooking and canning destroy folate.
- Tell patient to take only under medical supervision.
- After correcting anemia caused by folic acid deficiency, teach proper diet and give RDA supplements to prevent recurrence.

---

fomivirsen sodium
Vitravene
Antiviral (ophthalmic)
Pregnancy Risk Category: C

Local treatment of CMV retinitis in patients with AIDS who are intolerant of or have a contraindication to other treatment or who didn't respond well enough to previous treatment — **Adults:** induction dose 330 mcg (0.05 ml) by intravitreal injection every other wk for 2 doses. Subsequent maintenance dose 330 mcg (0.05 ml) by intravitreal injection once q 4 wk after induction.

- For use by intravitreal injection only.
- Provides localized therapy only to treated eye. Monitor patient for extraocular CMV disease or disease in other eye.
- Ocular inflammation (uveitis) may occur during induction dosing.
- Monitor light perception and optic nerve head perfusion postinjection.
- Monitor for increased IOP.

DRUG & CLASS	INDICATIONS & DOSAGES	NURSING CONSIDERATIONS
foscarnet sodium (phosphonoformic acid) Foscavir *Antiviral* Pregnancy Risk Category: C	*CMV retinitis in patients with AIDS* — **Adults:** initially, 60 mg/kg I.V. as induction treatment in patients with normal renal function. Give I.V. over 1 hr q 8 hr for 2 to 3 wk, depending on clinical response. Follow with maintenance infusion of 90 to 120 mg/kg q.d., given over 2 hr. *Mucocutaneous acyclovir-resistant herpes simplex virus infection* — **Adults:** 40 mg/kg I.V. Give I.V. infusion over 1 hr q 8 to 12 hr for 2 to 3 wk. ***Adjust-a-dose:*** Reduce dosage in renally impaired patients.	▪ ***I.V. use:*** Use infusion pump. To minimize renal toxicity, ensure adequate hydration before and during infusion. ▪ Can alter serum electrolytes; monitor levels. Assess for tetany and seizures associated with abnormal electrolyte levels. ▪ Monitor Hgb and Hct. ▪ Advise patient to report perioral tingling, numbness in extremities, and paresthesia. ▪ Instruct patient to alert nurse if discomfort occurs at I.V. insertion site.
fosinopril sodium Monopril *Antihypertensive* Pregnancy Risk Category: C (D in 2nd and 3rd trimesters)	*Hypertension* — **Adults:** initially, 10 mg P.O. q.d. Adjusted based on BP response at peak and trough levels. Usual dose 20 to 40 mg, up to 80 mg q.d. May be divided. *Heart failure* — **Adults:** initially, 10 mg P.O. q.d. Increase over several wk, up to 40 mg P.O. q.d.	▪ Monitor potassium intake and serum potassium and electrolyte levels. ▪ Monitor CBC with differential. ▪ Monitor BP for effect. ▪ Advise patient to report signs or symptoms of infection. ▪ Instruct patient to use caution in hot weather and during exercise. ▪ Contraindicated in renal artery stenosis.
fosphenytoin sodium Cerebyx *Anticonvulsant* Pregnancy Risk Category: D	*Status epilepticus* — **Adults:** 15 to 20 mg phenytoin sodium equivalent (PE)/kg I.V. at 100 to 150 mg PE/min as loading dose; then 4 to 6 mg PE/kg/day I.V. as maintenance dose. (May use phenytoin instead of fos-	▪ Drug should be prescribed and dispensed in PE units. Don't adjust recommended doses when substituting fosphenytoin for phenytoin, and vice versa. ▪ Before I.V. infusion, dilute in 5% dextrose

phenytoin as maintenance, using appropriate dose.)

Prevention and treatment of seizures during neurosurgery — **Adults:** loading dose 10 to 20 mg PE/kg I.M. or I.V. at infusion rate ≤ 150 mg PE/min. Maintenance dose: 4 to 6 mg PE/kg/day I.V.

Short-term substitution for P.O. phenytoin — **Adults:** same total daily dose equivalent as P.O. phenytoin sodium therapy; single daily dose I.M. or I.V. at infusion rate ≤ 150 mg PE/min. May require more frequent dosing.

or 0.9% NaCl to concentration 1.5 to 25 mg PE/ml.

- Monitor ECG, BP, and respirations.
- Severe CV complications most common in elderly or gravely ill patients.
- If rash appears, stop drug and notify doctor.
- ***ALERT*** Abrupt withdrawal may trigger status epilepticus.
- Warn patient that sensory disturbances may occur with I.V. use.
- Avoid use in patients with end-stage renal disease.

---

furosemide (frusemide‡)

Apo-Furosemide†, Lasix, Myrosemide, Novosemide†, Urex‡

Diuretic, antihypertensive

Pregnancy Risk Category: C

Acute pulmonary edema — **Adults:** 40 mg I.V. injected over 1 to 2 min; then 80 mg I.V. in 1 to 1½ hr, p.r.n.

Edema — **Adults:** 20 to 80 mg P.O. q.d. in morning, 2nd dose in 6 to 8 hr; carefully titrate up to 600 mg q.d., if needed. Or, 20 to 40 mg I.M. or I.V., increased by 20 mg q 2 hr until desired response achieved. Give I.V. dose over 1 to 2 min. **Infants and children:** 2 mg/kg P.O. q.d., increased by 1 to 2 mg/kg in 6 to 8 hr, if needed; carefully titrate to 6 mg/kg q.d., if needed.

Hypertension — **Adults:** 40 mg P.O. b.i.d. Adjust dosage according to response.

- ***I.V. use:*** Give by direct injection over 1 to 2 min. Or, dilute with D_5W, 0.9% NaCl, or lactated Ringer's solution, and infuse no faster than 4 mg/min to avoid ototoxicity. Use prepared infusion solution within 24 hr.
- Monitor weight, BP, and HR routinely.
- If oliguria or azotemia develops or worsens, may need to discontinue.
- Monitor I&O, and serum electrolyte, BUN, blood uric acid, and CO_2 levels frequently.
- Monitor potassium intake.
- May be poorly absorbed P.O. in severe heart failure. May need to be given I.V. even if patient receiving other oral medications.

DRUG & CLASS	INDICATIONS & DOSAGES	NURSING CONSIDERATIONS
gabapentin Neurontin *Anticonvulsant* Pregnancy Risk Category: C	*Adjunct treatment of partial seizures with and without secondary generalization in adults with epilepsy* — **Adults**: initially, 300 mg P.O. t.i.d. Increase p.r.n. and as tolerated to 1,800 mg q.d. in 3 divided doses. Doses $\leq$ 3,600 mg q.d. have been well tolerated. ***Adjust-a-dose:*** In patients with renal failure, adjust dose based on CrCl.	▪ Give 1st dose h.s. to minimize drowsiness, dizziness, fatigue, and ataxia. ▪ Stop or substitute alternative drug gradually, over $\geq$ 1 wk. ▪ ***ALERT*** Don't suddenly withdraw other anticonvulsants. ▪ Warn patient to avoid driving and operating heavy machinery until CNS effects known.
ganciclovir Cytovene *Antiviral* Pregnancy Risk Category: C	*CMV retinitis in immunocompromised patients, including those with AIDS and normal renal function* — **Adults:** induction: 5 mg/kg I.V. q 12 hr for 14 to 21 days; maintenance: 5 mg/kg I.V. q.d. for 7 days each wk, or 6 mg/kg q.d. for 5 days each wk. Or, 1,000 mg P.O. t.i.d. with food; or 500 mg P.O. q 3 hr while awake (6 times q.d.). *Prevention of CMV disease in advanced HIV infection and normal renal function* — **Adults:** 1,000 mg P.O. t.i.d. with food. *Prevention of CMV disease in transplant recipients with normal renal function* — **Adults:** 5 mg/kg I.V. q 12 hr for 1 to 2 wk, then 5 mg/kg q.d. for 7 days; or 6 mg/kg q.d. for 5 days q wk. ***Adjust-a-dose:*** Adjust dosage in patients with CrCl < 70 ml/min.	▪ ***I.V. use:*** Give infusion at constant rate over at least 1 hr. Too-rapid infusions increase toxicity. Use infusion pump. Don't give as bolus. ▪ Solution alkaline; use caution when preparing. ▪ Don't give S.C. or I.M. ▪ Obtain neutrophil and platelet counts q 2 days during twice-daily dosing and at least weekly thereafter. ▪ Explain importance of adequate hydration during therapy. ▪ Instruct patient to report adverse reactions promptly.

gatifloxacin
Tequin
Antibiotic
Pregnancy Risk Category: C

Acute bacterial exacerbation of chronic bronchitis caused by Streptococcus pneumoniae, Haemophilus influenzae, H. parainfluenzae, Moraxella catarrhalis, *or* Staphylococcus aureus; *complicated urinary tract infection caused by* Escherichia coli, Klebsiella pneumoniae, *or* Proteus mirabilis; *acute pyelonephritis caused by* E. coli — **Adults:** 400 mg I.V. or P.O. daily for 7 to 10 days.

Acute sinusitis caused by S. pneumoniae *or* H. influenzae — **Adults:** 400 mg I.V. or P.O. daily for 10 days.

Community-acquired pneumonia caused by S. pneumoniae, H. influenzae, H. parainfluenzae, M. catarrhalis, S. aureus, Mycoplasma pneumoniae, Chlamydia pneumoniae, *or* Legionella pneumophila — **Adults:** 400 mg I.V. or P.O. daily for 1 to 2 wk.

Adjust-a-dose: For patients with CrCl < 40 ml/min and those on hemodialysis or continuous peritoneal dialysis, initial dose is 400 mg I.V. or P.O. daily, and subsequent doses are 200 mg I.V. or P.O. daily. For patients on hemodialysis, give after hemodialysis session is complete.

Uncomplicated urethral gonorrhea in men and cervical gonorrhea or acute uncomplicated rectal infection in women caused by Neisseria gonorrhoeae — **Adults:** 400 mg P.O. as single dose daily.

- Monitor blood glucose in patients with diabetes.
- Monitor patients concurrently on digoxin for signs and symptoms of digoxin toxicity.
- Stop drug if patient has seizures, increased intracranial pressure, psychosis, or CNS stimulation leading to tremors, restlessness, light-headedness, confusion, hallucinations, paranoia, depression, nightmares, and insomnia.
- Monitor kidney function in patients with renal insufficiency.
- ***I.V. use:*** Dilute drug in single-use vials with D_5W or normal saline to a final concentration of 2 mg/ml before administration. Diluted solutions are stable for 14 days at room temperature or refrigerated. Frozen solutions, except 5% sodium bicarbonate, are stable for up to 6 mo. Thaw at room temperature. Solutions are stable for 2 wk after being removed from the freezer when stored at room temperature or under refrigeration. Don't mix with other drugs. Infuse over 60 min.

(continued)

DRUG & CLASS	INDICATIONS & DOSAGES	NURSING CONSIDERATIONS
gatifloxacin *(continued)*	*Uncomplicated urinary tract infection caused by* E. coli, K. pneumoniae, *or* P. mirabilis — **Adults:** 400 mg I.V. or P.O. as single dose or 200 mg I.V. or P.O. daily for 3 days.	
gemcitabine hydrochloride Gemzar *Antineoplastic* Pregnancy Risk Category: D	*Locally advanced or metastatic adenocarcinoma of pancreas and patients treated previously with fluorouracil* — **Adults:** 1,000 mg/m^2 I.V. over 30 min q wk ≤ 7 wk, unless toxicity develops. ***Adjust-a-dose:*** If absolute granulocyte count (AGC) 500/mm^3 to 999/mm^3 or platelet count 50,000/mm^3 to 9,999/mm^3, give 75% of dose. Withhold dose if AGC < 500/mm^3 or platelet count < 50,000/mm^3. Follow treatment course of 7 wk with 1 wk rest. Next dosage cycles consist of 1 infusion q wk for 3 or 4 consecutive wk. Adjust dosage for next cycles based on AGC and platelet count nadirs and degree of nonhematologic toxicity.	▪ Monitor patients before each dose with CBC (including differential) and platelet count. If bone marrow suppression, adjust therapy. Give full dose if AGC ≥ 1,000/mm^3 and platelet count ≥ 100,000/mm^3. ▪ Obtain baseline and periodic renal and hepatic lab test results. ▪ ***I.V. use:*** Don't reconstitute at concentration > 40 mg/ml. May further dilute resulting concentration with 0.9% NaCl injection, to as low as 0.1 mg/ml, p.r.n. Solution should be clear to light straw-colored and free from particulates. Stable for 24 hr at room temperature. Don't refrigerate reconstituted drug. ▪ Prolonging infusion time > 60 min or giving drug more frequently than q wk may increase toxicity. ▪ Careful hematologic monitoring required, especially of neutrophil and platelet counts. ▪ Monitor closely. Expect dosage modification according to toxicity and degree of myelosuppression. Age, gender, and renal impairment may predispose to toxicity.

gemfibrozil Lopid *Antilipemic* Pregnancy Risk Category: C	*Types IV and V hyperlipidemia unresponsive to diet and other drugs; reduction of CAD risk in patients with type IIb hyperlipidemia who can't tolerate or are refractory to bile acid sequestrants or niacin* — **Adults:** 1,200 mg P.O. q.d. in 2 divided doses, 30 min before morning and evening meals.	▪ Instruct patient to take 30 min before breakfast and dinner. ▪ Teach patient proper dietary management. ▪ Advise patient to avoid hazardous activities until CNS effects known. ▪ Tell patient to report signs of bile duct obstruction. ▪ Instruct patient to avoid alcohol.
gemtuzumab ozogamicin Mylotarg *Cancer chemotherapeutic* Pregnancy Risk Category: D	*CD33-positive acute myeloid leukemia in first relapse and who aren't considered candidates for cytotoxic chemotherapy* — **Adults ≥ 60 yr:** 9 mg/m^2 I.V. over 2 hr q 14 days for a total of 2 doses. Premedicate with diphenhydramine 50 mg P.O. and acetaminophen 650 to 1,000 mg P.O. 1 hr before infusion.	▪ A symptom complex of chills, fever, hypotension, hypertension, hyperglycemia, hypoxia, and dyspnea may occur during the first 24 hr after drug is given. ▪ ***ALERT*** Severe myelosuppression occurs in all patients given the recommended dose of this drug. Careful hematologic monitoring is required. ▪ ***ALERT*** Drug must be protected from direct and indirect sunlight and unshielded fluorescent light when the infusion is prepared and given. ▪ ***ALERT*** Don't give as an I.V. push or bolus. ▪ Give in 100 ml of sodium chloride injection. Place the 100-ml I.V. bag into an ultraviolet (UV)–protectant bag. The resulting drug solution in the I.V. bag should be used immediately. ▪ A separate I.V. line equipped with a low protein–binding 1.2-micron *(continued)*

DRUG & CLASS	INDICATIONS & DOSAGES	NURSING CONSIDERATIONS
gemtuzumab ozogamicin *(continued)*		terminal filter must be used to give the drug, which may be infused by central or peripheral line.
gentamicin sulfate (ophthalmic) Garamycin Ophthalmic, Genoptic, Gentacidin, Gentak, Ocu-Mycin *Ophthalmic antibiotic* Pregnancy Risk Category: C	*External ocular infections from susceptible organisms, especially* P. aeruginosa, Proteus, K. pneumoniae, E. coli, *other gram-negative organisms* — **Adults and children:** instill 1 to 2 drops in eye q 4 hr. In severe infections, up to 2 drops q hr. Or, apply ointment to lower conjunctival sac b.i.d. or t.i.d.	▪ Have culture taken before giving drug. Therapy may begin before results known. ▪ Apply light pressure on lacrimal sac for 1 min after instilling drops. ▪ If ophthalmic form given with systemic form, monitor serum gentamicin levels. ▪ Solution not for injection into conjunctiva or anterior chamber of eye. ▪ Ointment may cause blurred vision.
gentamicin sulfate (systemic) Cidomycin†, Garamycin, Gentamicin Sulfate ADD-Vantage, Jenamicin *Antibiotic* Pregnancy Risk Category: NR	*Serious infections from susceptible organisms* — **Adults:** 3 mg/kg/day in divided doses I.M. or I.V. infusion q 8 hr. For life-threatening infections, up to 5 mg/kg/day in 3 to 4 divided doses; reduce to 3 mg/kg/day as soon as indicated. **Children:** 6 to 7.5 mg/kg/day in divided doses q 8 hr I.M. or by I.V. infusion. **Neonates > 1 wk or infants:** 7.5 mg/kg/day in divided doses q 8 hr. *Meningitis* — **Adults:** systemic therapy as above; or 4 to 8 mg intrathecally q.d. **Children and infants > 3 mo:** systemic therapy as above; or 1 to 2 mg intrathecally q.d. *Endocarditis prophylaxis for GI or GU procedure or surgery* — **Adults:** 1.5 mg/kg I.M.	▪ Evaluate hearing before and during therapy. Notify doctor of tinnitus, vertigo, or hearing loss. ▪ ***I.V. use:*** For intermittent I.V. infusion, dilute with 50 to 200 ml D_5W or 0.9% NaCl injection and infuse over 30 min to 2 hr. After infusion, flush line with 0.9% NaCl or D_5W. ▪ Obtain blood for peak drug level 1 hr after I.M. injection and 30 min to 1 hr after I.V. infusion; for trough levels, draw blood just before next dose. Don't collect blood in heparinized tube. ▪ Monitor renal function (output, specific gravity, urinalysis, BUN, creatinine, and

	or I.V. 30 min before procedure or surgery. Maximum 80 mg. **Children:** 2 mg/kg I.M. or I.V. 30 min before procedure or surgery. Maximum 80 mg. After 8 hr, give half of initial dose.	CrCl). Notify doctor of signs of decreasing renal function. ▪ Give drug with ampicillin (vancomycin for patients allergic to penicillin) to prevent endocarditis. ▪ Trough levels > 2 mg/dl indicate nephrotoxicity and ototoxicity.
gentamicin sulfate (topical) Garamycin, G-Myticin *Topical antibiotic* Pregnancy Risk Category: C	*Treatment and prophylaxis of superficial skin infections from susceptible bacteria* — **Adults and children > 1 yr:** rub in small amount gently t.i.d. or q.i.d., with or without gauze dressing.	▪ Clean affected area before applying. Remove crusts before application for impetigo contagiosa. ▪ Prolonged use may cause overgrowth of nonsusceptible organisms.
glatiramer acetate for injection (formerly copolymer 1) Copaxone *Immune response modifier* Pregnancy Risk Category: B	*To reduce frequency of relapses in patients with relapsing-remitting multiple sclerosis* — **Adults:** 20 mg S.C. q.d.	▪ Use diluent provided. Gently swirl lyophilized material and diluent and allow to stand at room temperature until completely dissolved (about 5 min). ▪ Use immediately; drug does not contain preservatives. Discard unused drug. ▪ Immediate postinjection, transient and self-limiting reactions (flushing, chest pain, palpitations, anxiety, dyspnea, throat constriction, urticaria) may occur. ▪ Teach patient proper technique for self-injection.
glimepiride Amaryl *Antidiabetic* Pregnancy Risk Category: C	*Adjunct to diet and exercise to lower blood glucose in type 2 diabetes mellitus* — **Adults:** initially, 1 to 2 mg P.O. q.d. with breakfast. After reaching 2 mg, increase dosage in increments up to 2 mg q 1 to 2 wk,	▪ Monitor fasting blood glucose level periodically to determine therapeutic response. Monitor glycosylated Hgb, usually q 3 to 6 mo, to assess long-term glycemic control. *(continued)*

DRUG & CLASS	INDICATIONS & DOSAGES	NURSING CONSIDERATIONS
glimepiride *(continued)*	based on blood glucose response; maintenance 1 to 4 mg P.O. q.d., maximum 8 mg/day. *Adjunct to insulin therapy in type 2 diabetes mellitus combined with P.O. hypoglycemic agents* — **Adults:** 8 mg P.O. q.d. with breakfast; used with low-dose insulin. *Adjunct to metformin therapy in patients with type 2 diabetes mellitus whose hyperglycemia can't be managed by diet, exercise, and glimepiride or metformin alone* — **Adults:** 8 mg P.O. q.d. with 1st meal, with metformin. Adjust dosages based on patient's blood glucose response to determine minimum effective dosage of each drug. ***Adjust-a-dose:*** In renally impaired patients, give initial dose 1 mg P.O. q.d. with 1st meal. Adjust upward, p.r.n.	▪ Advise patient that drug relieves symptoms but doesn't cure diabetes. Explain potential risks and advantages of drug and other treatment methods. ▪ Stress importance of adhering to diet, exercise, and therapeutic regimen. Tell patient and family how and when to perform blood glucose self-monitoring, and teach them signs and symptoms of hyperglycemia and hypoglycemia. ▪ Hypoglycemia is most common complication. ▪ Drug contraindicated in diabetic ketoacidosis.
glipizide Glucotrol, Glucotrol XL, Minidiab‡ *Antidiabetic* Pregnancy Risk Category: C	*Adjunct to diet to lower blood glucose in type 2 diabetes mellitus* — **Adults:** usually 5 mg P.O. q.d. Maintenance: 10 to 15 mg. Maximum 40 mg q.d. Divide doses above 15 mg, except for extended-release tablets, give 5 mg P.O. q.d. Adjust in 5-mg increments q 3 mo for glycemic control. Maximum 20 mg/day. *To replace insulin therapy* — **Adults:** if insulin dosage > 20 units q.d., start at usual	▪ Give about 30 min before meals but give extended-release tablets with breakfast. ▪ During increased stress, patient may need insulin therapy. ▪ Patients switching from insulin therapy to P.O. antidiabetic require blood glucose monitoring at least t.i.d. before meals. ▪ Instruct patient about disease and importance of adhering to diet and therapeutic regimen. Tell how and when to perform

	dose plus 50% of insulin. If insulin dose < 20 units, may stop insulin on initiating glipizide. ***Adjust-a-dose:*** For liver disease, initial dose 2.5 mg P.O. q.d. Extended-release tablets: initially, 5 mg P.O. q.d.; adjust cautiously.	blood glucose self-monitoring, and teach them signs and symptoms of hypoglycemia and hyperglycemia.
glucagon *Antidiabetic, diagnostic agent* Pregnancy Risk Category: B	*Hypoglycemia* — **Adults and children > 20 kg (44 lb):** 0.5 to 1 mg S.C., I.M., or I.V.; may repeat q 5 to 20 min for 2 doses, p.r.n. For patient in deep coma, also give glucose 10% to 50% I.V. When response occurs, give more carbohydrate immediately. **Children ≤ 20 kg:** 0.025 mg S.C., I.M., or I.V.; may repeat within 25 min. For patient in deep coma, also give glucose 10% to 50% I.V. When response occurs, give more carbohydrate immediately. *Note:* May repeat in 15 min p.r.n. Give I.V. glucose if patient doesn't respond. When patient responds, give supplemental carbohydrate immediately. *Diagnostic aid for radiologic examination* — **Adults:** 0.25 to 2 mg I.V. or I.M. before radiologic procedure.	▪ ***I.V. use:*** Use only diluent supplied by manufacturer when preparing doses of ≤ 2 mg. For larger doses, dilute with sterile water for injection. ▪ For I.V. drip infusion, use dextrose solution. ▪ Arouse patient from coma as quickly as possible and give additional carbohydrates orally to prevent secondary hypoglycemic reactions. ▪ Unstable hypoglycemic diabetics may not respond to glucagon; give dextrose I.V. instead. ▪ Teach how to give drug properly and to recognize hypoglycemia.
glyburide (glibenclamide) DiaBeta, Glynase PresTab, Micronase *Antidiabetic* Pregnancy Risk Category: C	*Adjunct to diet to lower blood glucose in type 2 diabetes* — **Adults:** initially, 2.5 to 5 mg regular tablets P.O. q.d. with breakfast. In debilitated, malnourished, or elderly patients, start at 1.25 mg q.d. Usual maintenance: 1.25 to 20 mg q.d. as single or	▪ Micronized glyburide not bioequivalent to regular glyburide tablets. ▪ Instruct patient about nature of disease, importance of adhering to diet, therapeutic regimen, weight reduction, exercise, and personal hygiene programs, *(continued)*

DRUG & CLASS	INDICATIONS & DOSAGES	NURSING CONSIDERATIONS
glyburide *(continued)*	divided dose or micronized formulation. Initial dose 1.5 to 3 mg/day. In sensitive patients, start at 0.75 mg/day. Usual maintenance: 0.75 to 12 mg/day. Patients receiving > 6 mg/day may respond better to b.i.d. dosing. *To replace insulin therapy* — **Adults:** If insulin dose > 40 U/day, may start at 5 mg/day plus 50% of insulin dose; if < 20 U/day, give 2.5 to 5 mg/day; if 20 to 40 U/day, give 5 mg/day. In all patients, substitute glyburide and stop insulin abruptly. For micronized tablets, if insulin dose > 40 U/day, give 3 mg P.O. with 50% reduction in insulin; if 20 to 40 U/day, give 3 mg P.O. as single daily dose; if < 20 U/day, give 1.5 to 3 mg/day as single dose. ***Adjust-a-dose:*** In patients more sensitive to antidiabetic agents or those with adrenal or pituitary insufficiency, start at 1.25 mg q.d.	and avoiding infection. Explain how and when to perform blood glucose self-monitoring and teach how to recognize and intervene for hypoglycemia and hyperglycemia. ▪ Instruct patient to report hypoglycemic episodes to doctor immediately. ▪ Teach patient to carry candy or other simple sugars to treat mild hypoglycemic episodes. ▪ Patients switching from insulin to P.O. antidiabetics need blood glucose monitoring at least t.i.d. before meals. May need hospitalization during transition. ▪ Caution patient not to change dosage without doctor's consent and to report abnormal blood or urine glucose results. ▪ Don't give the drug if CrCl < 50 ml/min.
glycerin Fleet Babylax, Sani-Supp *Laxative (osmotic), lubricant* Pregnancy Risk Category: C	*Constipation* — **Adults and children ≥ 6 yr:** 2 to 3 g as rectal suppository or 5 to 15 ml as enema. **Children 2 to 5 yr:** 1 to 1.7 g as rectal suppository or 2 to 5 ml as enema.	▪ Advise patient to retain drug for ≥ 15 min. Usually acts within 1 hr. Entire suppository need not melt to be effective. ▪ Warn patient about adverse GI reactions.

goserelin acetate Zoladex *Luteinizing hormone–releasing hormone (LHRH; GnRH) analogue* Pregnancy Risk Category: X (endometriosis); D (breast cancer)	*Endometriosis*— **Adults:** 3.6 mg S.C. q 28 days into upper abdominal wall. For endometriosis: maximum duration of therapy 6 mo. *Advanced prostate CA* — 3.6 mg S.C. 8 wk before radiotherapy, followed in 28 days by 10.8 mg depot S.C. *Endometrial thinning before endometrial ablation* — **Adults:** 3.6 mg S.C., 1 or 2 times (with each depot given 4 wk apart). *Palliative treatment of advanced breast cancer in pre- and perimenopausal women* — **Adults:** 3.6 mg S.C. q 28 days into upper abdominal wall.	▪ After cleaning area and injecting local anesthetic, stretch skin with one hand while grasping barrel of syringe with other. Insert needle into S.C. fat; then change needle direction so it parallels abdominal wall. Push needle in until hub touches skin; then withdraw needle about 1 cm before depressing plunger completely. ▪ Don't aspirate after inserting needle. ▪ Implant comes in preloaded syringe. If package is damaged, don't use syringe. ▪ Make sure drug is visible in translucent container.
granisetron hydrochloride Kytril *Antiemetic, antinauseant* Pregnancy Risk Category: B	*Prevention of nausea and vomiting associated with emetogenic cancer chemotherapy* — **Adults and children 2 to 16 yr:** 10 mcg/kg I.V. infused over 5 min. Begin infusion within 30 min before chemotherapy: 2 mg once daily or 1 mg b.i.d. In the 2-mg once-daily regimen, give 2-mg tabs up to 1 hr before chemotherapy. In the 1-mg b.i.d. regimen, give 1st 1-mg tab up to 1 hr before chemotherapy; 2nd tab 12 hr after the first. *Prevention of nausea and vomiting from radiation, including total body irradiation and fractionated abdominal radiation* — **Adults:** 2 mg P.O. once daily within 1 hr of radiation.	▪ ***I.V. use:*** Dilute with 0.9% NaCl or D_5W to volume of 20 to 50 ml. ▪ Don't mix with other drugs. ▪ Stress importance of taking 2nd dose of oral drug 12 hr later for maximum effectiveness. ▪ Warn to report adverse reactions promptly.

DRUG & CLASS	INDICATIONS & DOSAGES	NURSING CONSIDERATIONS
griseofulvin microsize Fulcin‡, Fulvicin-U/F, Grifulvin V, Grisactin, Grisovin‡, Grisovin 500‡, Grisovin-FP† **griseofulvin ultramicrosize** Fulvicin P/G, Grisactin Ultra, Griseofulvin Ultramicrosize, Griseostatin‡, Gris-PEG *Antifungal* Pregnancy Risk Category: C	*Ringworm infections of skin, hair, nails* — **Adults:** 500 mg (microsize) P.O. q.d. in single or divided doses. Severe infections may need up to 1 g q.d. Or, 330 to 375 mg (ultramicrosize) P.O. q.d. in single or divided doses. **Children > 2 yr:** 125 to 250 mg (microsize) P.O. q.d. or 7.3 mg/kg (ultramicrosize) P.O. q.d. for child 13.1 to 22.7 kg (29 to 50 lb); or 250 to 500 mg (microsize) P.O. q.d. for child > 22.7 kg. *Tinea pedis; tinea unguium* — **Adults:** 0.75 to 1 g (microsize) P.O. q.d. Or, 660 to 750 mg (ultramicrosize) P.O. q.d. in divided doses. **Children > 2 yr:** 125 to 250 mg (microsize) P.O. q.d. or 7.3 mg/kg (ultramicrosize) P.O. q.d. for child 13.1 to 22.7 kg; or 250 to 500 mg (microsize) P.O. q.d. for child > 22.7 kg.	▪ Advise patient to take drug after high-fat meal. ▪ Inform patient that prolonged treatment may be needed to control infection and prevent relapse, even if symptoms abate in first few days. ▪ Instruct patient to keep skin clean and dry and to maintain good hygiene. ▪ Caution patient to avoid intense sunlight and alcoholic beverages. ▪ Instruct patient to notify doctor if fever, sore throat, or rash develops.
guaifenesin (glyceryl guaiacolate) Anti-Tuss, Glytuss, Halotussin, Humibid L.A., Neo-Spect†, Robitussin *Expectorant* Pregnancy Risk Category: C	*Expectorant* — **Adults and children ≥ 12 yr:** 100 to 400 mg P.O. q 4 hr, up to 2.4 g/day; or 600 to 1,200 mg extended-release capsules q 12 hr. Maximum 2,400 mg daily. **Children 6 to 11 yr:** 100 to 200 mg P.O. q 4 hr, maximum 1,200 mg/day. For extended-release capsules, 600 mg q 12 hr, maximum 1,200 mg/day. **Children 2 to 5 yr:** 50 to 100 mg P.O. q 4 hr. Maximum 600 mg/day. For extended-release capsules, 300 mg q 12 hr, maximum 600 mg/day.	▪ Explain that persistent cough may signal serious condition; instruct patient to contact doctor if cough lasts > 1 wk, recurs frequently, or is associated with high fever, rash, or severe headache. ▪ Advise patient to take with glass of water. ▪ Encourage deep-breathing exercises. ▪ If excessive amounts of drug are taken, nausea and vomiting may occur.

haloperidol
Apo-Haloperidol†, Haldol, Novo-Peridol†, Peridol†, Serenace‡
haloperidol decanoate
Haldol Decanoate, Haldol LA†
haloperidol lactate
Haldol
Antipsychotic
Pregnancy Risk Category: C

Psychotic disorders — **Adults and children ≥ 12 yr:** dosage varies. Initial range 0.5 to 5 mg P.O. b.i.d. or t.i.d.; or 2 to 5 mg I.M. q 4 to 8 hr. Maximum 100 mg P.O. q.d. **Children 3 to 11 yr:** 0.05 mg/kg to 0.15 mg/kg P.O. q.d. in 2 or 3 divided doses.
Chronic psychosis in patients who need prolonged therapy — **Adults:** 50 to 100 mg I.M. haloperidol decanoate q 4 wk.
Nonpsychotic behavior disorders and Tourette disorder — **Children 3 to 12 yr:** 0.05 mg/kg/day to 0.075 mg/kg/day P.O. in divided doses b.i.d. to t.i.d. Maximum 6 mg q.d.
Adjust-a-dose: In debilitated patients, give 0.5 to 2 mg P.O. b.i.d. or t.i.d; increase gradually, p.r.n.

- Don't give decanoate form I.V.
- Monitor for tardive dyskinesia, which may follow prolonged use.
- Warn patient to avoid activities that require alertness and psychomotor coordination until CNS effects known.
- Tell patient to avoid alcohol.
- Instruct patient to relieve dry mouth with sugarless gum or hard candy.
- Haloperidol decanoate injection should be given by deep I.M. injection with a 21-gauge needle. Maximum volume for injection is 3 ml.

---

heparin sodium
Hepalean†, Liquaemin Sodium, Uniparin‡
Anticoagulant
Pregnancy Risk Category: C

Dosage highly individualized, depending on disease state, age, and renal and hepatic status.
Full-dose continuous I.V. infusion therapy for deep vein thrombosis (DVT), MI, pulmonary embolism — **Adults:** initially, 5,000 U by I.V. bolus, then 750 to 1,500 U/hr by I.V. infusion with pump. Adjust hourly rate 8 hr after bolus dose and according to PTT. **Children:** initially, 50 U/kg I.V., then 25 U/kg/hr or 20,000 U/m^2 daily by I.V. infusion pump. Adjust dose according to PTT.
Full-dose S.C. therapy for DVT, MI, pul-

- Give low-dose injections sequentially between iliac crests in lower abdomen deep into S.C. fat. Inject slowly into fat pad. Leave needle in place for 10 sec after injection, then withdraw. Don't massage after S.C. injection. Watch for signs of bleeding at injection site. Alternate sites q 12 hr (right for morning, left for evening).
- ***I.V. use:*** Give I.V. using infusion pump. Check constant infusions regularly.
- During intermittent I.V. therapy, always draw blood ½ hr before *(continued)*

†Canadian ‡Australian

DRUG & CLASS	INDICATIONS & DOSAGES	NURSING CONSIDERATIONS
heparin sodium *(continued)*	*monary embolism* — **Adults:** initially, 5,000 U I.V. bolus and 10,000 to 20,000 U in concentrated solution S.C., then 8,000 to 10,000 U S.C. q 8 hr or 15,000 to 20,000 U in concentrated solution q 12 hr. *Fixed low-dose therapy for venous thrombosis, pulmonary embolism, atrial fibrillation with embolism, postoperative DVT, embolism prevention* — **Adults:** 5,000 U S.C. q 12 hr. In surgical patients, give 1st dose 2 hr before procedure, then 5,000 U S.C. q 8 to 12 hr for 5 to 7 days or until patient can walk. *Consumptive coagulopathy (such as disseminated intravascular coagulation)* — **Adults:** 50 to 100 U/kg by I.V. bolus or continuous I.V. infusion q 4 hr. **Children:** 25 to 50 U/kg by I.V. bolus or continuous I.V. infusion q 4 hr. If no improvement within 4 to 8 hr, discontinue.	next scheduled dose to avoid falsely elevated PTT. May draw blood for PTT after 8 hr of initiation of continuous I.V. therapy. Never draw blood for PTT from I.V. tubing of infusion or from infused vein; falsely elevated PTT will result. Always draw blood from opposite arm. ▪ Never piggyback other drugs into infusion line while infusion running. Never mix with another drug in same syringe when giving bolus. ▪ Measure PTT carefully and regularly. Anticoagulation present when PTT values 1.5 to 2 times control values. Monitor platelet count regularly. ▪ Treat severe overdose with protamine sulfate.
hydralazine hydrochloride Alphapress‡, Apo-Hydralazine†, Apresoline, Novo-Hylazin†, Nu-Hydral† *Antihypertensive* Pregnancy Risk Category: C	*Essential hypertension (orally); severe essential hypertension (parenterally)* — **Adults:** *P.O.:* 10 mg q.i.d.; increase gradually to 50 mg q.i.d. Maximum dosage 200 mg q.d., but some patients may need 300 to 400 mg q.d. *I.V.:* 10 to 20 mg repeated, p.r.n.; switch to P.O. as soon as possible. *I.M.:* 10 to 50 mg, repeated p.r.n.; switch to P.O. as soon as possible. **Children:** *P.O.:* 0.75 mg/kg/day divided into	▪ ***I.V. use:*** Give slowly and repeat as needed, usually q 4 to 6 hr. Color changes that occur in most infusion solutions don't indicate potency loss. Check with pharmacist for compatibility information. ▪ Monitor BP, pulse, and weight frequently. ▪ Elderly patients may be more sensitive to hypotensive effects. ▪ Call doctor immediately if symptoms of lupuslike syndrome develop.

	4 doses; increase gradually over 3 to 4 wk up to 7.5 mg/kg or 200 mg q.d. *I.V. or I.M.:* 1.7 to 3.5 mg/kg q.d. or 50 to 100 mg/m^2 q.d. in 4 to 6 divided doses. Initial parenteral dose shouldn't exceed 20 mg.	▪ Instruct patient to take oral form with meals to increase absorption. ▪ Advise patient to rise slowly and avoid sudden position changes to minimize orthostatic hypotension.
hydrochlorothiazide Apo-Hydro†, Aquazide-H, Diaqua, Dichlotride‡, Esidrix, HydroDIURIL, Microzide, Diuchlor†, Novo-Hydrazide†, Oretic *Diuretic, antihypertensive* Pregnancy Risk Category: B	*Edema* — **Adults:** 25 to 100 mg P.O. q.d. or intermittently. **Children 2 to 12 yr:** 37.5 to 100 mg P.O. q.d. in 2 divided doses. **Children 6 mo to 2 yr:** 2 to 2.2 mg/kg P.O. or 60 mg/m^2 q.d. in 2 divided doses. **Infants < 6 mo:** up to 3 mg/kg P.O. q.d. in 2 divided doses. Maximum 12.5 to 37.5 mg q.d. *Hypertension* — **Adults:** 25 to 50 mg P.O. q.d. as single dose or divided b.i.d. Adjust dose according to BP. Doses > 50 mg/day not required when combined with other antihypertensives.	▪ Monitor I&O, weight, BP, and serum electrolyte levels. ▪ Monitor serum creatinine, BUN, and serum uric acid regularly. Cumulative drug effects may occur with impaired renal function. ▪ Monitor elderly patients, who are especially susceptible to excessive diuresis. ▪ Monitor blood glucose level, especially in diabetic patients. ▪ In hypertension, therapeutic response may be delayed several wk.
hydrocortisone (systemic) Cortef, Hydrocortone **hydrocortisone acetate** Cortifoam, Hydrocortone Acetate **hydrocortisone sodium phosphate** Hydrocortone Phosphate **hydrocortisone sodium succinate**	*Severe inflammation; adrenal insufficiency* — **Adults:** 5 to 30 mg P.O. b.i.d., t.i.d., or q.i.d. (up to 80 mg q.i.d. in acute situations); or initially, 100 to 500 mg succinate I.M. or I.V., and then 50 to 100 mg I.M., as indicated; or 15 to 240 mg phosphate I.M. or I.V. q.d. in divided doses q 12 hr; or 5 to 75 mg acetate into joints or soft tissue. Dosage varies with size of joint. Local anesthetics often injected with dose. *Shock* — **Adults:** initially, 50 mg/kg succinate I.V., repeated in 4 hr. Repeat q 24 hr,	▪ May mask or exacerbate infections. ▪ Watch for depression or psychotic episodes. ▪ Diabetic patients may need increased insulin; monitor blood glucose level. ▪ Instruct patient to take oral form with milk or food. ▪ Warn patient on long-term therapy about cushingoid symptoms. ▪ ***ALERT*** Teach patient about symptoms of early adrenal insufficiency: fatigue, muscular weakness, joint pain, *(continued)*

DRUG & CLASS	INDICATIONS & DOSAGES	NURSING CONSIDERATIONS
hydrocortisone *(continued)* A-hydroCort, Solu-Cortef *Adrenocorticoid replacement* Pregnancy Risk Category: C	p.r.n. Or, 100 to 500 mg to 2 g q 2 to 6 hr until patient stabilized (usually ≤ 48 to 72 hr). **Children:** phosphate (I.M.) or succinate (I.M. or I.V.) 0.16 to 1 mg/kg or 6 to 30 mg/m^2 once daily or b.i.d.	fever, anorexia, nausea, dyspnea, dizziness, and fainting. ▪ Instruct patient to carry card identifying need for supplemental systemic glucocorticoids during stress. ▪ Warn patient about easy bruising.
hydrocortisone (topical) Acticort, CaldeCort, Cortef, Cortizone 5, Squibb-HC‡ **hydrocortisone acetate** CortaGel, Cortaid, Cortamed†, Hydrocortisone Acetate **hydrocortisone butyrate** Locoid **hydrocortisone valerate** Westcort Cream *Topical adrenocorticoid* Pregnancy Risk Category: C	*Inflammation from corticosteroid-responsive dermatoses; adjunctive topical management of seborrheic dermatitis of scalp* — **Adults and children:** clean area; apply cream, gel, lotion, ointment, or topical solution sparingly once daily to q.i.d. Spray aerosol onto affected area once daily to q.i.d. until acute phase controlled; then reduce dosage to 1 to 3 times q wk, p.r.n. *Inflammation associated with proctitis* — **Adults:** 1 applicator of rectal foam P.R. once daily or b.i.d. for 2 to 3 wk, then every other day, p.r.n.	▪ Gently wash skin before applying. To prevent skin damage, rub in gently, leaving thin coat. When treating hairy sites, part hair and apply directly to lesions. Don't apply near eyes, mucous membranes, or in ear canal; may be safely used on face, groin, armpits, and under breasts. ▪ Stop drug and tell doctor if skin infection, striae, atrophy, or fever develops. ▪ When using aerosol around face, cover patient's eyes and warn against inhaling spray. Don't spray for > 3 sec or < 6″ (15 cm). Apply to dry scalp after shampooing. No need to massage medication into scalp after spraying. ▪ Systemic absorption likely with use of occlusive dressings, prolonged treatment, or extensive body-surface treatment.
hydromorphone hydrochloride (dihydromorphinone hydrochloride)	*Moderate to severe pain* — **Adults:** 2 to 10 mg P.O. q 4 to 6 hr, p.r.n. or around the clock; or 1 to 4 mg I.M., S.C., or I.V. (slowly over ≥ 3 to 5 min) q 4 to 6 hr, p.r.n. or around	▪ Respiratory depression and hypotension possible with I.V. use. Give very slowly and monitor constantly. Keep resuscitation equipment available.

Dilaudid, Dilaudid-HP, Hydrostat *Analgesic, antitussive* Pregnancy Risk Category: C Controlled Substance Schedule: II	the clock; or 3-mg rectal suppository q 6 to 8 hr, or as doctor directs. (Give 1 to 14 mg Dilaudid-HP S.C. or I.M. q 4 to 6 hr.) *Cough* — **Adults and children > 12 yr:** 1 mg P.O. q 3 to 4 hr, p.r.n. **Children 6 to 12 yr:** 0.5 mg P.O. q 3 to 4 hr, p.r.n.	▪ Keep narcotic antagonist available. ▪ Tell patient to avoid alcohol. ▪ Dilaudid-HP highly concentrated. ▪ Tell patient to request drug or to take it before pain becomes intense. ▪ Warn outpatient to avoid hazardous activities until CNS effects known. ▪ Tell patient to take drug with food if GI upset occurs.
hydroxyzine embonate‡ Atarax **hydroxyzine hydrochloride** Apo-Hydroxyzine†, Atarax, Hyzine-50, Multipax†, Vistaquel, Vistaril, Vistazine 50 **hydroxyzine pamoate** Hy-Pam, Vamate, Vistaril *Anxiolytic, sedative, antipruritic, antiemetic, antispasmodic* Pregnancy Risk Category: C	*Anxiety; tension; hyperkinesia* — **Adults:** 50 to 100 mg P.O. q.i.d. **Children ≥ 6 yr:** 50 to 100 mg P.O. q.d. in divided doses. **Children < 6 yr:** 50 mg P.O. q.d. in divided doses. *Preoperative and postoperative adjunctive sedation; to control vomiting (excluding pregnancy); adjunct to asthma treatment* — **Adults:** 25 to 100 mg I.M. q 4 to 6 hr. **Children:** 1.1 mg/kg I.M. q 4 to 6 hr. *Pruritus from allergies* — **Adults:** 25 mg P.O. t.i.d. or q.i.d. . **Children ≥ 6 yr:** 50 to 100 mg P.O. q.d. in divided doses. **Children < 6 yr:** 50 mg P.O. q.d. in divided doses.	▪ Parenteral form (hydroxyzine hydrochloride) for I.M. use only; Z-track method preferred. Never give I.V. ▪ Aspirate I.M. injection carefully to prevent inadvertent intravascular injection. Inject deeply into large muscle mass. ▪ If patient receiving other CNS drugs, observe for oversedation. Warn patient to avoid hazardous activities that require alertness and psychomotor coordination until CNS effects known. ▪ Tell patient to avoid alcohol. ▪ To relieve dry mouth, suggest sugarless hard candy or gum.
hyoscyamine Cystospaz **hyoscyamine sulfate** Anaspaz, Bellaspaz,	*GI tract disorders caused by spasm; to diminish secretions and block cardiac vagal reflexes preoperatively; adjunct treatment for peptic ulcerations* — **Adults and children ≥ 12 yr:** 0.125 to 0.25 mg P.O. or S.L.	▪ Give 30 min to 1 hr before meals and dose at h.s. can be larger; give ≥ 2 hr after dinner. ▪ Monitor vital signs and urine output carefully. *(continued)*

DRUG & CLASS	INDICATIONS & DOSAGES	NURSING CONSIDERATIONS
hyoscyamine *(continued)* Cytospaz, ED-Spoz, Levbid, Levsin, Levsin Drops **hyoscyamine** Levsin S/L, Neoquess *Anticholinergic, antispasmodic* Pregnancy Risk Category: C	t.i.d. or q.i.d. before meals and h.s.; 0.375 mg to 0.75 mg P.O. (extended-release form) P.O. q 12 hr; or 0.25 to 0.5 mg (1 or 2 ml) I.M., I.V., or S.C. q 4 hr b.i.d. to q.i.d. Maximum 1.5 mg q.d. **Children < 12 yr:** dosage individualized according to weight.	▪ Injection may cause allergic reaction in certain patients. ▪ Monitor patient with cardiac history for tachycardia. ▪ Tell patient to avoid hazardous activities if adverse CNS effects occur, drink plenty of fluids, and report rash. ▪ Drug may reduce sweating, resulting possibly in heat stroke.
ibuprofen Aches-N-Pain, Actiprofen†, ACT-3‡, Advil, Children's Advil, Children's Motrin, Midol Maximum Strength Cramp Formula, Motrin, Motrin-IB Caplets, Motrin IB Tablets, Motrin Migraine Pain, Nu-Ibruprofen†, Nuprin Caplets, Nuprin Tablets, Pedia Profen *Nonnarcotic analgesic, antipyretic, anti-inflammatory* Pregnancy Risk Category: B; D in 3rd trimester	*Rheumatoid arthritis; osteoarthritis; arthritis* — **Adults:** 300 to 800 mg P.O. t.i.d. or q.i.d., not to exceed 3.2 g/day. *Mild to moderate pain; dysmenorrhea* — **Adults:** 400 mg P.O. q 4 to 6 hr, p.r.n. *Fever* — **Adults:** 200 to 400 mg P.O. q 4 to 6 hr. Don't give 1.2 g q.d. or > 3 days. **6 mo to 12 yr:** if fever < 102.5° F (39.2° C), 5 mg/kg P.O. q 6 to 8 hr. If > 102.5° F, 10 mg/kg q 6 to 8 hr. Maximum 40 mg/kg/day. *Juvenile arthritis* — **Children:** 20 to 40 mg/kg/day in 3 or 4 divided doses.	▪ Check renal and hepatic function periodically with long-term therapy. ▪ Changes in vision may occur. ▪ Instruct patient to take with food or milk to avoid GI upset; tell adult patient not to self-medicate for extended periods without consulting doctor. ▪ Caution patient that using with aspirin, alcohol, or corticosteroids may increase risk of adverse GI reactions. ▪ Teach patient signs and symptoms of GI bleeding, and tell him to contact doctor immediately if these occur. ▪ Don't give > 50 mg/kg/day to patient with juvenile arthritis.
ibutilide fumarate Corvert	*Rapid conversion of fibrillation or atrial flutter of recent onset to sinus rhythm* — **Adults ≥ 60 kg (132 lb):** 1 mg I.V. over 10	▪ Only skilled personnel should give drug. ▪ Before therapy, correct hypokalemia and hypomagnesemia.

Class III Antiarrhythmic
Pregnancy Risk Category: C

min. **Adults < 60 kg:** 0.01 mg/kg I.V. over 10 min. Stop infusion if arrhythmia ends or if ventricular tachycardia or marked prolongation of QT or QTc interval occurs. If arrhythmia doesn't end 10 min after stopping infusion, may give second 10-min infusion of equal strength.

- Adequately anticoagulate patients with atrial fibrillation of > 2 to 3 days' duration (generally for ≥ 2 wk).
- Monitor ECG continuously during and ≥ 4 hr after giving or until QTc interval returns to baseline.
- ***I.V. use:*** May give undiluted or diluted in 50 ml diluent.
- Streaking along the vein may indicate too rapid I.V. infusion rate.

---

idarubicin hydrochloride
Idamycin
Antineoplastic
Pregnancy Risk Category: D

Dosage and indications vary. Check treatment protocol with doctor.
Acute myeloid leukemia, including French-American-British classifications M1 through M7, with other approved antileukemic agents — **Adults:** 12 mg/m^2/day for 3 days by slow I.V. injection (over 10 to 15 min) with 100 mg/m^2/day of cytarabine for 7 days by continuous I.V. infusion; or as 25 mg/m^2 bolus (cytarabine); then 200 mg/m^2/day (cytarabine) for 5 days by continuous infusion. Second course may be given, p.r.n.
Adjust-a-dose: If patient experiences severe mucositis, delay until recovery complete, and reduce dose by 25%. Also reduce dose in hepatic or renal impairment. Don't give if bilirubin > 5 mg/dl.

- Cardiotoxicity is dose-limiting toxicity.
- Take preventive steps, such as adequate hydration, before treatment. Hyperuricemia may result from rapid lysis of leukemic cells; allopurinol may be ordered.
- ***ALERT:*** Don't give I.V. or I.M.
- Give over 10 to 15 min into free-flowing I.V. infusion of 0.9% NaCl or 5% dextrose solution running into large vein.
- Drug is a vesicant; tissue necrosis may result. If extravasation occurs, stop infusion immediately and notify doctor. Apply intermittent ice packs immediately for ½ hr, then for ½ hr q.i.d. for 4 days.
- Monitor hepatic and renal function tests and CBC frequently.
- Notify doctor if signs or symptoms of heart failure occur.

DRUG & CLASS	INDICATIONS & DOSAGES	NURSING CONSIDERATIONS
ifosfamide IFEX *Antineoplastic* Pregnancy Risk Category: D	*Testicular cancer* — **Adults:** 1.2 g/m^2/day I.V. for 5 consecutive days. Infuse each dose over ≥ 30 min. Repeat treatment q 3 wk or after patient recovers from hematologic toxicity. Give with protecting agent (mesna) to prevent hemorrhagic cystitis.	▪ Adequate fluid intake (2 L/day) essential before and for 72 hr after therapy. ▪ Assess for mental status changes. ▪ Don't give h.s. If cystitis develops, stop drug and notify doctor. ▪ Monitor CBC and renal function tests and LFTs. ▪ Tell patient to use contraceptives during therapy. ▪ Instruct patient to notify doctor of bleeding, bruising, fever, chills, sore throat, shortness of breath, seizures, and pain, sores in mouth or lips, or jaundice.
imipenem and cilastatin Primaxin IM, Primaxin IV *Antibiotic* Pregnancy Risk Category: C	*Serious lower respiratory tract, urinary tract, intra-abdominal, gynecologic, bone and joint, skin and soft-tissue infections; bacterial septicemia and endocarditis* — **Adults and children > 40 kg (88 lb):** 250 mg to 1 g by I.V. infusion q 6 to 8 hr. Maximum 50 mg/kg/day or 4 g/day, whichever is less. Or, 500 to 750 mg I.M. q 12 hr. Maximum 1,500 mg/day. **Children < 40 kg:** 60 mg/kg I.V. q.d. in divided doses. **Premature infants < 36 wk gestational age:** 20 mg/kg I.V. q 12 hr. ***Adjust-a-dose:*** Based on CrCl. Refer to package insert.	▪ Obtain culture and sensitivity tests before 1st dose. ▪ ***I.V. use:*** Give each 250- or 500-mg dose by I.V. infusion over 20 to 30 min. Infuse each 1-g dose over 40 to 60 min. If nausea occurs, may slow infusion. ▪ If seizures develop and persist, notify doctor. Drug should be discontinued. ▪ Monitor for superinfections and resistant infections.

imipramine hydrochloride Apo-Imipramine†, Impril†, Janimine, Melipramine‡, Norfranil, Tipramine, Tofranil **imipramine pamoate** Tofranil-PM *Antidepressant* Pregnancy Risk Category: D	*Depression* — **Adults:** 75 to 100 mg P.O. or I.M. q.d. in divided doses, increased in 25- to 50-mg increments. Maximum for outpatients 200 mg q.d.; 300 mg q.d. may be used for hospital patients. Entire dose may be given h.s. **Elderly and adolescent patients:** initially, 30 to 40 mg q.d.; usually not necessary to exceed 100 mg q.d. *Childhood enuresis* — **Children ≥ 6 yr:** 25 mg P.O. 1 hr before h.s. If no response within 1 wk, increase to 50 mg if child < 12 yr, and to 75 mg if child ≥ 12 yr. In either case, maximum 2.5 mg/kg/day.	▪ Reduce dosage in elderly, debilitated, or adolescent, or patients with aggravated psychotic symptoms. ▪ Don't withdraw abruptly. ▪ Discontinue gradually several days before surgery. ▪ Warn patient to avoid hazardous activities until CNS effects known. ▪ If signs of psychosis occur or increase, reduce dosage. Monitor for suicidal tendencies and allow only minimum drug supply. ▪ Instruct patient to avoid alcohol intake. ▪ Orthostatic hypotension may occur.
inamrinone Inocor *Inotropic, vasodilator* Pregnancy Risk Category: C	*Short-term management of heart failure* — **Adults:** initially, 0.75 mg/kg I.V. bolus over 2 to 3 min. Then start maintenance infusion of 5 to 10 mcg/kg/min. May give additional bolus of 0.75 mg/kg 30 min after therapy starts. Don't exceed 10 mg/kg/day. Dosage depends on clinical response.	▪ Primarily given to patients unresponsive to cardiac glycosides, diuretics, and vasodilators. ▪ ***ALERT*** Don't dilute with solution containing dextrose. Can be injected into free-flowing dextrose infusions through Y-connector or directly into tubing. ▪ Monitor BP and HR throughout infusion. ▪ Drug contains bisulfites; use with caution in sulfite-sensitive patients.
indapamide Lozide†, Lozol, Natrilix‡ *Diuretic, antihypertensive* Pregnancy Risk Category: B	*Edema* — **Adults:** initially, 2.5 mg P.O. q.d. in morning. Increase to 5 mg q.d. after 1 wk, if needed. *Hypertension* — **Adults:** initially, 1.25 mg	▪ Monitor I&O, weight, BP, serum electrolytes, BUN, creatinine, uric acid, and glucose. ▪ Watch for signs of hypokalemia. ▪ May use with *(continued)*

DRUG & CLASS	INDICATIONS & DOSAGES	NURSING CONSIDERATIONS
indapamide *(continued)*	P.O. q.d. in morning. Increase to 2.5 mg q.d. after 4 wk, p.r.n. Increase to 5 mg q.d. after 4 more wk, p.r.n.	potassium-sparing diuretic to prevent potassium loss. ▪ Monitor elderly patients closely.
indinavir sulfate Crixivan *Antiviral* Pregnancy Risk Category: C	*HIV infection, when antiretroviral therapy warranted* — **Adults:** 800 mg P.O. q 8 hr. Reduce to 600 mg P.O. q 8 hr in mild to moderate hepatic insufficiency from cirrhosis.	▪ Maintain adequate hydration during therapy (≥ 1.5 L fluids q 24 hr). ▪ Inform patient that drug won't cure HIV infection, may not prevent complications of HIV, and doesn't reduce risk of HIV transmission. ▪ Advise patient to report flank pain or dysuria. ▪ Take 1 hr before or 2 hr after meals.
indomethacin Apo-Indomethacin†, Indochron E-R, Indocid SR†, Indocin, Indocin SR, Novo-Methacin†, Rheumacin‡ **indomethacin sodium trihydrate** Apo-Indomethacin†, Indocid P.D.A.†, Indocin I.V., Novo-Methacin† *Nonnarcotic analgesic, antipyretic, anti-inflammatory* Pregnancy Risk Category: NR	*Moderate to severe rheumatoid arthritis or osteoarthritis; ankylosing spondylitis* — **Adults:** 25 mg P.O. or P.R. b.i.d. or t.i.d. with food or antacids; increase daily dose 25 or 50 mg q 7 days, up to 200 mg q.d. Or, SR capsule (75 mg): 75 mg P.O. to start, in morning or h.s.; then, 75 mg b.i.d., p.r.n. *Acute gouty arthritis* — **Adults:** 50 mg P.O. t.i.d. Reduce as soon as possible; then stop.	▪ Monitor carefully for bleeding and for reduced urine output with I.V. use. Don't give 2nd or 3rd scheduled I.V. dose if anuria or marked oliguria evident; instead, notify doctor. Monitor for bleeding in coagulation defects, in patients receiving anticoagulants, and in neonates. ▪ Causes sodium retention. Monitor for weight gain and increased BP. ▪ May mask signs and symptoms of infection. ▪ Give oral dosage with food, milk, or antacid if GI upset occurs. ▪ Don't crush extended release capsules.

inflximab
Remicade
Anti-inflammatory
Pregnancy Risk Category: C

Moderately to severely active Crohn's disease with inadequate response to conventional therapy — **Adults:** 5 mg/kg single I.V. infusion over ≥ 2 hr.

Reduction in number of draining enterocutaneous fistulas — **Adults:** 5 mg/kg I.V. infused over ≥ 2 hr. Give additional doses of 5 mg/kg at 2 and 6 wk after initial infusion.

Rheumatoid arthritis with inadequate response to methotrexate alone — **Adults:** 3 mg/kg I.V. infusion over ≥ 2 hr, then additional 3-mg/kg doses at 2 and 6 wk after 1st infusion; then q 8 wk thereafter. Give with methotrexate.

- Monitor for infusion-related reactions.
- Drug may affect normal immune responses.
- ***I.V. use:*** Prepare only in glass infusion bottle or polypropylene or polyolefin infusion bag; give through polyethylene-lined administration sets with in-line, sterile, nonpyrogenic, low-protein-binding filter (pore size ≤ 1.2 mm).
- Use reconstituted dose promptly; don't infuse in same I.V. line with other agents.

---

insulin aspart (rDNA origin) injection
NovoLog
Antidiabetic
Pregnancy Risk Category: C

Adults with diabetes mellitus, for the control of hyperglycemia — Dosage regimens of NovoLog are individualized and should be determined by the patient's prescriber according to patient's needs. Typical insulin dosage is 0.5 to 1.0 U/kg/day before meal S.C. in abdomen, thigh, or upper arm, with rotated sites of injection. Approximately 50% to 70% of this dose is provided with NovoLog and the remainder by an intermediate-acting or long-acting insulin. NovoLog has a rapid onset of action.

Adjust-a-dose: The dosage of NovoLog should be regularly adjusted according to the patient's blood glucose measurements.

- ***ALERT*** The warning signs of overdosage are fatigue, weakness, nervousness, confusion, headache, psychosis, dizziness, unconsciousness, rapid or shallow respirations, numb or tingling mouth, hunger, nausea, and skin pallor changes. Monitor serum glucose. Patient may need I.M. glucagon or I.V. glucose.
- When mixing and giving insulins, draw up drug into syringe first, and give immediately using insulin syringes only. Select injection site and rotate sites periodically to avoid lipodystrophies. Document injection site used.
- Give drug directly before meals. *(continued)*

DRUG & CLASS	INDICATIONS & DOSAGES	NURSING CONSIDERATIONS
insulin aspart *(continued)*	Close glucose monitoring and dosage adjustments of NovoLog may be necessary in patients with renal dysfunction and hepatic impairment.	▪ Observe injection sites for hypersensitivity reactions such as redness, swelling, itching, or burning. ▪ ***ALERT*** Don't give I.V. ▪ Monitor serum glucose levels regularly.
insulin glargine (rDNA) injection Lantus *Antidiabetic* Pregnancy Risk Category: C	*Management of type 1 diabetes mellitus in patients who require basal (long-acting) insulin for the control of hyperglycemia* — **Adults and children:** For patients taking once-daily NPH or ultralente human insulin, initiate Lantus at the same dose as the current insulin dose. For patients taking b.i.d. NPH human insulin, initiate Lantus at a dose that is 20% less than the current daily dose of insulin. Adjust dose based on patient response. *Management of type 2 diabetes mellitus in patients previously treated with oral antidiabetics* — **Adults:** 10 IU S.C. q.d. h.s. Adjust p.r.n. to total daily dose of 2 IU to 100 IU S.C. q.d. h.s.	▪ Give S.C. only; don't give I.V. ▪ As with any insulin, the desired serum glucose levels as well as the doses and timing of antidiabetics must be determined individually. Serum glucose monitoring is recommended for all patients with diabetes. ▪ The rate of absorption, onset, and duration of action may be affected by exercise and emotional stress. ▪ Lantus must not be diluted or mixed with any other insulin or solution. ▪ Hypoglycemia is the most common adverse effect of insulin. Early symptoms may be different or less pronounced in patients with long-standing diabetes, diabetic nerve disease, or intensified diabetes control. Monitor serum glucose closely in these patients because severe hypoglycemia may result before the patient develops symptoms. ▪ In elderly patients with diabetes, the initial dose, dose increments, and maintenance

dosage should be conservative to avoid hypoglycemic reactions, as hypoglycemia may be difficult to recognize in the elderly.

---

insulin injection (regular insulin, crystalline zinc insulin)
Humulin R, Novolin R, Regular (Conc.) Iletin II
insulin (lispro)
Humalog
insulin zinc suspension, prompt (semilente)
Semilente‡
isophane insulin suspension (NPH)
Humulin N, Humulin NPH‡, Novolin N, NPH Insulin
isophane insulin suspension with insulin injection
Humulin 50/50, Humulin 70/30, Novolin 70/30
insulin zinc suspension (lente)
Humulin L, Lente Insulin, Novolin L

Diabetic ketoacidosis (use regular insulin only) — **Adults:** 0.33 U/kg as I.V. bolus, then 0.1 U/kg/hr by continuous infusion. Continue infusion until blood glucose drops to 250 mg/dl, then begin S.C. insulin, adjusting dosage and intervals according to blood glucose level. Or, 50 to 100 U I.V. and 50 to 100 U S.C. immediately; then additional doses q 2 to 6 hr based on blood glucose levels. To prepare infusion, add 100 U regular insulin and 1 g albumin to 100 ml 0.9% NaCl. Insulin concentration will be 1 U/ml. **Children:** 0.1 U/kg as I.V. bolus, then 0.1 U/kg/hr by continuous infusion until blood glucose drops to 250 mg/dl; then start S.C. insulin. Or, 1 to 2 U/kg in 2 divided doses, one I.V. and other S.C., then 0.5 to 1 U/kg I.V. q 1 to 2 hr based on blood glucose levels.
Type 1 diabetes mellitus; adjunct to type 2 diabetes mellitus — **Adults and children:** adjust therapeutic regimen according to blood glucose levels.
Control of hyperglycemia in patients with type 1 diabetes mellitus, and of sulfonylureas in type 2 diabetes mellitus —

- Use regular insulin in circulatory collapse, diabetic ketoacidosis, or hyperkalemia. Don't use Humulin R insulin (concentrated), 500 U/ml I.V. Don't use intermediate or long-acting insulins for emergencies requiring rapid drug action.
- Lispro is for S.C. use and has rapid onset.
- May mix lispro insulin with Humulin N or Humulin U; give 15 min before meal.
- ***I.V. use:*** Use regular insulin only. Inject directly, at ordered rate, into vein through intermittent infusion device or into port close to I.V. access site. Intermittent infusion not recommended.
- Dosage expressed in USP units. Use syringes calibrated for specific insulin concentration.
- U-500 insulin available for patients requiring large doses.
- Monitor pregnant patients closely.
- When mixing regular insulin with intermediate or long-acting, always draw up regular insulin into syringe first.
- Rotate injection sites; chart to avoid overusing one area.
- Store in cool area.

(continued)

†Canadian ‡Australian

DRUG & CLASS	INDICATIONS & DOSAGES	NURSING CONSIDERATIONS
insulin injection *(continued)* **protamine zinc suspension (PZI) insulin zinc suspension, extended (ultralente)** Humulin U, Ultralente Insulin *Antidiabetic* Pregnancy Risk Category: NR	**Adults and children > age 3:** Inject S.C. within 15 min before or immediately after a meal. Adjust therapeutic regimen according to blood glucose levels.	
interferon alfa-2a, recombinant (rIFN-A) Roferon-A *Immunomodulator* Pregnancy Risk Category: C	*Hairy-cell leukemia* — **Adults:** induction, 3 million IU S.C. or I.M. q.d. for 16 to 24 wk. Maintenance, 3 million IU S.C. or I.M. 3 times/wk. *AIDS-related Kaposi's sarcoma* — **Adults:** induction, 36 million IU S.C. or I.M. q.d. for 10 to 12 wk. Maintenance, 36 million IU S.C. or I.M. 3 times/wk. *Philadelphia chromosome–positive chronic myelogenous leukemia* — **Adults:** initially, 3 million IU I.M. or S.C. q.d. for 3 days; then 6 million IU for 3 days, then 9 million IU for duration of treatment.	▪ Obtain allergy history. Contains phenol (preservative) and serum albumin (stabilizer). ▪ Give S.C. if platelet count < 50,000/mm^3. ▪ Give h.s. to minimize daytime drowsiness. ▪ Keep patient well hydrated, especially during initial treatment. ▪ Monitor for CNS adverse reactions, such as decreased mental status and dizziness. ▪ Different brands not equivalent; may require different dosage. ▪ Neurotoxicity and cardiotoxicity more common in elderly patients, especially those with underlying CNS or cardiac impairment.
interferon alfa-2b, recombinant (IFN-alpha 2) Intron A	*Hairy-cell leukemia* — **Adults:** 2 million IU/m^2 I.M. or S.C. 3 times/wk. *AIDS-related Kaposi's sarcoma* — **Adults:** 30 million IU/m^2 S.C. or I.M. 3 times/wk.	▪ Give S.C.if platelet count < 50,000/mm^3. ▪ Give h.s. to minimize daytime drowsiness. ▪ Keep patient well hydrated. ▪ Monitor for adverse CNS reactions.

Immunomodulator Pregnancy Risk Category: C	*Chronic hepatitis B* — **Adults:** 30 to 35 million IU q wk I.M. or S.C., given as 5 million IU q.d. or 10 million IU 3 times/wk for 16 wk. **Children ages 1 and older:** 3 million IU/m^2 S.C. 3 times/wk for 1st week; then increase to 6 million IU/m^2 S.C. 3 times/wk (maximum 10 million IU 3 times/wk) for 16 to 24 wk. *Malignant melanoma* — **Adults:** 20 million IU/m^2 I.V. infusion on 5 consecutive days/wk for 4 wk. Maintenance dose is 10 million IU/m^2 S.C. 3 times/wk for 48 wk. *Condylomata acuminata* — **Adults:** inject 1 million IU/lesion 3 times/wk for 3 wk intralesionally. *Chronic hepatitis C* — **Adults:** 3 million IU 3 times/wk S.C. or I.M. At 16 wk of treatment, extend therapy to 18 to 24 mo at 3 million IU 3 times/wk to improve sustained response.	▪ May increase bone marrow suppressant effects when used with blood dyscrasia–causing therapies. ▪ Flulike syndrome occurs in most patients 2 to 6 hr after dose; pretreatment with NSAIDs or acetaminophen to decrease symptoms.
interferon alfacon-1 Infergen *Immunomodulator* Pregnancy Risk Category: C	*Chronic hepatitis C viral infection* — **Adults:** 9 mcg S.C. 3 times/wk for 24 wk; for nonresponders or those who relapse, 15 mcg S.C. 3 times/wk for 6 mo. ***Adjust-a-dose:*** In patients intolerant to higher doses, may reduce dose to 7.5 mcg. Don't give doses < 7.5 mcg; decreased efficacy may result.	▪ Obtain laboratory work before therapy, 2 wk after initiation, and periodically thereafter (CBC, platelets; serum creatinine, albumin, bilirubin, thyroid-stimulating hormone, and thyroxine levels). ▪ Allow at least 48 hr between doses. ▪ Store drug in refrigerator at 36° to 46° F (2° to 8° C); don't freeze. May allow to reach room temperature just before use. Avoid vigorous shaking. Discard unused portion.

DRUG & CLASS	INDICATIONS & DOSAGES	NURSING CONSIDERATIONS
interferon beta-1a Avonex *Immunomodulator* Pregnancy Risk Category: C	*Relapsing forms of multiple sclerosis to slow progress of physical disability and decrease frequency of clinical exacerbation* — **Adults:** 30 mcg I.M. q wk.	▪ Monitor patient closely for depression and suicidal ideation. ▪ Monitor WBCs, platelet counts, and blood studies, including LFTs. ▪ To reconstitute, inject 1.1 ml supplied diluent (sterile water for injection) into vial and gently swirl to dissolve drug. Don't shake.
interferon beta-1b, recombinant Betaseron *Immunomodulator* Pregnancy Risk Category: C	*To reduce frequency of exacerbations in relapsing-remitting multiple sclerosis* — **Adults:** 8 million IU (0.25 mg) S.C. every other day.	▪ To reconstitute, inject 1.2 ml supplied diluent into vial and swirl to dissolve drug. ▪ Discard vials containing particulates or discolored solution. ▪ Inject immediately after preparation. ▪ Rotate injection sites. ▪ Monitor for depression.
interferon gamma-1b Actimmune *Immunomodulator* Pregnancy Risk Category: C	*To delay disease progression in patients with severe malignant osteopetrosis* — **Patients with body surface area > 0.5 m^2:** 50 mcg/m^2 (1 million IU/m^2) S.C. 3 times/wk. **Patients with body surface area ≤ 0.5 m^2:** 1.5 mcg/kg/dose S.C. 3 times/wk. *Chronic granulomatous disease* — **Adults with body surface area > 0.5 m^2:** 50 mcg/m^2 (1.5 million U/m^2) S.C. 3 times/wk. **Adults with body surface area ≤ 0.5 m^2:** 1.5 mcg/kg 3 times/wk.	▪ Premedicate with acetaminophen to minimize symptoms at start of therapy. ▪ Give in deltoid or anterior thigh. ▪ Refrigerate at once. Store vials at 36° to 46° F (2° to 8° C); don't freeze. Don't shake vial; avoid excessive agitation. Discard vials left at room temperature for > 12 hr. ▪ Discard unused portion.

ipecac syrup Ipecac Syrup *Emetic* Pregnancy Risk Category: C	*To induce vomiting in poisoning* — **Adults and children ≥ 12 yr:** 30 ml P.O.; then 200 to 300 ml water. **Children 1 to 11 yr:** 15 ml P.O.; then 240 to 480 ml water. **Children 6 mo to < 1 yr:** 5 to 10 ml P.O.; then 120 to 240 ml water. Repeat dose in patients > 1 yr if vomiting doesn't occur within 20 min.	▪ Usually induces vomiting within 20 to 30 min. ▪ If 2 doses don't induce vomiting, perform gastric lavage. ▪ No systemic toxicity with doses of ≤ 30 ml (1 oz) or less. ▪ Usually effective if < 1 hr has passed since antiemetic ingested.
ipratropium bromide **ipratropium bromide nasal spray** Atrovent *Bronchodilator* Pregnancy Risk Category: B	*Bronchospasm from COPD* — **Adults:** 1 to 2 inhalations q.i.d.; more may be needed. Don't exceed 12 inhalations in 24 hr. Or, use inhalation solution. Give 500 mcg dissolved in 0.9% NaCl by nebulizer q 6 to 8 hr. **Children 5 to 12 yr:** 125 to 250 mcg nebulizer solution dissolved in 0.9% NaCl given by nebulizer q 6 to 8 hr. *Symptomatic relief of rhinorrhea from allergies and the common cold* — **Children 6 to 11 yr:** 2 sprays (84 mcg) per nostril t.i.d. *Perennial rhinitis* — **Adults and children > 6 yr:** 2 sprays (42 mcg) of 0.03% nasal spray per nostril b.i.d. to t.i.d. *Common cold–induced rhinorrhea* — **Adults and children ≥ 12 yr:** 2 sprays (84 mcg) of 0.06% nasal spray per nostril t.i.d. to q.i.d. **Children 5 to 11 yr:** 2 sprays (84 mcg) per nostril t.i.d.	▪ If using face mask for nebulizer, avoid leakage around mask. ▪ ***ALERT*** Warn patient that drug doesn't treat acute bronchospasm. ▪ Teach patient to perform oral inhalation correctly: Clear nasal passages and throat. Breathe out as much as possible. Place mouthpiece well into mouth as dose is released, then inhale deeply. Hold breath for several seconds, then exhale slowly. If more than one inhalation is ordered, wait > 2 min before repeating. ▪ Atrovent inhalation solution can be mixed in the nebulizer with albuterol or metaproterenol if used within 1 hr. ▪ If patient also uses steroid inhaler, tell him to use ipratropium first, then wait 5 min before using steroid.

DRUG & CLASS	INDICATIONS & DOSAGES	NURSING CONSIDERATIONS
irbesartan Avapro *Antihypertensive* Pregnancy Risk Category: C (1st trimester); D (2nd and 3rd trimesters)	*Hypertension* — **Adults:** initially, 150 mg P.O. q.d., increased to maximum of 300 mg q.d. if needed. ***Adjust-a-dose:*** In volume- and salt-depleted patients, initially 75 mg P.O. q.d.	▪ ***ALERT*** Symptomatic hypotension may occur in volume- or salt-depleted patients. Correct cause of volume depletion before giving drug or lowering dose. ▪ May continue drug when BP has stabilized after transient hypotensive episode.
irinotecan hydrochloride Camptosar *Antineoplastic* Pregnancy Risk Category: D	*Metastatic carcinoma of colon or rectum that has recurred or progressed after fluorouracil therapy* — **Adults:** initially, 125 mg/m^2 I.V. infusion over 90 min. Recommended treatment 125 mg/m^2 I.V. q wk for 4 wk, then 2-wk rest. May repeat treatment course q 6 wk (4 wk on therapy, 2 wk off). May adjust subsequent doses down to 50 mg/m^2 or up to 150 mg/m^2 in 25- to 50-mg/m^2 increments, depending on tolerance. May give additional courses indefinitely if patient responds favorably or if disease remains stable, unless intolerable toxicity occurs.	▪ Pretreat with antiemetic therapy 30 min before irinotecan therapy. ▪ **I.V. use:** Don't add other drugs to infusion. ▪ If extravasation occurs, flush site with sterile water, apply ice, and notify doctor. ▪ ***ALERT*** Can induce severe diarrhea. Diarrhea occurring $\leq$ 24 hr of use may be relieved by atropine I.V., unless contraindicated. Late diarrhea (occurring after 24 hr) may be prolonged and life-threatening. Treat late diarrhea with loperamide. Monitor fluid status and serum electrolytes. ▪ Monitor WBC count with differential, Hgb, and platelet count before each dose. If low, doses may need to be reduced or held.
isoniazid (isonicotinic acid hydrazide, INH) Isotamine†, Laniazid, Nydrazid, PMS Isoniazid†	*Actively growing tubercle bacilli* — **Adults:** 5 to 10 mg/kg P.O. or I.M. q.d. in single dose, up to 300 mg/day, for 9 mo to 2 yr. **Infants and children:** 10 to 20 mg/kg P.O. or I.M. q.d. in single dose, up to 300 mg/day, for 18 mo to	▪ Always give with other antituberculotics to prevent development of resistant organisms. ▪ Monitor hepatic function closely. ▪ Tell patient to avoid alcoholic beverages,

Antituberculotic Pregnancy Risk Category: C	2 yr. Give with one other antituberculotic. *Prevention of tubercle bacilli in those exposed to TB or those with test results consistent with nonprogressive TB* — **Adults:** 300 mg P.O. q.d. in single dose, for 6 mo. **Infants and children:** 10 mg/kg P.O. q.d. in single dose, up to 300 mg/day, for 6 mo.	fish, and tyramine-containing products such as aged cheese, beer, and chocolate. ▪ Give pyridoxine to prevent peripheral neuropathy, especially in malnourished patients.
isoproterenol (isoprenaline) Dey-Dose Isoproterenol, Isuprel, Vapo-Iso **isoproterenol hydrochloride** Isuprel, Norisodrine Aerotrol **isoproterenol sulfate** Medihaler-Iso **isoproterenol** *Bronchodilator, cardiac stimulant* Pregnancy Risk Category: C	*Shock* — **Adults and children:** (hydrochloride) 0.5 to 5 mcg/min by continuous I.V. infusion titrated to response. Usual concentration 1 mg (5 ml) in 500 ml D_5W. *Bronchospasm during mild acute asthma attacks* — **Adults and children:** initially, 1 inhalation of sulfate form; repeat, p.r.n., after 2 to 5 min; maximum 6 inhalations per day. *Bronchospasm in COPD* — **Adults and children:** (hydrochloride) by handheld nebulizer; 5 to 15 deep inhalations of 0.5% solution. In adults needing stronger solution, 3 to 7 deep inhalations of 1% solution no more frequently than q 3 to 4 hr. *Heart block; ventricular arrhythmias* — **Adults:** (hydrochloride) 0.02 to 0.06 mg I.V. Subsequent doses 0.01 to 0.2 mg I.V. or 5 mcg/min I.V. titrated to response; or 0.2 mg I.M., then 0.02 to 1 mg I.M., p.r.n. **Children:** (hydrochloride): I.V. infusion of 2.5 mcg/min to 0.1 mcg/kg/min. Dosage based on response.	▪ ***I.V. use:*** Give by direct injection or infusion. For infusion, don't use with sodium bicarbonate injection. ▪ Correct volume deficit and hypotension before giving vasopressors. ▪ If HR > 110 with I.V. infusion, notify doctor. If HR > 130, ventricular arrhythmias may occur. ▪ When giving I.V. to treat shock, monitor BP, CVP, ECG, ABGs, and urine output. Adjust infusion rate according to results. ▪ May aggravate ventilation-perfusion abnormalities. ▪ May cause slight rise in systolic BP and slight to marked drop in diastolic BP. ▪ Don't use injection or inhalation solution if discolored or contains precipitate. ▪ If giving via inhalation with oxygen, make sure oxygen concentration won't suppress respiratory drive. ▪ Monitor patient for rebound bronchospasms when drug effects end.

DRUG & CLASS	INDICATIONS & DOSAGES	NURSING CONSIDERATIONS
isosorbide dinitrate Apo-ISDN†, Dilatrate-SR, Isonate, Isorbid, Isordil, Isordil Tembids, Isosorbide Tetradose, Isotrate, Sorbitrate **isosorbide mononitrate** Imdur, ISMO, Monoket *Antianginal, vasodilator* Pregnancy Risk Category: C	*Acute anginal attacks (S.L. and chewable tablets isosorbide dinitrate only); prophylaxis in situations likely to cause anginal attacks* — **Adults:** *S.L. form:* 2.5 to 10 mg under tongue, repeated q 5 to 10 min (maximum 3 doses for each 30-min period). Prophylaxis, 2.5 to 10 mg q 2 to 3 hr. *Chewable form:* 5 to 10 mg, p.r.n., for acute attack or q 2 to 3 hr for prophylaxis, but only after initial test dose of 5 mg. *Oral form (dinitrate):* 5 to 30 mg P.O. t.i.d. or q.i.d. for prophylaxis; 20 to 40 mg P.O. (SR form) q 6 to 12 hr. *Oral form (mononitrate, using Imdur):* 30 to 60 mg P.O. q.d. on arising; increased to 120 mg q.d. after several days. *Oral form (mononitrate, using ISMO or Monoket):* 20 mg P.O. b.i.d. with 2 doses given 7 hr apart.	▪ Monitor BP and intensity and duration of drug response. ▪ May cause headaches. Dose may be reduced temporarily, but tolerance usually develops. Give aspirin or acetaminophen. ▪ Inform patient that stopping abruptly may cause coronary vasospasm with increased anginal symptoms and potential risk of MI. ▪ Tell patient to take S.L. tablet at 1st symptoms of attack. Warn him not to confuse S.L. with P.O. form. ▪ To prevent tolerance, urge nitrate-free interval of 8 to 12 hr per day.
isotretinoin Accutane, Roaccutane‡ *Antiacne agent, keratinization stabilizer* Pregnancy Risk Category: X	*Severe recalcitrant nodular acne unresponsive to conventional therapy* — **Adults and adolescents:** 0.5 to 2 mg/kg P.O. q.d. in 2 divided doses for 15 to 20 wk.	▪ Monitor LFTs and serum lipid, blood glucose, and creatine kinase levels before and during therapy. ▪ If headache, nausea and vomiting, or visual disturbances occur, screen for papilledema.
isradipine DynaCirc	*Hypertension* — **Adults:** initially, 2.5 mg P.O. b.i.d., alone or with thiazide diuretic. If re-	▪ May cause symptomatic hypotension. ▪ Monitor BP closely.

Antihypertensive Pregnancy Risk Category: C	sponse inadequate after first 2 to 4 wk, adjust dosage 5 mg q.d. at 2- to 4-wk intervals, to maximum 20 mg q.d.	▪ Before surgery, inform anesthesiologist that patient takes calcium channel blocker.
itraconazole Sporanox *Antifungal* Pregnancy Risk Category: C	*Pulmonary, extrapulmonary blastomycosis; nonmeningeal histoplasmosis* — **Adults:** 200 mg P.O. q.d. Increase dose, p.r.n., in 100-mg increments. Maximum 400 mg q.d. Give doses > 200 mg q.d in 2 divided doses. *Aspergillosis* — **Adults:** 200 to 400 mg P.O. q.d. *Oropharyngeal and esophageal candidiasis* — **Adults:** 200 mg swished in mouth for several sec, then swallowed, q.d. for 1 to 4 wk. *Onychomycosis* — **Adults:** toenails with or without fingernail involvement: 200 mg P.O. q.d. for 12 consecutive weeks. Fingernails only: 200 mg b.i.d. (400 mg/day) for 1 wk. Therapies are separated by 3 wk without Sporanox.	▪ Perform baseline LFTs and monitor periodically. ▪ Teach patient to recognize and report signs and symptoms of liver disease (anorexia, dark urine, pale stools, unusual fatigue, or jaundice). ▪ Tell patient to take with food to ensure maximal absorption.
ketoconazole Nizoral *Antifungal* Pregnancy Risk Category: C	*Fungal infections from susceptible organisms* — **Adults:** 200 mg P.O. q.d. as single dose. Maximum 400 mg q.d. **Children ≥ 2 yr:** 3.3 to 6.6 mg/kg P.O. q.d. as single dose.	▪ To minimize nausea, divide daily dosage or give with meals. ▪ Monitor patient for elevated liver enzymes, persistent nausea, unusual fatigue, jaundice, dark urine, or pale stools. ▪ If antacids are required, separate doses by 2 hr.

DRUG & CLASS	INDICATIONS & DOSAGES	NURSING CONSIDERATIONS
ketoconazole (topical) Nizoral *Antifungal* Pregnancy Risk Category: C	*Tinea corporis, tinea cruris, tinea pedis, tinea versicolor from susceptible organisms; seborrheic dermatitis; cutaneous candidiasis* — **Adults:** cover affected and surrounding area with 2% cream q.d. for ≥ 2 wk; for seborrheic dermatitis, apply b.i.d. for 4 wk. Shampoo twice weekly for 4 wk, with ≥ 3 days between shampoos, p.r.n. *Topical treatment of tinea infestations* — **Adults and children:** Apply once daily or b.i.d. for about 2 wk; for tinea pedis, apply for 4 wk.	▪ Most patients show improvement soon after treatment begins. ▪ If condition worsens, may have to discontinue and redetermine diagnosis. ▪ For shampoo, wet hair, lather, and massage for 1 min. Rinse and repeat, leaving drug on scalp for 3 min before rinsing.
ketoprofen Actron, Orudi *Nonnarcotic analgesic, antipyretic, anti-inflammatory* Pregnancy Risk Category: B	*Rheumatoid arthritis and osteoarthritis* — **Adults:** 75 mg t.i.d. or 50 mg q.i.d. or 150 to 200 mg as extended-release q.d. Maximum 300 mg/day. *Mild to moderate pain; dysmenorrhea* — **Adults:** 25 to 50 mg P.O. q 6 to 8 hr, p.r.n. *Minor aches and pain or fever* — **Adults:** 12.5 mg q 4 to 6 hr, up to 75 mg in 24 hr.	▪ Check renal and hepatic function q 6 mo or p.r.n. ▪ May mask signs of infection. ▪ Full effect for arthritis may be delayed for 2 to 4 wk. ▪ Warn patient to avoid hazardous activities until CNS effects known. ▪ Give with food to minimize GI adverse effects.
ketorolac tromethamine (ophthalmic) Acular *Ophthalmic anti-inflammatory* Pregnancy Risk Category: C	*Relief of ocular itching caused by seasonal allergic conjunctivitis* — **Adults:** 1 drop instilled into conjunctival sac of each eye q.i.d.	▪ Apply light pressure to lacrimal sac 1 min after instillation. ▪ Store away from heat in dark, tightly closed container and protect from freezing.

ketorolac tromethamine (systemic)
Toradol
Analgesic
Pregnancy Risk Category: C

Short-term management of pain — **Adults < 65 yr:** 60 mg I.M. or 30 mg I.V. as single dose, or multiple doses of 30 mg I.M. or I.V. q 6 hr; maximum 120 mg/day. **Elderly ≥ 65 yr:** 30 mg I.M. or 15 mg I.V. as single dose, or multiple doses of 15 mg I.M. or I.V. q 6 hr; maximum 60 mg/day.

Adjust-a-dose: In renally impaired patients or those weighing > 50 kg (110 lb), give 30 mg I.M. or 15 mg I.V.

Short-term management of moderately severe, acute pain when switching from parenteral to oral therapy — **Adults < 65 yr:** 20 mg P.O. as single dose, then 10 mg P.O. q 4 to 6 hr; maximum 40 mg/day. **Elderly ≥ 65 yr, renally impaired patients, or those < 50 kg:** 10 mg P.O. as single dose; then 10 mg P.O. q 4 to 6 hr; maximum 40 mg/day.

- Limit duration of therapy to 5 days.
- Giving I.M. may cause injection site pain. Apply pressure over site after injection.
- Don't mix with morphine sulfate, meperidine hydrochloride, promethazine hydrochloride, or hydroxyzine hydrochloride.
- Inhibits platelet aggregation and can prolong bleeding time; carefully observe patients with coagulopathies and those taking anticoagulants. Won't alter platelet count, PTT, or PT.
- May mask signs and symptoms of infection.

labetalol hydrochloride
Normodyne, Presolol‡, Trandate
Antihypertensive
Pregnancy Risk Category: C

Hypertension — **Adults:** 100 mg P.O. b.i.d. with or without diuretic. May increase by 100 mg b.i.d. q 2 or 4 days until optimum response reached. Maintenance 200 to 600 mg b.i.d.

Hypertensive emergencies — **Adults:** infuse 0.5 to 2 mg/min and titrate; usual cumulative dose 50 to 200 mg. Or, by repeated I.V. injection: initially, 20 mg I.V. slowly over 2 min. Then repeat injections of 40 to 80 mg q 10 min to maximum 300 mg.

- ***I.V. use:*** Give injection with infusion control device. Monitor BP q 5 min for 30 min, q 30 min for 2 hr, then hourly for 6 hr. Keep patient supine for 3 hr.
- When given I.V. for hypertensive emergencies, produces rapid, predictable BP drop within 5 to 10 min.
- I.V. form incompatible with sodium bicarbonate injection.
- Masks common signs of shock.
- May mask signs of hypoglycemia.

DRUG & CLASS	INDICATIONS & DOSAGES	NURSING CONSIDERATIONS
lactulose Cephalac, Chronulac, Constulose, Duphalac, Enulose, Kristalose, Lactulax† *Laxative, hyperosmotic agent* Pregnancy Risk Category: B	*Constipation* — **Adults:** 10 to 20 g (15 to 30 ml) P.O. q.d., increased to 40 g/day, p.r.n. *Hepatic encephalopathy* — **Adults:** 20 to 30 g P.O. t.i.d. or q.i.d., until 2 or 3 soft stools q.d. Or, 300 ml diluted with 700 ml water or saline solution P.R. and retained for 40 to 60 min q 4 to 6 hr, p.r.n.	▪ To minimize sweet taste, dilute with water or juice or give with food. ▪ Monitor serum sodium for possible hypernatremia, especially when giving to treat hepatic encephalopathy. ▪ Be prepared to replace fluid loss. ▪ Dosage adjustment may be required q 1 to 2 days.
lamivudine Epivir, Epivir-HBV *Antiviral* Pregnancy Risk Category: C	*HIV infection with zidovudine* — **Adults ≥ 50 kg (110 lb); children ≥ 12 yr:** 150 mg P.O. b.i.d. **Adults < 50 kg:** 2 mg/kg P.O. b.i.d. **Children 3 mo to 11 yr:** 4 mg/kg P.O. b.i.d. Maximum 150 mg b.i.d. *Chronic hepatitis B virus (HBV) with evidence of hepatitis B viral replication and active liver inflammation* — **Adults:** 100 mg P.O. q.d. ***Adjust-a-dose:*** Reduce dosage in patients with CrCl < 50 ml/min.	▪ Monitor CBC, platelet count, and LFTs. ▪ Monitor patient for pancreatitis. ▪ Safety and effectiveness of treatment with Epivir-HBV > 1 yr not established. ▪ Test for HIV before starting and during treatment because formulation of lamivudine in Epivir-HBV is not appropriate for those infected with HBV and HIV. ▪ If lamivudine is given to patients with HBV and HIV, higher dose indicated for HIV therapy should be used as part of an appropriate combination regimen. ▪ Inform patient that drug doesn't cure HIV, won't prevent HIV complications, and doesn't reduce risk of HIV transmission.
lamivudine/zidovudine Combivir *Antiviral*	*HIV infection* — **Adults and children ≥ 12 yr weighing > 50 kg (110 lb):** 1 tablet P.O. b.i.d. ***Adjust-a-dose:*** Reduce dosage in patients	▪ Use cautiously in patients with bone marrow suppression. ▪ Notify doctor of signs of lactic acidosis or hepatotoxicity (abdominal pain, jaundice).

Pregnancy Risk Category: C	with CrCl < 50 ml/min	▪ Monitor for bone marrow toxicity. ▪ Assess fine motor skills and peripheral sensation for evidence of peripheral neuropathies.
lamotrigine Lamictal *Anticonvulsant* Pregnancy Risk Category: C	*Adjunct treatment for partial seizures caused by epilepsy* — **Adults:** 50 mg P.O. q.d. for 2 wk, then 100 mg q.d. in 2 divided doses for 2 wk. Usual maintenance dose 300 to 500 mg P.O. q.d. in 2 divided doses. For patients also taking valproic acid, 25 mg P.O. every other day. for 2 wk, then 25 mg P.O. q.d. for 2 wk. Maximum 150 mg P.O. q.d. in 2 divided doses. *Adjunct treatment for Lennox-Gaustaut syndrome* — **Adults and children > 12 yr:** (For patients taking valproic acid) 25 mg P.O. every other day. for 2 wk; then 25 mg P.O. q.d. for 2 wk; maintenance dose is 100 to 400 mg P.O. q.d. in 1 or 2 doses. (For patients taking antiepileptics without valproic acid) 50 mg P.O. q.d. for 2 wk; then 100 mg P.O. q.d. in 2 divided doses for 2 wk; maintenance dose is 300 to 500 mg P.O. q.d. in 2 divided doses. **Children 2 to 12 yr, weighing > 17 kg (37 lb):** (For patients taking valproic acid) 0.15 mg/kg/day P.O. in 1 or 2 doses for 2 wk. If calculated daily dose of lamotrigine is 2.5 to 5 mg, 5 mg of lamotrigine should be taken every other day; then 0.3 mg/kg/day P.O. in 1 or 2 doses for 2 wk.	▪ Don't stop abruptly. Instead, taper over ≥ 2 wk. Check adjunct anticonvulsant serum levels. ▪ Warn patient not to engage in hazardous activities until CNS effects known. ▪ Serious rashes requiring hospitalization and discontinuation of treatment have been reported. ▪ Photosensitivity reactions may occur. Advise patient to take precautions of sunscreen and protective clothing and to avoid direct sunlight exposure.

(continued)

DRUG & CLASS	INDICATIONS & DOSAGES	NURSING CONSIDERATIONS
lamotrigine *(continued)*	Maintenance dose is 1 to 5 mg/kg/day (maximum 200 mg/day in 1 to 2 doses). (For patients taking antiepileptics without valproic acid) 0.6 mg/kg/day P.O. in 2 divided doses for 2 wk; then 1.2 mg/kg/day P.O. in 2 divided doses for 2 wk. Maintenance dose is 5 to 15 mg/kg/day (maximum 400 mg/day in 2 divided doses). ***Adjust-a-dose:*** Lower maintenance doses in patients with severe renal impairment.	
lansoprazole Prevacid *Antiulcer agent* Pregnancy Risk Category: B	*Short-term treatment of active duodenal ulcer* — **Adults:** 15 mg P.O. q.d. before meals for 4 wk. *Short-term treatment of erosive esophagitis* — **Adults:** 30 mg P.O. q.d. before meals for up to 8 wk. If healing doesn't occur, may give for 8 more wk. *Short-term treatment of symptomatic gastroesophageal reflux disease* — **Adults**: 15 mg P.O. q.d. for up to 8 wk. *NSAID-associated ulcer in patients who still use NSAIDs* — **Adults:** 30 mg P.O. q.d. for up to 8 wk. *To reduce risk of NSAID-associated ulcer in patients with a history of gastric ulcer requiring NSAIDs* — **Adults:** 15 mg P.O. q.d. for up to 12 wk.	▪ Instruct patient to take before eating. ▪ May open capsules and sprinkle contents over applesauce. ▪ Breast-feeding may need to be stopped during therapy. ▪ Don't use as maintenance therapy for duodenal ulcer or erosive esophagitis. ▪ Monitor closely if also receiving ampicillin esters, digoxin, iron salts, or ketoconazole. ▪ May inhibit lansoprazole absorption.

latanoprost Xalatan *Antiglaucoma, ocular antihypertensive* Pregnancy Risk Category: C	*Increased IOP in patients with ocular hypertension or open-angle glaucoma who can't tolerate or who respond insufficiently to other IOP-lowering medications* — **Adults:** 1 drop in conjunctival sac of affected eye q.d. in evening.	▪ Don't give while patient is wearing contact lenses. Lenses may be inserted 15 min after drug administration. ▪ Exceeding recommended dosage may decrease IOP-lowering effects. ▪ May gradually change eye color, increasing amount of brown pigment in iris. ▪ If more than one topical ophthalmic drug is used, give drugs $\geq$ 5 min apart.
leflunomide Arava *Antiproliferative, anti-inflammatory* Pregnancy Risk Category: X	*To reduce signs and symptoms and to retard structural damage (X-ray erosions and joint space narrowing) in active rheumatoid arthritis* — **Adults:** 100 mg P.O. q 24 hr for 3 days, then 20 mg (maximum daily dose) P.O. q 24 hr. Dose may be decreased to 10 mg q.d. if higher dose not well-tolerated.	▪ Use cautiously in patients with renal insufficiency. ▪ ***ALERT*** Men planning to father a child should discontinue therapy and follow recommended leflunomide removal protocol. ▪ Monitor liver enzymes before starting therapy and monthly thereafter until stable.
letrozole Femara *Hormone, antineoplastic* Pregnancy Risk Category: D	*Metastatic breast cancer in postmenopausal women with disease progression after antiestrogen therapy* — **Adults:** 2.5 mg P.O. as a single daily dose.	▪ No dosage adjustment needed in renally impaired patients with CrCl $\geq$ 10 ml/min. ▪ Use cautiously in patients with severe liver impairment. ▪ May give without regard to meals.
leucovorin calcium (citrovorum factor, folinic acid) Wellcovorin *Vitamin, antidote* Pregnancy Risk Category: C	*Overdose of folic acid antagonist* — **Adults and children:** I.M. or I.V. dose equivalent to weight of antagonist given. *Leucovorin rescue after high methotrexate dose* — **Adults and children:** 10 mg/m^2 P.O., I.M., or I.V. q 6 hr until methotrexate levels $< 5 \times 10^{-8}$ M.	▪ ***I.V. use:*** When using powder for injection, reconstitute 50-mg vial with 5 ml, 100-mg vial with 10 ml, or 350-mg vial with 17 ml sterile or bacteriostatic water for injection. With doses > 10 mg/m^2, don't use diluents containing benzyl alcohol. ▪ Don't exceed 160 mg/min *(continued)*

DRUG & CLASS	INDICATIONS & DOSAGES	NURSING CONSIDERATIONS
leucovorin calcium *(continued)*	*Megaloblastic anemia caused by congenital enzyme deficiency* — **Adults and children:** 3 to 6 mg I.M. q.d. *Folate-deficient megaloblastic anemia* — **Adults and children:** up to 1 mg I.M. q.d.	when giving by direct injection. ▪ Don't confuse folinic acid with folic acid. ▪ Don't give along with systemic methotrexate. ▪ Give parenterally if patient has GI toxicity, nausea, and vomiting, and dose > 25 mg.
levalbuterol Xopenex *Short-acting sympathomimetic bronchodilator* Pregnancy Risk Category: C	*Treatment or prevention of bronchospasm in patients with reversible obstructive airway disease* — **Adults and children ≥ 12 yr:** 0.63 mg t.i.d. by nebulization. **Elderly:** Safety and efficacy of drug may differ in patients < 65 yr and patients ≥ 65 yr. Start patients ≥ 65 yr at 0.63 mg. ***Adjust-a-dose:*** Patients with more severe asthma who don't respond adequately to dose of 0.63 mg may benefit from dosage of 1.25 mg t.i.d.	▪ ***ALERT*** Can produce life-threatening paradoxical bronchospasm. If this occurs, stop immediately. ▪ Can produce clinically significant CV effects and ECG changes; use with caution in patients with CV disorders, especially coronary artery insufficiency, arrhythmias, and hypertension. ▪ Protect unit-dose vials from light and excessive heat. ▪ Keep unopened vials in foil pouch. After foil pouch is opened, use vials within 2 wk. ▪ Discard vial if solution is not colorless.
levetiracetam Keppra *Anticonvulsant* Pregnancy RiskCategory: C	*Adjunct treatment for partial seizures* — **Adults:** initially, 500 mg b.i.d. Dosage can be increased by 500 mg b.i.d., p.r.n., for seizure control at 2-wk intervals to maximum dose of 1,500 mg b.i.d. ***Adjust-a-dose:*** For patients with renal failure, if CrCl is > 80, give 500 to 1,500 mg q	▪ Reduce dosage in patients with poor renal function. ▪ Leukopenia and neutropenia have been reported with drug use. Use cautiously in immunocompromised patients (such as those with cancer or HIV infection). ▪ Seizures can occur if drug is stopped

	12 hr; if CrCl is 50 to 80, give 500 to 1,000 mg q 12 hr; if CrCl is 30 to 50, give 250 to 750 mg q 12 hr; if CrCl is < 30, give 250 to 500 mg q 12 hr. For dialysis patients, give 500 to 1,000 mg q 24 hr. A 250- to 500-mg dose should be given after dialysis.	abruptly. Tapering is recommended. ▪ Monitor patients closely for dizziness, which may lead to falls, especially in elderly population. ▪ Use only with other anticonvulsants; not recommended for monotherapy.
levobunolol hydrochloride Betagan *Antiglaucoma agent* Pregnancy Risk Category: C	*Chronic open-angle glaucoma and ocular hypertension* — **Adults:** 1 to 2 drops q.d. (0.5%) or b.i.d. (0.25%).	▪ Apply light pressure to lacrimal sac for 1 min after instilling. ▪ Don't let dropper touch eye or surrounding tissue. ▪ If patient is taking other ophthalmic topical drugs, give ≥ 5 min apart.
levodopa Larodopa *Antiparkinsonian* Pregnancy Risk Category: C	*Parkinsonism* — **Adults:** initially, 0.5 to 1 g P.O. once daily, b.i.d., t.i.d., or q.i.d. with food; increase by ≤ 0.75 g daily q 3 to 7 days, as tolerated; usual optimal dose 3 to 6 g q.d. divided into 3 doses. Don't exceed 8 g daily. Significant therapeutic response may take 6 mo.	▪ Report muscle twitching. ▪ With long-term therapy, test regularly for diabetes and acromegaly; periodically monitor renal, liver, and hematopoietic function. ▪ Multivitamins, fortified cereals, and OTC medications may block drug effects.
levodopa-carbidopa Sinemet, Sinemet CR *Antiparkinsonian* Pregnancy Risk Category: C	*Idiopathic Parkinson's disease; postencephalitic parkinsonism; symptomatic parkinsonism resulting from carbon monoxide or manganese intoxication* — **Adults:** 1 tablet 25 mg carbidopa/100 mg levodopa P.O. t.i.d.; then increase by 1 tablet q.d. or every other day p.r.n., up to 8 tablets q.d. May substitute 25 mg carbidopa/250 mg levodopa or 10 mg carbidopa/100 mg levodopa tablet p.r.n. to	▪ ***ALERT*** Muscle twitching and blepharospasm may be early signs of overdose. ▪ Discontinue levodopa at least 8 hr before starting levodopa-carbidopa. ▪ Therapeutic and adverse reactions more rapid with levodopa-carbidopa than with levodopa alone. Monitor vital signs, especially while adjusting dosage. ▪ Tell patient not to crush *(continued)*

DRUG & CLASS	INDICATIONS & DOSAGES	NURSING CONSIDERATIONS
levodopa-carbidopa *(continued)*	obtain maximum response. Optimum dosage determined by individual titration. Patients treated with conventional tablets may receive extended-release tablets; dosage calculated on current levodopa intake. Extended-release tablet dosage should initially amount to 10% more levodopa per day, increased p.r.n. and as tolerated to 30% more per day. Give in divided doses at intervals of 4 to 8 hr.	or chew sustained-release tablets, although they may be broken in half. ▪ With long-term therapy, patient should be tested regularly for diabetes and acromegaly and for liver, renal, and hematopoietic function.
levofloxacin Levaquin *Antibiotic* Pregnancy Risk Category: C	*Acute maxillary sinusitis from susceptible organisms* — **Adults:** 500 mg P.O. or I.V. q.d. for 10 to 14 days. *Acute exacerbation of chronic bronchitis from susceptible organisms* — **Adults:** 500 mg P.O. or I.V. q.d. for 7 days. *Community-acquired pneumonia from susceptible organisms* — **Adults:** 500 mg P.O. or I.V. q.d. for 7 to 14 days. *Mild to moderate skin infections from susceptible organisms* — **Adults:** 500 mg P.O. or I.V. q.d. for 7 to 10 days. *UTIs from susceptible organisms* — **Adults:** 250 mg P.O. or I.V. q.d. for 10 days. *Acute pyelonephritis from* E. coli — **Adults:** 250 mg P.O. or I.V. q.d. for 10 days. *Mild to moderate uncomplicated urinary tract infection from* Escherichia coli, Klebsiella pneumoniae, *or* Staphylococcus sapro-	▪ ***I.V. use:*** Give injection by I.V. infusion only. Dilute drug in single-use vials according to manufacturer's instructions. Reconstituted solution should be clear and slightly yellow. Don't mix with other medications. Infuse over 60 min. ▪ Discontinue and notify doctor if symptoms of excessive CNS stimulation occur. Institute seizure precautions. Use cautiously in renal impairment. ▪ Notify doctor if diarrhea occurs. ▪ Monitor blood glucose level and renal, hepatic, and hematopoietic studies. ▪ If patient is taking antacids, give 1 hr before or 2 hr after.

	phyticus—**Adults:** 250 mg P.O. daily. *Complicated skin and skin-structure infections from methicillin-sensitive* Staphylococcus aureus, Enterococcus faecalis, Streptococcus pyogenes, *or* Proteus mirabilis — **Adults:** 750 mg P.O. or I.V. infusion over 90 min q 24 hr for 7 to 14 days.	
levonorgestrel Norplant System *Contraceptive* Pregnancy Risk Category: X	*Prevention of pregnancy* — **Women:** 6 capsules implanted subdermally in midportion of upper arm, about 8 cm above elbow crease, during first 7 days of menses. Capsules placed in fanlike position, 15° apart (total of 75°). Contraceptive efficacy lasts for 5 yr.	▪ Irregular bleeding may mask symptoms of cervical or endometrial cancer. ▪ Expect implant to be removed if patient develops active thrombophlebitis or thromboembolic disease, will be immobilized for significant time, or jaundice develops.
levothyroxine sodium (T_4 or L-thyroxine sodium) Eltroxin†, Levo-T, Levothroid, Levoxine, Levoxyl, Synthroid *Thyroid hormone replacement* Pregnancy Risk Category: A	*Myxedema coma* — **Adults:** 200 to 500 mcg I.V.; if no response in 24 hr, give 100 to 300 mcg I.V. Maintenance dose 50 to 200 mcg I.V. q.d. *Thyroid hormone replacement* — **Adults:** initially, 50 mcg P.O. q.d., increased by 25 to 50 mcg P.O. q.d. q 2 to 4 wk. Maximum dose 200 mcg/day. May give I.V. or I.M. if unable to take P.O., but initial parenteral dose should be 50% of established oral dose. **Elderly:** 12.5 to 50 mcg P.O. q.d. Increase by 12.5 to 25 mcg at 2- to 8-wk intervals, p.r.n. **Children > 12 yr:** over 150 mcg or 2 to 3 mcg/kg/day. **Children 6 to 12 yr:** 100 to 150 mcg, or 4 to 5 mcg/kg/day. **Children 1 to 5 yr:** 75 to 100 mcg or 5 to 6 mcg/kg/day.	▪ ***ALERT*** Rapid replacement in arteriosclerotic patients may trigger angina, coronary occlusion, or CVA; use cautiously. ▪ ***I.V. use:*** Prepare I.V. dose immediately before injection. Don't mix with other solutions. Inject into vein over 1 to 2 min. ▪ Monitor BP and HR closely. Normal serum T_4 levels should occur within 24 hr; then threefold increase in serum liothyronine (T_3) in 3 days. ▪ When switching *to* T_3, stop T_4 and begin T_3. Increase dose in small increments after residual effects of T_4 disappear. When switching *from* T_3, start T_4 several days before withdrawing T_3. ▪ Discontinue 4 wk before *(continued)*

DRUG & CLASS	INDICATIONS & DOSAGES	NURSING CONSIDERATIONS
levothyroxine sodium *(continued)*	**Children 6 to 12 mo:** 50 to 75 mcg or 6 to 8 mcg/kg/day. **Children < 6 mo:** 25 to 50 mcg or 8 to 10 mcg/kg/day.	radioactive iodine uptake studies.
lidocaine hydrochloride (lignocaine hydrochloride) LidoPen Auto-Injector, Xylocaine *Ventricular antiarrhythmic, local anesthetic* Pregnancy Risk Category: B	*Ventricular arrhythmias from MI, cardiac manipulation, or cardiac glycosides* — **Adults:** 50 to 100 mg (1 to 1.5 mg/kg) by I.V. bolus at 25 to 50 mg/min. Repeat bolus dose q 5 to 10 min until arrhythmias subside or adverse reactions develop. Don't exceed 300-mg total bolus over 1-hr period. Simultaneously, begin constant infusion of 20 to 50 mcg/kg/min (1 to 4 mg/min). **Elderly:** reduce dose and rate of infusion by 50%. **Children:** 0.5 to 1 mg/kg by I.V. bolus, then infusion of 20 to 50 mcg/kg/min. ***Adjust-a-dose:*** In patients with heart failure or renal or liver disease or in those weighing < 50 kg (110 lb), reduce dosage.	▪ ***I.V. use:*** Patient must be on cardiac monitor. Use infusion control device. Don't exceed rate of 4 mg/min. Seizures may be first clinical sign of toxicity. Therapeutic levels 2 to 5 mcg/ml. ▪ If signs of toxicity occur, stop drug immediately and notify doctor. Keep oxygen and resuscitative equipment available. ▪ Stop infusion and notify doctor if arrhythmias worsen or ECG changes appear. ▪ Give I.M. injections in deltoid muscle only. ▪ Monitor patient response, especially BP, and electrolyte, BUN, and creatinine levels.
lindane GBH†, G-well, Kwellada†, Scabene *Scabicide, pediculicide* Pregnancy Risk Category: B	*Parasitic infestation (scabies, pediculosis)* — **Adults and children:** apply thin layer of cream or lotion over entire skin surface (with special attention to folds, creases, interdigital spaces, and genital area) for scabies, or to hairy areas for pediculosis. After 8 to 12 hr, wash off drug. Repeat in 1 wk if mites appear or new lesions develop. Apply shampoo undiluted to affected area and work into lather for 4 to 5 min.	▪ Apply topical corticosteroids or give oral antihistamines for pruritus. ▪ Don't apply to face, eyes, or mucous membranes, or areas with open cuts or extensive excoriation. ▪ Place hospitalized patient in isolation, with special linen-handling precautions. ▪ Wash drug off skin and notify doctor immediately if skin irritation or hypersensitivity develops.

- In case of accidental contact with eyes, flush with water and notify doctor.
- Inform patient that sexual partners must also be treated.
- Wear gloves when applying.
- Patient shouldn't bathe before applying; if patient bathes, let skin dry and cool thoroughly before using.

---

linezolid
Zyvox
Antibiotic
Pregnancy Risk Category: C

Vancomycin-resistant Enterococcus faecium *infections, including cases with concurrent bacteremia* — **Adults:** 600 mg I.V. or P.O. (tablets or suspension) q 12 hr for 14 to 28 days.
Nosocomial pneumonia caused by Staphylococcus aureus *(methicillin-susceptible [MSSA] and methicillin-resistant [MRSA] strains), or* Streptococcus pneumoniae *(penicillin-susceptible strains only)* — **Adults:** 600 mg I.V. or P.O. (tablets or suspension) q 12 hr for 10 to 14 days.
Complicated skin and skin structure infections caused by S. aureus *(MSSA and MSRA),* Streptococcus pyogenes, *or* Streptococcus agalactiae — **Adults:** 600 mg I.V. or P.O. (tablets or suspension) q 12 hr for 10 to 14 days.
Uncomplicated skin and skin-structure infections caused by S. aureus *(MSSA only) or* S. pyogenes — **Adults:** 400 mg P.O. (tablets or suspension) q 12 hr for 10 to 14 days.

- Get samples for culture and sensitivity testing before starting linezolid therapy. Sensitivity results should be used to guide subsequent therapy.
- Reconstitute the oral suspension according to the manufacturer's instructions. The reconstituted suspension should be stored at room temperature and used within 21 days.
- Superinfection may occur. Consider this diagnosis and institute appropriate measures in patients who develop secondary infections.
- ***I.V. use:*** Inspect for particulate matter and leaks.
- Infuse over 30 to 120 min. Don't infuse linezolid in a series connection.
- Linezolid is compatible with the following I.V. solutions: 5% dextrose injection, USP; 0.9% sodium chloride injection, USP; and lactated Ringer's injection, USP.
- Don't inject additives into *(continued)*

DRUG & CLASS	INDICATIONS & DOSAGES	NURSING CONSIDERATIONS
linezolid *(continued)*	*Community-acquired pneumonia caused by* S. pneumoniae *(penicillin-susceptible strains only), including case with concurrent bacteremia, or* S aureus*(MSSA only)* — **Adults**: 600 mg I.V. or P.O. (tablets or suspension) q 12 hr for 10 to 14 days.	the infusion bag. Give concomitant I.V. medications separately or via a separate I.V. line to avoid physical incompatibilities. If a single I.V. line is used, flush line before and after linezolid infusion with a compatible solution.
liothyronine sodium (T_3) Cyronine, Cytomel, *Thyroid hormone replacement* Pregnancy Risk Category: A	*Cretinism* — **Children:** 5 mcg P.O. q.d. with 5-mcg increase q 3 to 4 days, p.r.n. *Myxedema* — **Adults:** initially, 5 mcg P.O. q.d., increased by 5 to 10 mcg q 1 or 2 wk. Maintenance dose 50 to 100 mcg q.d. *Myxedema coma; premyxedema coma* — **Adults:** initially, 10 to 20 mcg I.V. for known or suspected CV disease; 25 to 50 mcg I.V. for patients without known CV disease. *Nontoxic goiter* — **Adults:** initially, 5 mcg P.O. q.d.; increase by 5 to 10 mcg q.d. q 1 to 2 wk. May increase by 12.5 or 25 mcg q.d. q 1 to 2 wk. Maintenance: 75 mcg q.d. *Thyroid hormone replacement* — **Adults:** initially, 25 mcg P.O. q.d., increased by 12.5 to 25 mcg q 1 to 2 wk, p.r.n. Maintenance: 25 to 75 mcg q.d. **Elderly:** 5 mcg q.d., increased in 5-mcg daily increments.	▪ Rapid replacement in patients with arteriosclerosis may trigger angina, coronary occlusion, or CVA; use cautiously. In patients with CAD, observe carefully for possible coronary insufficiency. ▪ Alters thyroid function tests. Monitor PT; decreased anticoagulant dosage usually required. ▪ When switching *from* levothyroxine (T_4), stop that drug and start T_3 at low dosage. Increase dosage in small increments after residual effects of T_4 disappear. When switching *to* T_4, start T_4 several days before withdrawing T_3. ▪ Discontinue 7 to 10 days before radioactive iodine uptake studies.
lisinopril Prinivil, Zestril *Antihypertensive*	*Hypertension* — **Adults:** initially, 5 to 10 mg P.O. q.d. Most patients well controlled on 20 to 40 mg q.d. as single dose.	▪ Monitor BP often. If drug doesn't adequately control BP, may add diuretic. ▪ Monitor WBC with differential before ther-

Pregnancy Risk Category: C (1st trimester); D (2nd and 3rd trimesters)	***Adjust-a-dose:*** In patients receiving a diuretic, give 5 mg P.O. q.d. *Adjunct treatment in heart failure (with diuretics and cardiac glycosides)* — **Adults:** initially, 5 mg P.O. q.d. Most patients well controlled on 5 to 20 mg q.d. as single dose. *Acute MI* — **Adults:** initially, 5 mg P.O., followed by 5 mg in 24 hr, 10 mg in 48 hr, and then 10 mg q.d. for 6 wk. In patients with low systolic BP (≤ 120) when treatment starts or during first 3 days after MI, reduce to 2.5 mg P.O. If systolic BP ≤ 100, may reduce daily maintenance dose from 5 mg to 2.5 mg.	apy, every 2 wk for 3 mo, and then periodically. Monitor serum electrolytes. ▪ When used in acute MI, patient should receive standard treatment, as appropriate (thrombolytics, aspirin, beta blockers). ▪ Angioedema (including laryngeal edema) may occur, especially after first dose. Advise patient to report breathing difficulty or swelling of face, eyes, lips, or tongue. ▪ Light-headedness may occur, especially in first few days. Tell patient to rise slowly and report symptoms. Advise to stop drug and call doctor immediately if fainting occurs.
lithium carbonate Carbolith†, Eskalith CR, Lithane, Lithicarb‡, Lithobid, Lithonate, Lithotabs **lithium citrate** Cibalith-S *Antimanic agent, antipsychotic* Pregnancy Risk Category: D	*Prevention or control of mania* — **Adults:** 300 to 600 mg P.O. up to q.i.d., or 900 mg (Eskalith CR tablets) P.O. q 12 hr; increase on basis of serum levels to achieve optimal dosage.	▪ Serum drug level measurements are crucial to safe use. Monitor weekly to monthly during maintenance therapy. ▪ Monitor electrolyte levels and baseline ECG, thyroid, and renal studies. ▪ Instruct patient to inform doctor of adverse effects. ▪ May alter glucose tolerance in diabetics. ▪ Check fluid I&O. Weigh daily; check for edema or sudden weight gain. ▪ Warn ambulatory patient to avoid hazardous activities until CNS effects known. ▪ Give with food or milk to lessen GI upset.
lomefloxacin hydrochloride Maxaquin	*Acute bacterial exacerbations of chronic bronchitis, uncomplicated UTI (cystitis), and complicated UTI from susceptible or-*	▪ Obtain culture and sensitivity tests before 1st dose. Begin therapy pending results. ▪ Photosensitization and *(continued)*

†Canadian ‡Australian

DRUG & CLASS	INDICATIONS & DOSAGES	NURSING CONSIDERATIONS
lomefloxacin hydrochloride *(continued)* *Broad-spectrum antibiotic* Pregnancy Risk Category: C	*ganisms* — **Adults:** 400 mg P.O. q.d. for 10 to 14 days. ***Adjust-a-dose:*** In patients with CrCl of 10 to 40 ml/min, give loading dose of 400 mg P.O. on day 1, followed by 200 mg q.d. for duration of therapy. *Prophylaxis of UTI after transrectal prostate biopsy* — **Adults:** 400 mg P.O. as single dose 1 to 6 hr before procedure.	phototoxicity may occur. ▪ Prolonged use may cause overgrowth of resistant organisms. ▪ Warn patient to avoid hazardous tasks until CNS effects known. ▪ Drug interactions possible with antacids, sucralfate, cimetidine, probenecid, warfarin, or cyclosporine. Give these ≥ 4 hr before or 2 hr after lomefloxacin.
lomustine (CCNU) CeeNU *Antineoplastic* Pregnancy Risk Category: D	*Brain tumor; Hodgkin's disease* — **Adults and children:** 100 to 130 mg/m² P.O. as single dose q 6 wk. Reduce dosage according to degree of bone marrow suppression. Don't repeat doses until WBC count > 4,000/mm³ and platelet count > 100,000/mm³.	▪ Give 2 to 4 hr after meals for more complete absorption. ▪ Monitor CBC weekly. Usually not given more often than q 6 wk; bone marrow toxicity cumulative and delayed, usually occurring 4 to 6 wk after drug is taken. ▪ Periodically monitor LFT results.
loperamide Imodium A-D, Kaopectate II Caplets *Antidiarrheal* Pregnancy Risk Category: B	*Acute, nonspecific diarrhea* — **Adults and children > age 12:** initially, 4 mg P.O., then 2 mg after each unformed stool. Maximum 16 mg q.d. **Children 9 to 11 yr:** 2 mg t.i.d. on 1st day. **Children 6 to 8 yr:** 2 mg b.i.d. on 1st day. **Children 2 to 5 yr:** 1 mg t.i.d. on 1st day. Maintenance dose ⅓ to ½ of initial dose.	▪ In acute diarrhea, tell patient to stop and call doctor if no improvement within 48 hr. In chronic diarrhea, tell him to stop and call doctor if no improvement after taking 16 mg q.d. for ≥ 10 days. ▪ Advise patient with acute colitis to stop drug immediately.
loracarbef Lorabid *Antibiotic* Pregnancy Risk Category: B	*Acute bacterial exacerbations of chronic bronchitis* — **Adults and children ≥ 13:** 400 mg P.O. q 12 hr for 7 days. *Pharyngitis; sinusitis; tonsillitis* — **Adults and**	▪ Obtain specimen for culture and sensitivity tests before 1st dose. ▪ Monitor patient for superinfection. ▪ To reconstitute powder for oral suspen-

	children ≥ **13 yr:** 200 mg P.O. q 12 hr for 10 days. **Children 6 mo to 12 yr:** 15 mg/kg P.O. q.d. in divided doses q 12 hr for 10 days. *Acute otitis media* — **Children 6 mo to 12 yr:** 15 mg/kg (oral suspension) P.O. q 12 hr for 10 days. *Skin and skin-structure infections* — **Adults and children** ≥ **13 yr:** 200 mg P.O. q 12 hr. **Children 6 mo to 12 yr:** 7.5 mg P.O. q 12 hr for 7 days. ***Adjust-a-dose:*** In patients with CrCl of 10 to 49 ml/min, give 50% usual dose at same interval; for CrCl < 10 ml/min, give usual dose q 3 to 5 days.	sion, add 30 ml water in 2 portions to 50-ml bottle or 60 ml water in 2 portions to 100-ml bottle; shake after each addition. After reconstitution, store oral suspension for 14 days at 59° to 86° F (15° to 30° C). ▪ Monitor patient for seizures. If seizures occur, stop and notify doctor. Give anticonvulsants.
loratadine Claratyne‡, Claritin *Antihistaminic* Pregnancy Risk Category: B	*Symptomatic treatment of seasonal allergic rhinitis* — **Adults and children** ≥ **6 yr:** 10 mg P.O. q.d. **Children 2 to 5 yr:** 5 mg P.O. q.d. *Chronic idiopathic urticaria* — **Children 2 to 5 yr:** 5 mg P.O. q.d. ***Adjust-a-dose:*** In patients with liver failure or glomerular filtration rate < 30 ml/min, initially, give 10 mg every other day.	▪ May affect allergy skin tests results. ▪ Tell patient to stop drug 7 days before allergy skin tests to preserve test accuracy.
lorazepam Apo-Lorazepam†, Ativan, Lorazepam Intensol, Novo-Lorazem†, Nu-Loraz† *Anxiolytic, sedative-hypnotic* Pregnancy Risk Category: D	*Anxiety; agitation; irritability* — **Adults:** 2 to 6 mg P.O. q.d. in divided doses. Maximum 10 mg/day. Or, 0.05 mg/kg up to 4 mg I.M. q.d. in divided doses, or 0.044 to 0.05 mg/kg up to 4 mg I.V. q.d. in divided doses. *Insomnia from anxiety* — **Adults:** 2 to 4 mg P.O. h.s.	▪ Monitor respirations q 5 to 15 min and before each repeated I.V. dose. Have resuscitation equipment and oxygen available. ▪ ***I.V. use:*** Give slowly, > 2 mg/min. Dilute with equal volume of sterile water for injection, 0.9% NaCl for injection, or D_5W. ▪ Reduce dose in elderly or *(continued)*

†Canadian ‡Australian

DRUG & CLASS	INDICATIONS & DOSAGES	NURSING CONSIDERATIONS
lorazepam *(continued)* Controlled Substance Schedule: IV	*Preoperative sedation* — **Adults:** 0.05 mg/kg I.M. 2 hr before procedure. Maximum 4 mg. Or, 0.044 mg/kg (maximum total dose 2 mg) I.V., 15 to 20 min before surgery. In adults < 50 yr, may give 0.05 mg/kg (maximum 4 mg) if increased lack of recall of preoperative events desired.	debilitated patients. ▪ Inject I.M. doses deeply into muscle. ▪ With repeated or prolonged therapy, monitor liver, renal, and hematopoietic function studies periodically. ▪ Possibility of abuse and addiction exists. ▪ Don't withdraw abruptly after long-term use; withdrawal symptoms may occur. ▪ Instruct patient to avoid alcohol.
losartan potassium Cozaar *Antihypertensive* Pregnancy Risk Category: C (1st trimester), D (2nd and 3rd trimesters)	*Hypertension* — **Adults:** initially, 25 to 50 mg P.O. q.d. Maximum 100 mg q.d., given once daily or b.i.d. ***Adjust-a-dose:*** In patients with hepatic impairment and intravascular volume depletion, initially, give 25 mg.	▪ If pregnancy suspected, notify doctor. ▪ Monitor BP closely to evaluate effectiveness. ▪ Closely monitor patient with severe heart failure; acute renal failure possible. ▪ Tell patient to avoid sodium substitutes. ▪ Regularly assess renal function.
lovastatin (mevinolin) Mevacor *Cholesterol-lowering agent, antilipemic* Pregnancy Risk Category: X	*Reduction of LDL and total cholesterol in primary hypercholesterolemia (types IIa and IIb)* — **Adults:** initially, 20 mg P.O. q.d. with evening meal. For patients with cholesterol > 300 mg/dl, initial dose 40 mg. Range 20 to 80 mg q.d. in single or divided doses. *Prevention of CAD in patients without symptomatic CV disease and with elevated total LDL and cholesterol and decreased HDL cholesterol* — **Adults:** 20 mg P.O. q.d. with evening meal; dosing range is 10 to 80 mg q.d. in single or divided doses.	▪ Initiate only after diet and other nonpharmacologic therapies prove ineffective. Patient should be on low-cholesterol diet. ▪ Obtain LFT results at start of therapy and periodically thereafter. ▪ Inform women that drug contraindicated during pregnancy. ▪ Advise patient to have periodic eye exams.

	Adjust-a-dose: Reduce dosage in patients with CrCl < 30 ml/min.	
loxapine hydrochloride Loxapac†, Loxitane, Loxitane C, Loxitane IM **loxapine succinate** Loxapac†, Loxitane *Antipsychotic* Pregnancy Risk Category: C	*Psychotic disorders* — **Adults:** 10 mg P.O. b.i.d. to q.i.d., rapidly increased to 60 to 100 mg P.O. q.d. for most patients; dosage varies among individuals. If patient can't take oral dose, 12.5 to 50 mg I.M. q 4 to 6 hr or longer, both dose and interval depending on patient response. Don't give > 250 mg/day.	▪ Obtain baseline BP before therapy and monitor regularly. ▪ Dilute liquid concentrate with orange or grapefruit juice just before giving. ▪ Monitor for tardive dyskinesia. May treat acute dystonic reactions with diphenhydramine. ▪ Monitor for neuroleptic malignant syndrome. ▪ Warn patient to avoid hazardous activities until CNS effects known.
Lyme disease vaccine (recombinant OspA) LYMErix *Vaccine* Pregnancy Risk Category: C	*Active immunization against Lyme disease* — **Adults and children ≥ 15 yr:** 30 mcg I.M.; repeat dose at 1 and 12 mo after 1st dose. Safety and efficacy based on giving 2nd and 3rd doses several wk before *Borrelia burgdorferi* transmission season.	▪ Review history for vaccine adverse reactions. Have epinephrine available. ▪ Vaccine should be turbid white suspension; if not, discard. Discard any unused vaccine. ▪ Give I.M. injection in deltoid region.
magaldrate (aluminum-magnesium complex) Antiflux†, Losopan, Riopan *Antacid* Pregnancy Risk Category: C	*Antacid* — **Adults:** 480 to 960 mg P.O. (or 5 to 10 ml P.O. of suspension) with water between meals and h.s.; or 1 to 2 chewable tablets (chewed before swallowing) between meals and h.s.	▪ Monitor serum magnesium in mild renal impairment. Symptomatic hypermagnesemia usually occurs only in severe renal failure. ▪ Not typically used in renal failure to help control hypophosphatemia. ▪ Very low sodium content; good choice for patients on restricted sodium intake.

DRUG & CLASS	INDICATIONS & DOSAGES	NURSING CONSIDERATIONS
magnesium chloride Slow-Mag **magnesium sulfate** *Anticonvulsant* Pregnancy Risk Category: B	*Mild hypomagnesemia* — **Adults:** 1 g I.V. by piggyback or I.M. q 6 hr for 4 doses, depending on serum magnesium level. Or, 3 g P.O. q 6 hr for 4 doses. *Severe hypomagnesemia (serum magnesium 0.8 mEq/L or less, with symptoms)* — **Adults:** 2 to 5 g I.V. in 1 L solution over 3 hr. Subsequent doses depend on serum magnesium levels. *Magnesium supplementation* — **Adults:** 54 to 483 mg/day in divided doses.	▪ ***I.V. use:*** Inject I.V. bolus dose slowly, using infusion pump for continuous infusion. Maximum infusion rate 150 mg/min. ▪ When giving I.V. for severe hypomagnesemia, watch for respiratory depression and signs of heart block. Respirations should be > 16 before giving dose. ▪ Monitor I&O. ▪ Test knee-jerk and patellar reflexes before each additional dose. If absent, notify doctor and withhold drug until reflexes return. ▪ Incompatible with alkalis.
magnesium citrate (citrate of magnesia) Citroma, Citro-Mag†, Citro-Nesia, Evac-Q-Mag **magnesium hydroxide (milk of magnesia)** Milk of Magnesia, Phillips' Milk of Magnesia **magnesium sulfate (epsom salts)** *Antacid, antiulcer agent, laxative* Pregnancy Risk Category: B	*Constipation; to evacuate bowel before surgery* — **Adults and children ≥ 12 yr:** 11 to 25 g magnesium citrate P.O. q.d.; 2.4 to 4.8 g (30 to 60 ml) magnesium hydroxide P.O. q.d.; 10 to 30 g magnesium sulfate P.O. q.d. **Children 6 to 11 yr:** 5.5 to 12.5 g magnesium citrate P.O. q.d.; 1.2 to 2.4 g (15 to 30 ml) magnesium hydroxide P.O. q.d.; 5 to 10 g magnesium sulfate P.O. q.d. **Children 2 to 5 yr:** 2.7 to 6.25 g magnesium citrate P.O. q.d.; 0.4 to 1.2 g (5 to 15 ml) magnesium hydroxide P.O. q.d.; 2.5 to 5 g magnesium sulfate P.O. q.d. *Note:* All doses may be single or divided. *Antacid* — **Adults:** 5 to 15 ml milk of magnesia P.O. t.i.d. or q.i.d.	▪ Produces watery stools in 3 to 6 hr. Time doses so drug won't interfere with scheduled activities or sleep. ▪ Before giving for constipation, determine if patient has adequate fluid intake, exercise, and diet. ▪ Chill magnesium citrate before use to make more palatable. ▪ Shake suspension well; give with large amount of water when used as laxative. ▪ May accumulate in patients with renal insufficiency. ▪ Monitor serum electrolyte levels during prolonged use.

magnesium oxide Mag-Ox 400, Maox 420, Uro-Mag *Antacid, laxative* Pregnancy Risk Category: B	*Antacid* — **Adults:** 140 mg P.O. with water or milk after meals and h.s. *Laxative* — **Adults:** 4 g P.O. with water or milk, usually h.s. *Oral replacement therapy in mild hypomagnesemia* — **Adults:** 400 to 840 mg P.O. q.d.	▪ Monitor serum magnesium. With prolonged use and renal impairment, watch for symptoms of hypermagnesemia (hypotension, nausea, vomiting, depressed reflexes, respiratory depression, and coma). ▪ If diarrhea occurs, use another drug.
magnesium salicylate Doan's, Magan, Mobidin, Momentum Muscular Backache Formula, Bayer Select Maximum Strength Backache Pain Relief Formula *Nonnarcotic analgesic, antipyretic, anti-inflammatory* Pregnancy Risk Category: NR	*Arthritis* — **Adults:** 545 mg to 1.2 g P.O. t.i.d. or q.i.d. *Mild pain or fever* — **Adults and children > 11 yr:** 300 to 600 mg P.O. q 4 hr, not to exceed 3.5 g/day.	▪ Don't give to children or teenagers with chickenpox or flulike illness. ▪ ***ALERT*** Febrile, dehydrated children can develop toxicity rapidly. ▪ Therapeutic level in arthritis 10 to 30 mg/100 ml. With chronic therapy, mild toxicity may occur at 20 mg/100 ml. ▪ Monitor Hgb and PT in long-term, high-dose treatment.
magnesium sulfate *Anticonvulsant* Pregnancy Risk Category: A	*Prevention or control of seizures in preeclampsia or eclampsia* — **Adults:** 4 g I.V. in 250 ml D_5W and 4 to 5 g deep I.M. each buttock; then 4 g deep I.M. alternate buttock q 4 hr, p.r.n. Or, 4 g I.V. loading dose, then 1 to 2 g/hr as I.V. infusion. Maximum 40 g/day. *Hypomagnesemia; seizures* — **Adults:** 1 to 2 g (as 10% solution) I.V. over 15 min, then 1 g I.M. q 4 to 6 hr, per response and drug levels. *Seizures, hypomagnesemia associated with acute nephritis in children* — **Children**: 0.2 ml/kg 50% solution I.M. q 4 to 6 hr, p.r.n., or 100 to 200 mg/kg 1% to 3% solution I.V.	▪ ***I.V. use:*** If necessary, dilute to maximum concentration of 20%. Infuse no faster than 150 mg/min (1.5 ml/min of 10% solution or 0.75 ml/min of 20% solution). Compatible with D_5W. ▪ Monitor vital signs q 15 min when giving I.V. Watch for respiratory depression and signs of heart block. ▪ Keep I.V. calcium gluconate on hand to reverse magnesium intoxication; however, use cautiously in patients undergoing digitalization. ▪ Check serum magnesium *(continued)*

DRUG & CLASS	INDICATIONS & DOSAGES	NURSING CONSIDERATIONS
magnesium sulfate *(continued)*	slowly. *Management of paroxysmal atrial tachycardia* — **Adults:** 3 to 4 g I.V. over 30 sec. *Management of life-threatening ventricular arrhythmias* — **Adults:** 1 to 6 g I.V. over several min, then I.V. infusion of 3 to 20 mg/min for 5 to 48 hr.	level after repeated doses. Absence of knee-jerk and patellar reflexes signals impending toxicity. ▪ Observe neonates for signs of magnesium toxicity, including neuromuscular or respiratory depression, when I.V. form given to toxemic mothers within 24 hr before delivery.
mannitol Osmitrol *Diuretic* Pregnancy Risk Category: B	*Marked oliguria or suspected inadequate renal function* — **Adults and children > 12 yr:** 1st test dose of 200 mg/kg or 12.5 g as 25% I.V. solution over 3 to 5 min. Response adequate if 30 to 50 ml urine/hr excreted over 2 to 3 hr; if inadequate, give 2nd test dose. If still inadequate, discontinue. *Oliguria* — **Adults and children > 12 yr:** 50 to 100 g I.V. as 5% to 25% solution over 1½ to several hr.	▪ To redissolve crystallized solution, warm bottle in hot water and shake vigorously. Cool to body temperature before giving. ▪ ***I.V. use:*** Give as intermittent or continuous infusion, using in-line filter. Direct injection not recommended. ▪ Monitor vital signs, CVP, and I&O q hr. Check weight, renal function, and serum and urine sodium and potassium daily.
mebendazole Vermox, Mebendazole *Anthelmintic* Pregnancy Risk Category: C	*Pinworm* — **Adults and children > 2 yr:** 100 mg P.O. as single dose; repeat if infection persists 2 to 3 wk later. *Roundworm; whipworm; hookworm* — **Adults and children > 2 yr:** 100 mg P.O. b.i.d. for 3 days; repeat if infection persists 3 wk later.	▪ Tablets may be chewed, swallowed whole, or crushed and mixed with food. ▪ Give to all family members, as prescribed, to decrease risk of spreading infection.
mechlorethamine hydrochloride (nitrogen mustard) Mustargen	*Chronic lymphocytic leukemia; Hodgkin's disease; bronchogenic cancer* — **Adults:** 0.4 mg/kg I.V. as single dose or in divided doses of 0.1 to 0.2 mg/kg/day. Give through run-	▪ Prepare immediately before infusion. Very unstable solution. Inspect before using; use within 15 min. Discard unused solution. ▪ If extravasation occurs, apply cold com-

Antineoplastic Pregnancy Risk Category: D	ning I.V. infusion. Give subsequent courses when patient recovers hematologically from previous course (usually 3 to 6 wk).	presses and infiltrate area with isotonic sodium thiosulfate. ▪ Neurotoxicity increases with dose and patient age. ▪ Watch for signs of infection and bleeding.
meclizine hydrochloride Antivert, Antrizine, Bonamine†, Dramaine Less Drowsy Formula, D-Vert, Meni-D, Vergon *Antiemetic, antivertigo agent* Pregnancy Risk Category: B	*Vertigo* — **Adults:** 25 to 100 mg P.O. q.d. in divided doses. Dosage varies with response. *Motion sickness* — **Adults:** 25 to 50 mg P.O. 1 hr before travel, then q.d. for duration of trip.	▪ May mask symptoms of ototoxicity, brain tumor, or intestinal obstruction. ▪ Advise patient to avoid hazardous activities that require alertness until CNS effects known.
medroxyprogesterone acetate Amen, Curretab, Cycrin, Depo-Provera, Provera *Antineoplastic* Pregnancy Risk Category: X	*Abnormal uterine bleeding caused by hormonal imbalance* — **Adults:** 5 to 10 mg P.O. q.d. for 5 to 10 days starting on 16th day of menstrual cycle. If patient also has received estrogen, 10 mg P.O. q.d. for 10 days starting on 16th day of cycle. *Secondary amenorrhea* — **Adults:** 5 to 10 mg P.O. q.d. for 5 to 10 days. *Endometrial or renal cancer* — **Adults:** 400 to 1,000 mg I.M. q wk. *Contraception in women* — **Adults:** 150 mg I.M. q 3 mo; give 1st injection during first 5 days of menstrual cycle.	▪ Don't use as test for pregnancy; may cause birth defects and masculinization of female fetus. ▪ I.M. injection may be painful. Monitor sites for sterile abscess. Rotate injection sites. ▪ Tell patient to report unusual symptoms immediately and to stop drug and call doctor if visual disturbances or migraines occur. ▪ FDA regulations require that patient read package insert before 1st dose for information on possible side effects. Also give verbal information.
megestrol acetate Megace, Megostat‡	*Breast cancer* — **Adults:** 40 mg P.O. q.i.d. *Endometrial cancer* — **Adults:** 40 to 320 mg P.O. q.d. in divided doses.	▪ Advise patient to stop breast-feeding during therapy; infant toxicity possible. ▪ Advise women of childbearing *(continued)*

†Canadian ‡Australian

DRUG & CLASS	INDICATIONS & DOSAGES	NURSING CONSIDERATIONS
megestrol acetate *(continued)* *Antineoplastic* Pregnancy Risk Category: D	*Unexplained significant weight loss* — **Adults:** 800 mg P.O. (oral suspension) q.d.	age to use effective contraception during therapy. ▪ Inform patient that therapeutic response isn't immediate.
meloxicam Mobic *Anti-inflammatory, analgesic* Pregnancy Risk Category: C	*Relief of the signs and symptoms of osteoarthritis* — **Adults:** 7.5 mg P.O. q.d. May increase p.r.n. to maximum dose of 15 mg daily.	▪ ***ALERT*** Patients may be allergic to meloxicam or may have allergic-like reactions if they're hypersensitive to aspirin or other NSAIDs. ▪ Patients with a history of ulcers or GI bleeding are at higher risk for GI bleeding while taking NSAIDs such as meloxicam. Other risk factors for GI bleeding include treatment with corticosteroids or anticoagulants, longer duration of NSAID treatment, smoking, alcoholism, older age, and poor overall health. ▪ Monitor for signs and symptoms of overt and occult bleeding. ▪ May cause fluid retention; closely monitor patients with hypertension, edema, or heart failure. ▪ May be hepatotoxic; elevations of ALT or AST should be monitored if they occur. If signs and symptoms of liver disease or other systemic signs occur (such as eosinophilia or rash), stop the drug. ▪ As with any NSAID, use cautiously in elderly patients.

melphalan (L-phenylalanine mustard) Alkeran *Antineoplastic* Pregnancy Risk Category: D	*Multiple myeloma* — **Adults:** initially, 6 mg P.O. q.d. for 2 to 3 wk; then stop drug for up to 4 wk, or until WBC and platelet counts begin to rise again; then maintenance of 2 mg q.d. Or, 16 mg/m^2 by I.V. infusion over 15 to 20 min q 2 wk for 4 doses. After toxicity recovery, give q 4 wk. ***Adjust-a-dose:*** In patients with renal insufficiency, reduce dose up to 50%. *Nonresectable advanced ovarian cancer* — **Adults:** 0.2 mg/kg P.O. q.d. for 5 days. Repeat q 4 to 5 wk.	▪ ***I.V. use:*** Immediately before giving, reconstitute with 10 ml of sterile diluent supplied by manufacturer. Shake vigorously until solution clear. ▪ Promptly dilute and give; reconstituted product begins to degrade within 30 min. Give within 60 min of reconstitution. Don't refrigerate reconstituted product. ▪ Avoid skin contact with I.V. formulations. ▪ Give oral form on empty stomach. ▪ Monitor serum uric acid and CBC. ▪ To prevent bleeding, avoid all I.M. injections when platelet count < 100,000/mm^3.
meningococcal polysaccharide vaccine Menomune-A/C/Y/W-135 *Bacterial vaccine* Pregnancy Risk Category: C	*Meningococcal meningitis prophylaxis* — **Adults and children ≥ 2 yr:** 0.5 ml S.C.	▪ Obtain history of allergies and reaction to immunization. ▪ Keep epinephrine 1:1,000 available to treat anaphylaxis. ▪ Stress importance of avoiding pregnancy for 3 mo after vaccination. Offer contraception information.
meperidine hydrochloride (pethidine hydrochloride) Demerol *Analgesic, anesthesia adjunct* Pregnancy Risk Category: C Controlled Substance Schedule: II	*Moderate to severe pain* — **Adults:** 50 to 150 mg P.O., I.M., I.V., or S.C. q 3 to 4 hr. **Children:** 1.1 to 1.8 mg/kg P.O., I.M., I.V., or S.C. q 3 to 4 hr, or 175 mg/m^2 q.d. in 6 divided doses. Maximum single dose ≤ 100 mg. **Elderly:** Don't give to treat chronic pain because drug may cause seizures. *Preoperatively* — **Adults:** 50 to 100 mg I.M., I.V., or S.C. 30 to 90 min before	▪ Monitor respiratory and CV status. Don't give if respirations < 12, if respiratory rate or depth decreases, or if pupil change occurs. ▪ ***I.V. use:*** Give slowly by direct I.V. injection. May also give by slow infusion. ▪ Keep narcotic antagonist (naloxone) available when giving I.V. ▪ Watch for withdrawal *(continued)*

†Canadian ‡Australian

DRUG & CLASS	INDICATIONS & DOSAGES	NURSING CONSIDERATIONS
meperidine hydrochloride *(continued)*	surgery. **Children:** 1 to 2.2 mg/kg I.M., I.V., or S.C. up to adult dose 30 to 90 min before surgery. Don't exceed adult dosage.	symptoms if drug stopped abruptly after long-term use.
mercaptopurine (6-mercaptopurine, 6-MP) Purinethol *Antineoplastic* Pregnancy Risk Category: D	*Acute myeloblastic leukemia; chronic myelocytic leukemia* — **Adults:** 80 to 100 mg/m^2 P.O. q.d. up to 5 mg/kg/day. **Children:** 70 mg/m^2 P.O. q.d. *Acute lymphoblastic leukemia* — **Children:** 70 mg/m^2 P.O. q.d. **Maintenance for adults and children:** 1.5 to 2.5 mg/kg/day. ***Adjust-a-dose:*** In renally impaired patients, reduce dosage to avoid increased accumulation.	▪ Watch for hepatic dysfunction, which is reversible on discontinuation. If hepatic tenderness occurs, stop drug and notify doctor. ▪ Watch for signs of bleeding or infection. ▪ To prevent bleeding, avoid all I.M. injections when platelet count $< 100,000/mm^3$.
meropenem Merrem IV *Antibiotic* Pregnancy Risk Category: B	*Complicated appendicitis and peritonitis from susceptible organisms; bacterial meningitis (children only) from susceptible organisms* — **Adults:** 1 g I.V. q 8 hr over 15 to 30 min as I.V. infusion or over 3 to 5 min as I.V. bolus injection. Maximum 2 g I.V. q 8 hr. **Children ≥ 3 mo and ≤ 110 lb (50 kg):** 20 to 40 mg/kg q 8 hr over 15 to 30 min as I.V. infusion or over 3 to 5 min as I.V. bolus injection. Maximum 2 g I.V. q 8 hr. **Children > 110 lb (50 kg):** 2 g I.V. q 8 hr for meningitis. ***Adjust-a-dose:*** Adults with impaired renal function:	▪ Obtain specimen for culture and sensitivity test before giving 1st dose. ▪ Monitor for superinfection. ▪ ***ALERT*** Serious and occasionally fatal hypersensitivity reactions reported. Determine if patient is hypersensitive to antibiotics. ▪ If seizures occur, stop infusion and notify doctor. ▪ Assess organ system functions periodically during prolonged therapy. ▪ Reduce dosage in patients with renal insufficiency.

CrCl	Dose	Dosing interval
26-50 ml/min	1 g (usual dose)	q 12 hr
10-25 ml/min	½ usual dose	q 12 hr
< 10 ml/min	½ usual dose	q 24 hr

---

mesalamine
Rowasa
Anti-inflammatory
Pregnancy Risk Category: B

Active mild to moderate distal ulcerative colitis, proctitis, or proctosigmoiditis — **Adults:** 500 mg P.R. (suppository) b.i.d. or 4 g (retention enema) once daily, preferably h.s. for 3 to 6 wk. Rectal form should be retained overnight (for about 8 hr).

- Monitor periodic renal function studies with long-term therapy, as ordered.
- May cause hypersensitivity reactions in patients sensitive to sulfites.
- Instruct to stop if fever or rash occurs.
- Advise patient to carefully follow instructions supplied with medication.

---

mesna
Mesnex, Dromitexan
Uroprotectant
Pregnancy Risk Category: B

Prophylaxis of hemorrhagic cystitis in patients receiving ifosfamide — **Adults:** dosage varies with amount of ifosfamide given; calculated as 20% of ifosfamide dose at time given. Usual dose 240 mg/m² as I.V. bolus with ifosfamide; repeat at 4 and 8 hr after ifosfamide given.

- ***I.V. use:*** Prepare solution by diluting commercially available ampules with D_5W solution, dextrose 5% and 0.9% NaCl for injection, 0.9% NaCl for injection, or lactated Ringer's to obtain final solution of 20 mg mesna/ml.
- Monitor urine samples daily in patients receiving mesna for hematuria.

---

mesoridazine besylate
Serentil, Serentil Concentrate
Antipsychotic
Pregnancy Risk Category: NR

Alcoholism — **Adults and children > 12 yr:** 25 mg P.O. b.i.d. Maximum 200 mg daily.
Behavioral problems associated with chronic organic mental syndrome — **Adults and children > 12 yr:** 25 mg P.O. t.i.d. to maximum 300 mg daily.
Psychoneurotic manifestations (anxiety) — **Adults and children > 12 yr:** 10 mg P.O. t.i.d. to maximum 150 mg daily.
Schizophrenia — **Adults and children**

- Obtain baseline BP before starting.
- Watch for tardive dyskinesia. Treat acute dystonic reactions with diphenhydramine.
- Assess for neuroleptic malignant syndrome.
- Withhold dose and notify doctor if patient develops jaundice, symptoms of blood dyscrasia, or persistent extrapyramidal reactions (> several hours).
- Arrange for weekly bilirubin tests during 1st month; periodic blood *(continued)*

†Canadian ‡Australian

DRUG & CLASS	INDICATIONS & DOSAGES	NURSING CONSIDERATIONS
mesoridazine besylate *(continued)*	**> 12 yr:** initially, 50 mg P.O. t.i.d. or 25 mg I.M., repeated in 30 to 60 min, p.r.n. Maximum oral dose 400 mg daily; maximum I.M. dose 200 mg daily.	tests (CBC and LFT); and ophthalmic tests. ▪ Wear gloves when preparing solutions, and avoid contact with skin and clothing.
metaproterenol sulfate Alupent, Dey-Dose Metaproterenol, Dey-Lute Metaproterenol, Metaprel *Bronchodilator* Pregnancy Risk Category: C	*Acute episodes of bronchial asthma* — **Adults and children ≥ 12 yr:** 2 to 3 inhalations. Don't repeat inhalation more often than q 3 to 4 hr. Maximum 12 inhalations/day. *Bronchial asthma and reversible bronchospasm* — **Adults and children > 9 yr or > 27 kg (60 lb):** 20 mg P.O. q 6 to 8 hr. **Children 6 to 9 yr or < 27 kg:** 10 mg P.O. q 6 to 8 hr. Or, via IPPB or nebulizer: **Adults and children ≥ 12 yr:** 0.2 to 0.3 ml of 5% solution diluted in 2.5 ml of 0.45% or 0.9% NaCl, or 2.5 ml commercially available 0.4% or 0.6% solution q 4 hr, p.r.n. **Children 6 to 11 yr:** 0.1 to 0.2 ml of 5% solution diluted in 0.9% NaCl to final volume of 3 ml q 4 hr, p.r.n.	▪ May use tablets and aerosol together. ▪ Inhalant solution can be given by IPPB with drug diluted in 0.45% or 0.9% NaCl or with hand nebulizer at full strength. ▪ If patient also uses steroid inhaler, tell him to use bronchodilator, then wait 5 min before using steroid. ▪ Warn patient to stop immediately and notify doctor if paradoxical bronchospasm occurs. ▪ Instruct patient to notify doctor if drug ineffective or to request dosage adjustment.
metformin hydrochloride Glucophage *Antidiabetic* Pregnancy Risk Category: B	*Adjunct to diet to lower blood glucose in type 2 diabetes mellitus* — **Adults:** initially, 500 mg P.O. b.i.d. with morning and evening meals, or 850 mg P.O. q.d. with morning meal. With 500-mg form, increase dosage 500 mg weekly to maximum 2,500 mg P.O. daily in divided doses, p.r.n. With	▪ Monitor renal function. If renal impairment detected, expect to switch to different antidiabetic. ▪ Give with meals. ▪ Monitor blood glucose level regularly to evaluate effectiveness. ▪ Monitor blood glucose level closely during

	850-mg form, increase dosage 850 mg every other wk to maximum 2,550 mg P.O. daily in divided doses, p.r.n. ***Adjust-a-dose:*** In elderly or debilitated patients, give lower dose.	times of increased stress because patient may need insulin therapy. ▪ Don't give to patients with acute or chronic metabolic acidosis, including diabetic ketoacidosis.
methadone Dolophine, Methadose, Physeptone‡ *Analgesic, narcotic detoxification adjunct* Pregnancy Risk Category: C Controlled Substance Schedule: II	*Severe pain* — **Adults:** 2.5 to 10 mg P.O., I.M., or S.C. q 3 to 4 hr, p.r.n. *Narcotic withdrawal syndrome* — **Adults:** 15 to 40 mg P.O. q.d. (highly individualized). Maintenance 20 to 120 mg P.O. q.d. Adjust dosage, p.r.n. Daily doses > 120 mg require special state and federal approval.	▪ Oral liquid form legally required in maintenance programs. Completely dissolve tablets in 120 ml orange juice or powdered citrus drink. ▪ For parenteral use; give I.M. ▪ Give around-the-clock for severe, chronic pain.
methamphetamine Desoxyn, Desoxyn Gradumets *CNS stimulant, short-term adjunctive anorexigenic, sympathomimetic amine* Pregnancy Risk Category: C Controlled Substance Schedule: II	*Attention deficit disorder with hyperactivity* — **Children ≥ 6 yr:** 2.5 to 5 mg P.O. once daily or b.i.d.; increase in 5-mg increments weekly, p.r.n. Usual effective dose 20 to 25 mg q.d. *Short-term adjunct in exogenous obesity* — **Adults:** 2.5 to 5 mg P.O. b.i.d. to t.i.d., 30 min before meals; or 10 to 15 mg long-acting tablets P.O. q.d. before breakfast.	▪ Not for first-line treatment of obesity. Use as anorexigenic prohibited in some states. ▪ When used for obesity, be sure patient on weight-reduction program. ▪ If tolerance to anorexigenic effect develops, notify doctor. ▪ Don't use long-acting form for initiation of dosage or until the adjusted daily dose is equal to or greater than the dosage provided in a long-acting tablet.
methimazole Tapazole *Antihyperthyroid agent* Pregnancy Risk Category: D	*Hyperthyroidism* — **Adults:** if mild, 15 mg P.O. q.d.; if moderately severe, 30 to 45 mg q.d.; if severe, 60 mg q.d. All given in 3 equally divided doses q 8 hr. Maintenance 5 to 30 mg q.d. **Children:** 0.4 mg/kg/day P.O.	▪ Monitor hepatic function and CBC . ▪ Doses > 30 mg/day increase risk of agranulocytosis. ▪ Watch for signs of hypothyroidism. ▪ Discontinue and notify *(continued)*

DRUG & CLASS	INDICATIONS & DOSAGES	NURSING CONSIDERATIONS
methimazole *(continued)*	divided q 8 hr. Maintenance 0.2 mg/kg/day divided q 8 hr.	doctor of severe rash or enlarged cervical lymph nodes. ▪ Advise patient not to take OTC cough medicines.
methocarbamol Robaxin *Skeletal muscle relaxant* Pregnancy Risk Category: NR	*Adjunct in acute, painful musculoskeletal conditions* — **Adults:** 1.5 g P.O. q.i.d. for 2 to 3 days. Maintenance 4 to 4.5 g P.O. q.d. in 3 to 6 divided doses. Or, 1 g I.M. or I.V. Maximum 3 g q.d. I.M. or I.V. for 3 consecutive days. *Supportive therapy in tetanus management* — **Adults:** 1 to 2 g I.V. push or 1 to 3 g as infusion q 6 hr. **Children:** 15 mg/kg I.V. q 6 hr.	▪ Parenteral form irritates veins; may cause fainting or phlebitis or aggravate seizures if injected rapidly. Keep patient supine during infusion. Avoid infiltration. ▪ Give I.M. deeply, only into upper outer quadrant of buttock, with maximum 5 ml in each buttock. Don't give S.C. ▪ Warn patient to avoid activities that require alertness until CNS effects known. ▪ ***I.V. use:*** May be injected, undiluted, directly into the vein at a maximum rate of 3 ml/min.
methotrexate (amethopterin, MTX) **methotrexate sodium** Folex PFS, Mexate-AQ, Rheumatrex *Antineoplastic* Pregnancy Risk Category: X	*Trophoblastic tumors (choriocarcinoma, hydatidiform mole)* — **Adults:** 15 to 30 mg P.O. or I.M. q.d. for 5 days. Repeat after ≥ 1 wk, according to response or toxicity. *Acute lymphocytic leukemia* — **Adults and children:** 3.3 mg/m^2/day P.O., I.M., or I.V. for 4 to 6 wk or until remission; then 20 to 30 mg/m^2 P.O. or I.M. weekly in 2 divided doses or 2.5 mg/kg I.V. q 14 days. *Meningeal leukemia* — **Adults and children:** 12 mg/m^2 or less (maximum 15 mg) intrathecally q 2 to 5 days until CSF normal, then 1 additional dose.	▪ Reconstitute solutions without preservatives just before use; discard unused drug. ▪ Leucovorin rescue necessary with high-dose (> 100 mg) protocols; start 24 hr after methotrexate therapy begins. ▪ Rash, redness, or ulcerations in mouth or adverse pulmonary reactions may signal serious complications. ▪ Monitor pulmonary function tests periodically. ▪ Monitor I&O daily. Encourage intake of 2 to 3 L daily. ▪ Watch for infection or bleeding.

methylcellulose Citrucel, Cologel *Bulk-forming laxative* Pregnancy Risk Category: C	*Chronic constipation* — **Adults:** maximum 6 g q.d., divided into 0.45 to 3 g/dose. **Children 6 to 12 yr:** maximum 3 g/day, divided into 0.45 to 1.5 g/dose.	▪ Especially useful in debilitated patients and in those with postpartum constipation, irritable bowel syndrome, diverticulitis, and colostomies.
methyldopa Aldomet, Apo-Methyldopa†, Dopamet†, Novomedopa† **methyldopate hydrochloride** Aldomet, Aldomet Ester Injection‡ *Antihypertensive* Pregnancy Risk Category: B	*Hypertension; hypertensive crisis* — **Adults:** initially, 250 mg P.O. b.i.d. to t.i.d. in first 48 hr. Then increase, p.r.n., q 2 days. Maintenance 500 mg to 3 g/day in 2 to 4 divided doses; maximum: 3 g/day. Or, 250 to 500 mg I.V. q 6 hr, diluted in D_5W and given over 30 to 60 min; maximum dose 1 g q 6 hr. **Children:** 10 mg/kg P.O. q.d. in 2 to 4 divided doses; or 20 to 40 mg/kg I.V. q.d. in 4 evenly divided doses. Dosage increased q.d., p.r.n. Maximum daily dose 65 mg/kg or 3 g.	▪ ***I.V. use:*** Add dose to 100 ml of D_5W or a concentration of 10 mg/ml. Infuse slowly over 30 to 60 min. ▪ Observe for and report involuntary choreoathetoid movements. ▪ After dialysis, monitor patient for hypertension and notify doctor if necessary. ▪ Monitor Coombs' test results. ▪ Monitor LFTs and CBC with differential. ▪ Caution patient not to stop taking suddenly but to contact doctor if adverse reactions occur.
methylergonovine maleate Methergine *Oxytocic* Pregnancy Risk Category: C	*Prevention and treatment of postpartum hemorrhage caused by uterine atony or subinvolution* — **Adults:** 0.2 mg I.M. q 2 to 4 hr; for excessive uterine bleeding or other emergencies, 0.2 mg I.V. over 1 min while BP and uterine contractions monitored. After initial I.M. or I.V. dose, 0.2 mg P.O. q 6 to 8 hr for 2 to 7 days. Decrease dosage if severe cramping occurs.	▪ ***I.V. use:*** Don't routinely give I.V. If necessary, give slowly over 1 min with BP monitoring. May dilute I.V. dose to 5 ml with 0.9% NaCl. Contractions begin immediately after I.V. use and continue for up to 45 min. ▪ Monitor and record BP, pulse rate, and uterine response; report sudden changes.
methylphenidate hydrochloride PMS-Methylphenidate†	*Attention deficit hyperactivity disorder* — **Children ≥ 6 yr:** initial dose, 5 to 10 mg P.O. q.d. before breakfast and lunch, increased	▪ May trigger Tourette's syndrome in children. ▪ Observe for signs of excessive stimulation. ▪ Monitor BP.

(continued)

†Canadian ‡Australian

DRUG & CLASS	INDICATIONS & DOSAGES	NURSING CONSIDERATIONS
methylphenidate hydrochloride *(continued)* *CNS stimulant, analeptic* Pregnancy Risk Category: NR Controlled Substance Schedule: II	in 5- to 10-mg increments weekly, p.r.n., up to 2 mg/kg or 60 mg q.d. Usual effective dose 20 to 30 mg. *Narcolepsy* — **Adults:** 10 mg P.O. b.i.d. or t.i.d. 30 to 45 min before meals. Dose varies with patient needs; average 40 to 60 mg/day.	▪ Monitor height and weight in children on long-term therapy. May delay growth spurt, but children will attain normal height when drug stopped. ▪ Monitor for tolerance or psychological dependence. ▪ Give 30 to 45 minutes before meals.
methylprednisolone Medrol **methylprednisolone acetate** depMedalone, Depoject, Depo-Medrol, Depopred, Duralone, Medralone **methylprednisolone sodium succinate** A-methaPred, Solu-Medrol *Anti-inflammatory, immunosuppressant* Pregnancy Risk Category: C	*Multiple sclerosis* — **Adults:** 200 mg P.O. q.d. for 1 wk, then 80 mg every other day for 1 mo. *Severe inflammation or immunosuppression* — **Adults:** 2 to 60 mg P.O. q.d. in 4 divided doses; 10 to 80 mg acetate I.M. q.d., or 10 to 250 mg succinate I.M. or I.V. up to q 4 hr; or 4 to 40 mg acetate into smaller joints or 20 to 80 mg acetate into larger joints. **Children:** 0.03 to 0.2 mg/kg succinate or 1 to 6.25 mg/m^2 I.M. once daily or b.i.d. *Shock* — **Adults:** 100 to 250 mg succinate I.V. q 2 to 6 hr; or 30 mg/kg I.V. initially; repeated q 4 to 6 hr, p.r.n. Continue therapy for 2 to 3 days or until patient stable.	▪ Give oral dose with food when possible. Critically ill patients may require concomitant antacid or H_2-receptor antagonist. ▪ ***I.V. use:*** Use only methylprednisolone sodium succinate; never give acetate form I.V. Reconstitute according to manufacturer's directions. ▪ Give direct injection over at least 1 min. Give massive doses over at least 10 min. If used for continuous infusion, change solution q 24 hr. ▪ May mask or exacerbate infections. ▪ Watch for depression or psychotic episodes. ▪ Diabetic patients may need increased insulin.
methyltestosterone Android, Oreton Methyl, Testred, Virilon *Androgen replacement*	*Breast cancer in women* — **Adults:** 50 to 200 mg P.O. q.d.; or 25 to 100 mg buccally q.d. *Male hypogonadism* — **Adults:** 10 to 50 mg	▪ In children, obtain wrist bone X-rays before therapy to establish bone maturation level. ▪ Check Hgb, Hct, cholesterol, calcium, and

Pregnancy Risk Category: X Controlled Substance Schedule: III	P.O. q.d.; or 5 to 25 mg buccally q.d. Evaluate semen q 3 to 4 mo. *Androgen deficiency* — **Adults:** 10 to 50 mg P.O. q.d.	cardiac and liver function. ▪ Stop therapy if disease progresses.
metoclopramide hydrochloride Apo-Metoclop†, Clopra, Maxolon, Octamide, Reclomide, Reglan *Antiemetic, GI stimulant* Pregnancy Risk Category: B	*Prevention or reduction of nausea and vomiting associated with cancer chemotherapy* — **Adults:** 1 to 2 mg/kg I.V. 30 min before cancer chemotherapy, then repeated q 2 hr for 2 doses, then q 3 hr for 3 doses. *Prevention of postoperative nausea and vomiting* — **Adults:** 10 to 20 mg I.M. near end of procedure; then q 4 to 6 hr, p.r.n. *To facilitate small-bowel intubation and to aid in radiologic exams* — **Adults and children > 14 yr:** 10 mg I.V. as single dose over 1 to 2 min. **Children 6 to 14 yr:** 2.5 to 5 mg I.V. **Children < 6 yr:** 0.1 mg/kg I.V. *Gastroesophageal reflux* — **Adults:** 10 to 15 mg P.O. q.i.d., p.r.n., 30 min before meals and h.s.	▪ ***I.V. use:*** Give lower doses (≤ 10 mg) by direct injection over 1 to 2 min. Dilute doses > 10 mg in 50 ml compatible diluent; infuse over ≥ 15 min. Protection from light unnecessary if mixture given ≤ 24 hr. ▪ Compatible with D_5W, 0.9% NaCl for injection, D_5W in 0.45% NaCl, or lactated Ringer's injection. ▪ Use diphenhydramine 25 mg I.V. to counteract extrapyramidal adverse effects caused by high doses. ▪ Advise patient to avoid activities requiring alertness for 2 hr after each dose. ▪ Monitor BP in patient receiving I.V. form.
metolazone Mykrox (prompt-release), Zaroxolyn (extended-release) *Diuretic, antihypertensive* Pregnancy Risk Category: B	*Edema in heart failure or renal disease* — **Adults:** 5 to 20 mg (extended-release) P.O. q.d. *Hypertension* — **Adults:** 2.5 to 5 mg (extended-release) P.O. q.d. Maintenance based on BP. Or 0.5 mg (prompt-release) P.O. q.d. in morning; increased to 1 mg P.O. q.d.	▪ To prevent nocturia, give in morning. ▪ Monitor I&O, weight, BP, and electrolytes. ▪ Watch for signs of hypokalemia, such as muscle weakness and cramps. ▪ Advise patient to avoid sudden posture changes.

†Canadian ‡Australian

DRUG & CLASS	INDICATIONS & DOSAGES	NURSING CONSIDERATIONS
metoprolol succinate Toprol XL **metoprolol tartrate** Apo-Metoprolol†, Lopresor SR†, Lopressor, Minax‡ *Antihypertensive, adjunctive treatment for acute MI* Pregnancy Risk Category: C	*Hypertension* — **Adults:** 100 mg P.O. in single or divided doses (may increase q wk); maintenance 100 to 450 mg q.d. in 2 or 3 divided doses. Or, 50 to 100 mg extended-release tablets q.d. (maximum 400 mg/day). *Early intervention in acute MI* — **Adults:** three 5-mg (tartrate) I.V. boluses q 2 min. Then, 15 min after last dose, 25 to 50 mg P.O. q 6 hr for 48 hr. Maintenance 100 mg P.O. b.i.d. *Angina pectoris* — **Adults:** initially, 100 mg P.O. q.d. in 2 divided doses. Maintenance 100 to 400 mg q.d.	▪ Check apical pulse before giving. If < 60, withhold dose and call doctor immediately. ▪ Masks common signs of hypoglycemia. Monitor blood glucose level closely in diabetic patients. ▪ Masks common signs of shock. Monitor BP frequently. ▪ May precipitate asthma attacks. Monitor for breathing difficulties. ▪ Dosage may be increased q wk.
metronidazole (systemic) Apo-Metronidazole†, Flagyl, Flagyl ER, Flagyl 375, Metrozine‡, Neo-Metric†, PMS Metronidazole†, Protostat, Trikacide† **metronidazole hydrochloride** Flagyl I.V. RTU, Metro I.V., Novonidazol† *Antibacterial, antiprotozoal, amebicide* Pregnancy Risk Category: B	*Intestinal amebiasis* — **Adults:** 750 mg P.O. t.i.d. for 5 to 10 days. **Children:** 30 to 50 mg/kg/day (in 3 doses) for 10 days. *Trichomoniasis* — **Adults:** 250 mg P.O. t.i.d. or 375 mg P.O. b.i.d. for 7 days or 2 g P.O. in single dose; 4 to 6 wk should elapse between courses of therapy. **Children:** 5 mg/kg dose P.O. t.i.d. for 7 days. *Refractory trichomoniasis* — **Adults:** 250 or 500 mg P.O. b.i.d. for 10 or 7 days, respectively. *Bacterial infections from anaerobic microorganisms* — **Adults:** loading dose 15 mg/kg I.V. infused over 1 hr. Maintenance dose 7.5	▪ ***I.V. use:*** Infuse over ≥ 1 hr. Don't give I.V. push. ▪ Record number and character of stools when used to treat amebiasis. Should be used only after *T. vaginalis* confirmed by wet smear or culture or *E. histolytica* identified. Asymptomatic sexual partners of patients treated for *T. vaginalis* should be treated simultaneously to avoid reinfection. ▪ Instruct patient to take oral form with food. ▪ ***ALERT*** Tell patient to avoid alcohol or alcohol-containing medications during therapy and for ≥ 48 hr afterward.

	mg/kg I.V. or P.O. q 6 hr. Give 1st maintenance dose 6 hr after loading dose. Maximum 4 g/day. *Prevention of postoperative infection in contaminated or potentially contaminated colorectal surgery* — **Adults:** 15 mg/kg I.V. infused over 30 to 60 min 1 hr before surgery. Then, 7.5 mg/kg I.V. infused over 30 to 60 min at 6 and 12 hr after initial dose.	▪ Inform patient that metallic taste and dark or reddish brown urine may occur. ▪ Don't refrigerate neutralized diluted solution; precipitation may occur. If Flagyl I.V. RTU refrigerated, crystals may form; these disappear after solution warms to room temperature.
metronidazole (topical) MetroGel, MetroGel-Vaginal Metro Lotion, Noritate *Antiprotozoal, antibacterial* Pregnancy Risk Category: B	*Acne rosacea* — **Adults:** apply thin film to affected area b.i.d., morning and evening. Frequency and duration of therapy adjusted after response evaluated. *Bacterial vaginosis* — **Adults:** 1 applicatorful once daily or b.i.d. for 5 days.	▪ Avoid using topical gel around eyes. Clean area before use and wait 15 to 20 min before applying drug. Cosmetics may be used after applying drug. ▪ If local reactions occur, tell patient to apply less frequently or to stop and contact doctor. ▪ Daily doses should be given h.s.
mexiletine hydrochloride Mexitil *Ventricular antiarrhythmic* Pregnancy Risk Category: C	*Refractory life-threatening ventricular arrhythmias, including ventricular tachycardia and PVCs* — **Adults:** 200 mg P.O. q 8 hr. May increase dose q 2 to 3 days in increments of 50 to 100 mg q 8 hr. Or, loading dose of 400 mg with maintenance dose of 200 mg q 8 hr. Maximum no more than 1,200 mg/day.	▪ When switching from lidocaine, stop infusion when 1st mexiletine dose given. Keep infusion line open until arrhythmia controlled. ▪ ***ALERT*** Tremor is an early toxicity sign, progressing to dizziness and later to ataxia and nystagmus. ▪ Monitor BP, HR, and heart rhythm often.
mezlocillin sodium Mezlin	*Systemic infections from susceptible strains of gram-positive and especially gram-negative organisms* — **Adults:** 200 to 300 mg/kg/day I.V. or I.M. in 4 to 6 divided doses. Usual dose	▪ ***ALERT*** Before giving, ask about previous allergic reactions to penicillin. ▪ Obtain specimen for culture and sensitivity tests before 1st dose. *(continued)*

DRUG & CLASS	INDICATIONS & DOSAGES	NURSING CONSIDERATIONS
mezlocillin sodium *(continued)* *Antibiotic* Pregnancy Risk Category: B	3 g q 4 hr or 4 g q 6 hr. For serious infections, may give up to 24 g/day. **Children > 1 mo and ≤ 12 yr:** 50 mg/kg I.V. or I.M. q 4 hr. For serious infections, may give to 300 mg/kg/day in 4 to 6 divided doses.	▪ Don't give > 2 g per I.M. injection. ▪ May cause thrombocytopenia. Check CBC and platelet counts frequently. ▪ Monitor serum potassium level.
miconazole nitrate Micatin, Monistat-Derm Cream and Lotion, Femizol, Monistat, M-Zole, *Antifungal* Pregnancy Risk Category: C	*Tinea pedis; tinea cruris; tinea corporis* — **Adults and children:** apply or spray sparingly b.i.d. for 2 to 4 wk. *Vulvovaginal candidiasis* — **Adults:** 1 applicatorful or 100 mg suppository (Monistat 7) inserted intravaginally h.s. for 7 days; repeat course, if necessary. Or, 200 mg suppository (Monistat 3) intravaginally h.s. for 3 days.	▪ Concurrent use of intravaginal forms and certain latex products, such as vaginal contraceptive diaphragms, not recommended. ▪ Instruct patient to avoid sexual intercourse during vaginal treatment. ▪ Caution patient to discontinue if sensitivity or chemical irritation occurs.
midazolam hydrochloride Hypnovel‡, Versed *Preoperative sedative, agent for conscious sedation, adjunct for induction of general anesthesia, amnesic agent* Pregnancy Risk Category: D Controlled Substance Schedule: IV	*Preoperative sedation* — **Adults:** 0.07 mg to 0.08 mg/kg I.M. 1 hr before surgery. *Conscious sedation before short diagnostic procedures* — **Adults:** 1 to 2 mg by slow I.V. injection before procedure. *Induction of general anesthesia* — **Adults:** 0.15 to 0.35 mg/kg over 20 to 30 sec. Additional increments of 25% initial dose may be needed. Maximum: 0.6 mg/kg. **Unpremedicated adults ≥ 55 yr:** initially, 0.3 mg/kg. ***Adjust-a-dose:*** In debilitated patients, initial dose 0.2 to 0.25 mg/kg.	▪ May mix in same syringe with morphine sulfate, meperidine, atropine sulfate, or scopolamine. ▪ ***I.V. use:*** Give slowly over ≥ 2 min, and wait ≥ 2 min when titrating. ▪ I.V. dose may cause respiratory depression and respiratory arrest. ▪ Monitor BP, HR, heart rhythm, respirations, airway integrity, and SaO_2. ▪ Have oxygen and resuscitation equipment available.

midodrine hydrochloride ProAmatine *Vasopressor, antihypertensive* Pregnancy Risk Category: C	*Symptomatic orthostatic hypotension unresponsive to standard clinical care* — **Adults:** 10 mg P.O. t.i.d. Suggested dosing schedule: 1st dose when arising in morning; 2nd dose at midday; 3rd dose in late afternoon (no later than 6 p.m.). Use cautiously in abnormal renal function; initially, 2.5-mg doses recommended.	▪ Monitor supine and sitting BP; notify doctor if supine BP increases excessively. ▪ Tell patient to take during day when he can be upright and doing daily activities. Space doses ≥ 3 hr apart. Tell him not to take after evening meal or within 4 hr before h.s. ▪ Perform renal and hepatic function tests before and during therapy, as ordered. ▪ Instruct patient to consult doctor before taking OTC medications.
miglitol Glyset *Antidiabetic* Pregnancy Risk Category: B	*To improve glycemic control in patients with type 2 diabetes mellitus when hyperglycemia can't be managed by diet alone, or combined with a sulfonylurea when diet plus either miglitol or sulfonylurea alone don't adequately control hyperglycemia* — **Adults:** initially, 25 mg P.O. t.i.d. at the start (with the first bite) of each main meal. Dose may be increased after 4 to 8 wk to a maintenance dose of 50 mg P.O. t.i.d. and further increased after 3 mo, based on the glycosylated hemoglobin level, to a maximum of 100 mg P.O. t.i.d.	▪ Use cautiously in patients also receiving insulin or oral sulfonylureas because miglitol may increase the hypoglycemic potential of insulin or sulfonylureas. Risk of hypoglycemia increases when miglitol and insulin or a sulfonylurea are used together; drug dosages may have to be adjusted. Monitor patients for increased frequency of hypoglycemia. ▪ Monitor blood glucose level regularly, especially during increased stress, as with infection, fever, surgery, and trauma. ▪ Besides checking glucose levels regularly, monitor glycosylated hemoglobin q 3 mo, to evaluate long-term glycemic control. ▪ Instruct patient to take with the first bite of each main meal. ▪ Treat mild to moderate hypoglycemia with a form of dextrose such *(continued)*

DRUG & CLASS	INDICATIONS & DOSAGES	NURSING CONSIDERATIONS
miglitol *(continued)*		as glucose tablets or gel. Severe hypoglycemia may require I.V. glucose or glucagon.
milrinone lactate Primacor *Inotropic vasodilator* Pregnancy Risk Category: C	*Short-term treatment of heart failure* — **Adults:** initial loading dose 50 mcg/kg I.V., given slowly over 10 min, then continuous I.V. infusion of 0.375 to 0.75 mcg/kg/min. Adjust infusion dose according to clinical and hemodynamic responses. ***Adjust-a-dose:*** If CrCl ≤ 50 ml/min, titrate dose to maximum clinical effect, not to exceed 1.13 mg/kg/day.	• Improved cardiac output may enhance urine output. Potassium loss may predispose patient to digitalis toxicity. • Monitor fluid and electrolyte status, BP, HR, and renal function. Excessive BP decrease requires discontinuing or slowing rate of infusion.
minocycline hydrochloride Apo-Minocycline†, Dynacin, Minocin, Minocin IV, Vectrin *Antibiotic* Pregnancy Risk Category: NR	*Infections from susceptible gram-negative and gram-positive organisms* — **Adults:** initially, 200 mg I.V.; then 100 mg I.V. q 12 hr. Maximum 400 mg/day. Or, 200 mg P.O. initially; then 100 mg P.O. q 12 hr. Can use 100 or 200 mg P.O. initially, then 50 mg q.i.d. **Children > 8 yr:** initially, 4 mg/kg P.O. or I.V.; then 2 mg/kg q 12 hr. Given I.V. in 500- to 1,000-ml solution without calcium over 6 hr. *Gonorrhea in patients allergic to penicillin* — **Adults:** initially, 200 mg P.O.; then 100 mg q 12 hr for ≥ 4 days. *Syphilis in patients allergic to penicillin* — **Adults:** initially, 200 mg P.O.; then 100 mg q 12 hr for 10 to 15 days.	• Obtain specimen for culture and sensitivity tests before 1st dose. May begin therapy pending test results. • With large doses or prolonged therapy, monitor for superinfection, especially in high-risk patients. • Check tongue for signs of candidal infection. Stress good oral hygiene. • May cause tooth discoloration in children < 8 yr. Observe for brown pigmentation; inform doctor if present. • Thrombophlebitis may occur with I.V. administration. Avoid extravasation. Switch to oral therapy as soon as possible. • Tell patient to take oral form with full glass

	Meningococcal carrier state — **Adults:** 100 mg P.O. q 12 hr for 5 days. *Uncomplicated urethral, endocervical, rectal infection caused by* C. trachomatis — 100 mg P.O. b.i.d. for ≥ 7 days.	of water or with food. ▪ Tell patient not to take within 1 hr of h.s. ▪ Take at least 2 hours after antacids. ▪ Avoid exposure to direct sunlight, and wear sunscreen and protective clothing.
minoxidil (oral) Loniten *Antihypertensive* Pregnancy Risk Category: C	*Severe hypertension* — **Adults:** initially, 5 mg P.O. q.d. Effective dosage range 10 to 40 mg q.d. Maximum 100 mg q.d. **Children < 12 yr:** 0.2 mg/kg P.O. (maximum 5 mg) q.d. Effective dosage range 0.25 to 1 mg/kg q.d. Maximum 50 mg/day.	▪ Closely monitor BP and HR at start of therapy. Elderly patients may be more sensitive to hypotensive effects. ▪ Removed by hemodialysis. Give dose after dialysis. ▪ Monitor fluid I&O. Check for weight gain and edema.
mirtazapine Remeron *Tetracyclic antidepressant* Pregnancy Risk Category: C	*Depression* — **Adults:** initially, 15 mg P.O. h.s. Maintenance 15 to 45 mg q.d. Dosage adjustments at intervals of 1 to 2 wk. Maximum dose is 45 mg/day.	▪ Caution patient not to perform hazardous activities if sleepy. ▪ Instruct patient not to use alcohol or other CNS depressants. ▪ Monitor closely for signs of dependence; not known if drug causes physical or psychological dependence.
misoprostol Cytotec *Antiulcer agent, gastric mucosal protectant* Pregnancy Risk Category: X	*Prevention of NSAID-induced gastric ulcer in elderly or debilitated patients at high risk for complications from gastric ulcer and in patients with history of NSAID-induced ulcer* — **Adults:** 200 mcg P.O. q.i.d. with food; if not tolerated, may decrease to 100 mcg P.O. q.i.d. Give last dose h.s. Give for duration of NSAID therapy.	▪ Provide oral and written warnings about dangers to fetus. Ensure that patient can comply with contraception and has negative serum pregnancy test result within 2 wk of starting drug. ▪ Advise patient not to begin therapy until 2nd or 3rd day of next menstrual period.

DRUG & CLASS	INDICATIONS & DOSAGES	NURSING CONSIDERATIONS
mitomycin (mitomycin-C) Mutamycin *Antineoplastic* Pregnancy Risk Category: NR	Dosage and indications vary. Check treatment protocol with doctor. *Disseminated adenocarcinoma of stomach or pancreas* — **Adults:** 20 mg/m^2 as I.V. single dose. Repeat cycle after 6 to 8 wk, when WBC and platelet counts return to normal.	▪ Stop infusion immediately and notify doctor if extravasation occurs. Extravasation may cause necrosis. ▪ Monitor for dyspnea with cough. ▪ Watch for signs of infection and bleeding.
modafinil Provigil *Wakefulness-promoting agent* Pregnancy Risk Category: C	*Improvement of wakefulness in patients with excessive daytime sleepiness associated with narcolepsy* — **Adults:** 200 mg P.O. q.d., given as single dose in morning. Although doses of 400 mg q.d. as single dose have been well tolerated, may be no additional benefit with doses > 200 mg. **Elderly:** Lower dose may be needed because of reduced elimination of drug and its metabolites. ***Adjust-a-dose:*** In patients with severe hepatic impairment, reduce dose by 50%.	▪ May increase risk of pregnancy when using steroidal contraceptives, including depot or implantable contraceptives, during and for 1 mo after stopping therapy. ▪ Advise patient to inform doctor if taking or planning to take a prescription or OTC drug. ▪ Advise patients to report rash, hives, or related allergic phenomenon. ▪ Safety and efficacy not determined for patient with severe renal impairment; avoid use.
molindone hydrochloride Moban *Antipsychotic* Pregnancy Risk Category: NR	*Psychotic disorders* — **Adults:** initially, 50 to 75 mg P.O. q.d., increased to 100 to 225 mg/day in 3 or 4 days. Maintenance doses as follows: mild severity, 5 to 15 mg P.O. t.i.d. to q.i.d.; moderate severity, 10 to 25 mg P.O. t.i.d. or q.i.d.; extreme severity, 225 mg/day P.O. **Elderly:** Start therapy with lowest dose.	▪ Monitor for tardive dyskinesia. ▪ Assess for neuroleptic malignant syndrome. ▪ May treat acute dystonic reactions with diphenhydramine. ▪ Warn patient to avoid hazardous activities until CNS effects known. Drowsiness and dizziness usually subside after first few wk.

montelukast sodium Singulair *Antiasthmatic* Pregnancy Risk Category: B	*Prevention and treatment of chronic asthma* — **Adults and children ≥ 15 yr:** 10 mg (film-coated tablet) P.O. q.d. in evening. **Children 6 to 14 yr:** 5 mg (chewable tablet) P.O. q.d. in evening. *Prevention and long-term treatment of asthma* — **Children ages 2 to 5:** 4-mg chewable tablet P.O. q.d. h.s.	▪ Don't abruptly substitute drug for inhaled or oral corticosteroids. ▪ Drug isn't indicated for use in patients with acute asthmatic attacks or status asthmaticus or as monotherapy for management of exercise-induced bronchospasm. Patient should continue appropriate rescue medication for acute exacerbations.
moricizine hydrochloride Ethmozine *Antiarrhythmic* Pregnancy Risk Category: B	*Life-threatening ventricular arrhythmias* — **Adults:** dosages individualized. Therapy should begin in hospital. Most patients respond to 600 to 900 mg P.O. q.d. in divided doses q 8 hr. Daily dose increased q 3 days by 150 mg.	▪ Determine electrolyte status and correct imbalances before therapy. ▪ Notify doctor if chest pain or discomfort or fever occurs.
morphine hydrochloride Morphitec†, M.O.S.† **morphine sulfate** Astramorph, Astramorph PF, Duramorph, Epimorph†, Infumorph 200, MSIP, Morphine H.P.†, MS Contin, Oramorph SR, RMS Roxanol **morphine tartrate†** *Opioid* Pregnancy Risk Category: C Controlled Substance Schedule: II	*Severe pain* — **Adults:** 5 to 20 mg S.C. or I.M., or 2.5 to 15 mg I.V. q 4 hr, p.r.n.; or 10 to 30 mg P.O. or 10 to 20 mg P.R. q 4 hr, p.r.n. When given by continuous I.V., loading dose of 15 mg I.V. may be followed by continuous infusion of 0.8 to 10 mg/hr. May also give 15 to 30 mg controlled-release tablets P.O. q 8 to 12 hr. As epidural injection, 5 mg; then, if adequate pain relief not obtained within 1 hr, additional doses of 1 to 2 mg. Maximum total epidural dose shouldn't exceed 10 mg/24 hr. **Children:** 0.1 to 0.2 mg/kg S.C. or I.M. q 4 hr. Maximum single dose 15 mg.	▪ Keep narcotic antagonist (naloxone) and resuscitation equipment available. ▪ When given epidurally, monitor for respiratory depression up to 24 hr after injection. ▪ Monitor circulatory, respiratory, bowel, and bladder functions carefully. May cause transient BP decrease. May worsen or mask gallbladder pain. ▪ May cause CNS depression, hypotension, urine retention, nausea, vomiting, or ileus. Withhold dose and notify doctor if respirations < 12. ▪ Tell patient not to crush, break, or chew controlled-release tablets.

†Canadian ‡Australian

DRUG & CLASS	INDICATIONS & DOSAGES	NURSING CONSIDERATIONS
moxifloxacin hydrochloride Avelox *Antibiotic* Pregnancy Risk Category: C	*Acute bacterial sinusitis from* Streptococcus pneumoniae, Haemophilus influenzae, *or* Moraxella catarrhalis — **Adults:** 400 mg P.O. q.d. for 10 days. *Acute bacterial exacerbation of chronic bronchitis from* S. pneumoniae, H. influenzae, H. parainfluenzae, Klebsiella pneumoniae, Staphylococcus aureus, *or* M. catarrhalis — **Adults:** 400 mg P.O. q.d. for 5 days. *Mild to moderate community-acquired pneumonia from* S. pneumoniae, H. influenzae, Mycoplasma pneumoniae, Chlamydia pneumoniae, *or* M. catarrhalis — **Adults:** 400 mg P.O. q.d. for 10 days.	▪ Drug may be given without regard to meals. Give at same time each day. ▪ ***ALERT*** Monitor patient for CNS events, including seizures, dizziness, confusion, tremors, hallucinations, depression, and suicidal thoughts or acts. If these reactions occur, stop drug and institute appropriate measures. ▪ Serious hypersensitivity reactions, including anaphylaxis, have occurred in patients receiving fluoroquinolones. Stop moxifloxacin and begin supportive measures as indicated. ▪ Rupture of the Achilles and other tendons has been associated with fluoroquinolones. If pain, inflammation, or rupture of a tendon occurs, moxifloxacin should be stopped. ▪ ***ALERT*** Give moxifloxacin 4 hr before or 8 hr after antacids, sucralfate, or didanosine chewable buffered tablets or pediatric powder for oral solution, and products containing iron or zinc.
mupirocin Bactroban *Topical antibacterial* Pregnancy Risk Category: B	*Impetigo* — **Adults and children:** apply to affected areas t.i.d. for 1 to 2 wk.	▪ Wash and dry affected area thoroughly. Apply thin film, rubbing in gently. ▪ If no improvement in 3 to 5 days, tell patient to notify doctor immediately. ▪ Warn patient about local adverse reactions.

mycophenolate mofetil CellCept **mycophenolate mofetil hydrochloride** CellCept Intravenous *Immunosuppressant* Pregnancy Risk Category: C	*To prevent organ rejection in allogenic heart or kidney transplant patients* — **Adults:** 1 g P.O. or I.V. b.i.d. (kidney transplant) or 1.5 g P.O. or I.V. b.i.d. (heart transplant) within 72 hr after transplant, together with corticosteroids and cyclosporine. *For use with cyclosporine and corticosteroids to prevent organ rejection in heart transplant patients* — **Adults:** 1.5 g P.O. or I.V. b.i.d. with cyclosporine and corticosteroids. *For use with cyclosporine and corticosteroids to prevent organ rejection in allogeneic liver transplant patients*— **Adults:** 1 g I.V. b.i.d. over ≥ 2 hr or 1.5 g P.O. b.i.d. ***Adjust-a-dose:*** In patients with severe chronic renal impairment outside of immediate transplant period, avoid doses > 1 g b.i.d. If neutropenia occurs, interrupt or reduce dose.	▪ Don't open or crush capsule. Avoid inhaling powder in capsule or letting it contact skin or mucous membranes. If contact occurs, wash with soap and water and rinse eyes with plain water. ▪ Stress importance of not stopping therapy without consulting doctor. ▪ Monitor CBC regularly. ▪ May have teratogenic effects. Tell woman to use contraception during therapy and for 6 wk after stopping drug. ▪ Dilute infusion to 6 mg/dl in D_5W and infuse over ≥ 2 hr.
nabumetone Relafen *Antarthritic* Pregnancy Risk Category: C	*Rheumatoid arthritis; osteoarthritis* — **Adults:** initially, 1,000 mg P.O. q.d. as single dose or in divided doses b.i.d. Maximum 2,000 mg/day.	▪ May lead to reversible renal impairment. ▪ May cause serious GI toxicity. Teach patient about signs and symptoms of GI bleeding. ▪ With long-term therapy, monitor renal and liver function, CBC, and Hct.
nadolol Corgard *Antihypertensive, antianginal* Pregnancy Risk Category: C	*Long-standing angina pectoris* — **Adults:** 40 mg P.O. q.d. Increased in 40- to 80-mg increments q 3 to 7 days until response optimum. Maintenance 40 to 80 mg q.d. Dosage up to 160 to 240 mg q.d. may be needed. *Hypertension* — **Adults:** 40 mg P.O. q.d. In-	▪ Check apical pulse before giving. If < 60, withhold dose and call doctor. Monitor BP frequently. If severe hypotension occurs, give vasopressor. ▪ Masks signs of shock and hyperthyroidism. *(continued)*

DRUG & CLASS	INDICATIONS & DOSAGES	NURSING CONSIDERATIONS
nadolol *(continued)*	crease in 40- to 80-mg increments until response optimum. Maintenance 40 to 80 mg q.d. Doses of 320 mg q.d. may be needed. ***Adjust-a-dose:*** In renally impaired patients, adjust dosage interval according to creatinine clearance .	▪ Stopping drug abruptly can exacerbate angina and trigger MI. Reduce dosage gradually over 1 to 2 wk.
nafcillin sodium Nallpen, Unipen *Antibiotic* Pregnancy Risk Category: B	*Systemic infections from penicillinase-producing staphylococci* — **Adults:** 2 to 4 g P.O. q.d. in divided doses q 6 hr; or 2 to 12 g I.M. or I.V. q.d. in divided doses q 4 to 6 hr. **Children:** 25 to 50 mg/kg P.O. q.d. in divided doses q 6 hr. **Neonates:** 25 mg/kg I.V. b.i.d.	▪ Ask about allergic reactions to penicillin. Obtain specimen for culture and sensitivity tests before 1st dose. ▪ Give P.O. 1 to 2 hr before or 2 to 3 hr after meals. ▪ Give > 1 hr before bacteriostatic antibiotics.
nalbuphine hydrochloride Nubain *Analgesic, anesthesia adjunct* Pregnancy Risk Category: NR	*Moderate to severe pain* — **Adults:** For typical (70-kg [154-lb]) person, give 10 to 20 mg S.C., I.M., or I.V. q 3 to 6 hr, p.r.n. Maximum 160 mg/day. *Adjunct to balanced anesthesia* — **Adults:** 0.3 to 3 mg/kg I.V. over 10 to 15 min, then maintenance doses of 0.25 to 0.50 mg/kg in single I.V. dose, p.r.n.	▪ ***ALERT*** Causes respiratory depression, which can be reversed with naloxone. Monitor circulatory and respiratory status and bladder and bowel function. ▪ Acts as narcotic antagonist; may trigger withdrawal syndrome. ▪ ***I.V. use:*** Inject slowly over ≥ 2 to 3 min into vein or into I.V. line containing compatible, free-flowing I.V. solution.
naloxone hydrochloride Narcan *Narcotic antagonist* Pregnancy Risk Category: B	*Narcotic-induced respiratory depression* — **Adults:** 0.4 to 2 mg I.V., S.C., or I.M. repeated q 2 to 3 min, p.r.n. If no response after 10 mg, reconsider diagnosis of narcotic-induced toxicity. **Children:** 0.01 mg/kg I.V., then 2nd	▪ Abrupt reversal of opiate-induced CNS depression may result in nausea, vomiting, diaphoresis, tachycardia, tachypnea, CNS excitement, and increased BP. ▪ ***ALERT*** Monitor respiratory depth and

	dose of 0.1 mg/kg I.V., p.r.n. If I.V. route not available, may give I.M. or S.C. in divided doses. **Neonates:** 0.01 mg/kg I.V., I.M., or S.C. May repeat dose q 2 to 3 min, p.r.n. *Postoperative narcotic depression* — **Adults:** 0.1 to 0.2 mg I.V. q 2 to 3 min, p.r.n. May repeat dosage within 1 to 2 hr, p.r.n. **Children:** 0.005 to 0.01 mg I.V. Repeat q 2 to 3 min, p.r.n. **Neonates (asphyxia neonatorum):** 0.01 mg/kg I.V. into umbilical vein. May repeat q 2 to 3 min.	rate. Be prepared to provide oxygen, ventilation, and other resuscitation measures. ▪ ***I.V. use:*** Be prepared to give continuous I.V. infusion. If 0.02 mg/ml not available, may dilute adult concentration (0.4 mg) by mixing 0.5 ml with 9.5 sterile water or 0.9% NaCl for injection to make neonatal concentration (0.02 mg/ml). ▪ Narcotic duration of action may exceed that of naloxone; patient may relapse into respiratory depression.
naltrexone hydrochloride Depade, ReVia *Narcotic detoxification adjunct* Pregnancy Risk Category: C	*Adjunct for maintenance of opioid-free state in detoxified individuals* — **Adults:** 25 mg P.O. If no withdrawal signs < 1 hr, give additional 25 mg. When patient on 50 mg q 24 hr, may use flexible maintenance schedule. *Treatment of alcohol dependence* — **Adults:** 50 mg P.O. q.d.	▪ Treatment for opioid dependency should not begin until patient receives naloxone challenge. If signs of withdrawal persist, don't give naltrexone. ▪ ***ALERT*** Patient must be completely opioid-free before taking, or severe withdrawal symptoms may occur.
naphazoline hydrochloride (ophthalmic) AK-Con, Allerest, Clear Eyes, Naphcon, Naphcon Forte, Optazine‡, VasoClear, Vasocort Regular *Decongestant, vasoconstrictor* Pregnancy Risk Category: C	*Ocular congestion, irritation, itching* — **Adults:** 1 drop 0.1% solution instilled q 3 to 4 hr, or 1 drop 0.012% to 0.03% solution up to q.i.d.	▪ Wash hands before and after instilling. Apply light pressure on lacrimal sac. Don't touch dropper tip to eye or surrounding tissue. ▪ Notify doctor if photophobia, blurred vision, pain, or lid edema develops. ▪ Instruct patient not to use OTC preparations > 72 hr without consulting doctor.

DRUG & CLASS	INDICATIONS & DOSAGES	NURSING CONSIDERATIONS
naproxen Inza 250‡, Naprosyn, Naprosyn SR†‡, Novo-Naprox† **naproxen sodium** Aleve, Anaprox, Anaprox DS, Apo-Napro-Na†, Naprelan, Naprogesic‡, Synflex† *Nonnarcotic analgesic, antipyretic, anti-inflammatory* Pregnancy Risk Category: B	*Rheumatoid arthritis; osteoarthritis; ankylosing spondylitis; pain; dysmenorrhea; tendinitis; bursitis* — **Adults:** 250 to 500 mg (naproxen) b.i.d.; maximum 1.5 g/day. Or, 750 to 1,000 mg controlled-release (Naprelan) b.i.d.; or 275 to 550 mg naproxen sodium b.i.d. *Juvenile arthritis* — **Children:** 10 mg/kg P.O. in 2 divided doses. *Acute gout* — **Adults:** 750 mg (naproxen) P.O., then 250 mg q 8 hr until attack subsides. Or, 825 mg naproxen sodium, then 275 mg q 8 hr until attack subsides; or 1,000 to 1,500 mg/day controlled-release (Naprelan) on 1st day, then 1,000 mg q.d. *Mild to moderate pain* — **Adults:** 500 mg (naproxen) P.O., then 250 mg q 6 to 8 hr, up to 1.25 g/day. Or, 550 mg naproxen sodium, then 275 mg q 6 to 8 hr, up to 1.375 g/day; or 1,000 mg controlled-release (Naprelan) q.d.	▪ May lead to reversible renal impairment, especially in preexisting renal failure, liver dysfunction, or heart failure, and in elderly patients and patients taking diuretics. ▪ ***ALERT*** Serious GI toxicity, including peptic ulcers and bleeding, can occur despite absence of GI symptoms. Teach patient about signs and symptoms of GI bleeding. Tell him to contact doctor immediately if they occur. ▪ Caution that use with aspirin, alcohol, or corticosteroids may increase risk of adverse GI reactions. ▪ May mask signs and symptoms of infection. ▪ Warn against activities that require mental alertness until CNS effects known. ▪ Advise patient to take with food or milk to minimize GI upset. Instruct to take each dose with full glass of water or other fluid. ▪ If patient taking for arthritis, inform him that full therapeutic effect may take 2 to 4 wk.
naratriptan hydrochloride Amerge *Antimigraine agent* Pregnancy Risk Category: C	*Acute migraine headache attacks with or without aura* — **Adults:** 1 or 2.5 mg P.O. as single dose. If headache returns or if response only partial, may repeat dose after 4 hr; maximum 5 mg within 24 hr. ***Adjust-a-dose:*** In patients with renal or hepatic impairment, use lower initial dose. Maximum 2.5 mg/24 hr.	▪ Use cautiously in patients with risk factors for CAD unless CV evaluation shows patient doesn't have cardiac disease. ▪ Can cause coronary artery vasospasm and increase risk of cerebrovascular events. ▪ Don't use for prophylactic therapy in managing hemiplegic or basilar migraine.

nefazodone hydrochloride Serzone *Antidepressant* Pregnancy Risk Category: C	*Depression* — **Adults:** initially, 200 mg q.d. P.O. in 2 divided doses. Increase in increments of 100 to 200 mg q.d. at intervals of ≥ 1 wk, p.r.n. Usual range 300 to 600 mg q.d. Full effect may take several wk. **Elderly:** 50 mg P.O. b.i.d. ***Adjust-a-dose:*** In debilitated patients, initially, 50 mg, P.O. b.i.d.	▪ Separate from MAO inhibitor dosage by ≥ 2 wk. ▪ Monitor patient for suicidal tendencies. ▪ Warn patient not to engage in hazardous activity until CNS effects known.
nelfinavir mesylate Viracept *Antiviral* Pregnancy Risk Category: B	*HIV infection when antiretroviral therapy warranted* — **Adults:** 750 mg P.O. t.i.d. **Children 2 to 13 yr:** 20 to 30 mg/kg/dose P.O. t.i.d. Maximum 750 mg t.i.d.	▪ Monitor LFT results. ▪ Give oral powder to children unable to take tablets. Mixing with acidic foods or juice creates a bitter taste. ▪ Give with meals or light snack.
neomycin sulfate (oral) Mycifradin, Neo-fradin, Neosulf‡, Neo-Tabs *Antibiotic* Pregnancy Risk Category: NR	*Infectious diarrhea caused by* E. coli — **Adults:** 50 mg/kg q.d. P.O. in 4 divided doses for 2 to 3 days; maximum 3 g q.d. **Children:** 50 to 100 mg/kg/day P.O. divided q 4 to 6 hr for 2 to 3 days. *Suppression of intestinal bacteria preoperatively* — **Adults:** 1 g P.O. q hr for 4 doses, then 1 g q 4 hr for balance of 24 hr. Saline cathartic should precede therapy. **Children:** 50 to 100 mg/kg/day P.O. divided q 4 to 6 hr. First dose should follow saline cathartic.	▪ Monitor renal function (output, specific gravity, urinalysis, BUN, creatinine level, and CrCl). Notify doctor of signs of decreasing renal function. ▪ Evaluate hearing before, during, and after prolonged therapy. ▪ For preoperative disinfection, provide low-residue diet and cathartic immediately before giving P.O.
neomycin sulfate (topical) Mycifradin†, Myciguent *Antibiotic* Pregnancy Risk Category: C	*Prevention or treatment of superficial bacterial infections* — **Adults and children:** rub into affected area once daily to t.i.d.	▪ More absorption occurs on abraded areas. ▪ Watch for signs of hypersensitivity and ototoxicity. ▪ If no improvement or if condition worsens, tell patient to stop using and notify doctor.

†Canadian ‡Australian

DRUG & CLASS	INDICATIONS & DOSAGES	NURSING CONSIDERATIONS
neostigmine bromide, neostigmine methylsulfate Prostigmin *Muscle stimulant* Pregnancy Risk Category: C	*Symptomatic control of myasthenia gravis* — **Adults:** 0.5 mg S.C. or I.M. P.O. dose from 15 to 375 mg/day. Later dosages individualized. **Children:** 7.5 to 15 mg P.O. t.i.d. to q.i.d. *Diagnosis of myasthenia gravis* — **Adults:** 0.022 mg/kg I.M. 30 min after atropine I.M. **Children:** 0.025 to 0.04 mg/kg I.M. after atropine S.C. *Postoperative abdominal distention and bladder atony* — **Adults:** 0.5 to 1 mg I.M. or S.C. q 3 hr for 5 doses after bladder has emptied. *Antidote for nondepolarizing neuromuscular blocking agents* — **Adults:** 0.5 to 2 mg I.V. slowly. Repeat, p.r.n., to total of 5 mg. Before antidote dose, give atropine I.V.	▪ In myasthenia gravis, schedule doses before periods of fatigue. ▪ ***I.V. use:*** Give at slow, controlled rate, ≤ 1 mg/min in adults and 0.5 mg/min in children. ▪ Monitor vital signs frequently, especially respirations. Have atropine injection available and be prepared to give; provide respiratory support, p.r.n. ▪ Monitor and document response after each dose. Optimum dosage hard to judge. Observe closely for improvement in strength, vision, and ptosis 45 to 60 min after each dose. ▪ Resistance to drug may occur.
nevirapine Viramune *Antiviral* Pregnancy Risk Category: C	*Adjunctive treatment in patients with HIV-1 infection* — **Adults:** 200 mg P.O. q.d. for first 14 days, then 200 mg P.O. b.i.d. Used in combination with nucleoside analogue antiretroviral agents. **Children ages 8 and older:** 4 mg/kg P.O. q.d. for first 14 days; then 4 mg/kg P.O. b.i.d. (not to exceed 400 mg/day). **Children ages 2 mo to 7 yr:** 4 mg/kg P.O. q.d. for first 14 days; then 7 mg/kg P.O. b.i.d. (not to exceed 400 mg/day).	▪ Monitor LFTs. ▪ If therapy interrupted for > 7 days, restart as if giving for 1st time. ▪ Advise women not to use hormonal birth control methods. ▪ Notify doctor if severe rash occurs.

niacin (vitamin B_3, nicotinic acid) Niac, Niacor, Nico-400, Nicobid, Nicolar **niacinamide (nicotinamide)** *Vitamin B_3, antilipemic, peripheral vasodilator* Pregnancy Risk Category: C	*Pellagra* — **Adults:** 300 to 500 mg P.O., S.C., I.M., or I.V. q.d. in divided doses, depending on severity of deficiency. **Children:** up to 300 mg P.O. q.d. in divided doses, depending on severity of deficiency. *Hyperlipidemias, especially with hypercholesterolemia (niacin only)* — **Adults:** 1 to 2 g P.O. t.i.d. with or after meals, increased at intervals to 6 g q.d.	▪ ***I.V. use:*** Give no faster than 2 mg/min. ▪ Give aspirin to reduce flushing response p.r.n. ▪ Stress that niacin is potent medication, not just vitamin, and may cause serious adverse effects. Explain importance of adhering to therapeutic regimen. ▪ Monitor hepatic function and blood glucose level early in therapy. ▪ Give with meals.
nicardipine Cardene, Cardene IV, Cardene SR *Antianginal, antihypertensive* Pregnancy Risk Category: C	*Chronic stable angina, hypertension* — **Adults:** initially, 20 mg P.O. t.i.d. (immediate-release only). Adjust to response q 3 days. Usual range 20 to 40 mg t.i.d. Usual range 30 to 60 mg (SR) b.i.d. *Short-term management of hypertension* — **Adults:** if unable to take oral nicardipine, give 5 mg/hr I.V. infusion, titrated to 2.5 mg/hr q 15 min to maximum 15 mg/hr.	▪ ***I.V. use:*** When switching to P.O. therapy other than nicardipine, initiate when infusion stopped. If P.O. nicardipine to be used, give first dose of t.i.d. regimen 1 hr before infusion stopped. ▪ Measure BP frequently during initial therapy. Check for orthostatic hypotension. Adjust rate if hypotension or tachycardia occurs. ▪ Tell patient to report chest pain immediately.
nicotine polacrilex (nicotine resin complex) Nicorette, Nicorette DS, Nicotrol NS *Smoking cessation aid* Pregnancy Risk Category: X	*Relief of nicotine withdrawal symptoms in patients undergoing smoking cessation* — **Adults**: initially, one 2-mg square; highly dependent patients should start with 4-mg. Chew 1 piece of gum slowly and intermittently for 30 min whenever urge occurs. Most require 9 to 12 pieces daily during first mo. For patients using 4-mg squares, maximum 20 pieces daily. For patients using 2-mg squares, maximum 30 pieces daily.	▪ Instruct patient to chew gum slowly and intermittently (chew several times; then place between cheek and gum) for about 30 min. Fast chewing tends to produce more adverse reactions. ▪ Most likely to benefit smokers with high physical nicotine dependence.

DRUG & CLASS	INDICATIONS & DOSAGES	NURSING CONSIDERATIONS
nicotine transdermal system Habitrol, Nicoderm, Nicotrol, ProStep *Smoking cessation aid* Pregnancy Risk Category: D	*Relief of nicotine withdrawal symptoms in patients undergoing smoking cessation* — **Adults:** initially, 1 transdermal system, delivering largest available nicotine dose in series, applied q.d. to nonhairy body part. For Habitrol, Nicoderm, and ProStep, patch should be kept on 24 hr, then removed and new system applied to alternate skin site. For Nicotrol, patch should be applied on awakening and removed h.s. After 4 to 12 wk, taper to next lowest dose in series, then in 2 to 4 wk to lowest system in series being used. Stop drug in 2 to 4 wk.	▪ To reduce exposure to nicotine, avoid unnecessary contact with system. Wash hands with water alone; soap may enhance absorption. ▪ Teach patient proper disposal to prevent accidental poisoning of children or pets. ▪ Warn patient not to smoke. ▪ Advise patient to apply patch promptly. Patch should not be altered in any way (folded or cut) before application.
nifedipine Adalat, Adalat CC, Adapine‡, Apo-Nifed†, Nu-Nifed†, Procardia, Procardia XL *Antianginal* Pregnancy Risk Category: C	*Prinzmetal's (variant) angina* — **Adults:** starting dose 10 mg P.O. t.i.d. Usual effective range 10 to 20 mg t.i.d. Maximum 180 mg/day. *Hypertension* — **Adults:** 30 or 60 mg P.O. q.d. Adjust over 7 to 14 days. Don't give > 90 mg (for Adalat CC) or 120 mg (for Procardia XL) q.d.	▪ When rapid response to drug desired, have patient bite and swallow capsule. ▪ Monitor BP and ECG continuously. ▪ Patient may briefly develop anginal exacerbation.
nilutamide Anandron†, Nilandron *Antiandrogen* Pregnancy Risk Category: C	*Adjunct therapy with surgical castration for treatment of metastatic prostate cancer* — **Adults:** 6 tablets (50 mg each) P.O. q.d. for total of 300 mg/day for 30 days; then 3 tablets q.d. for total of 150 mg/day thereafter.	▪ Begin on same day or day after surgical castration, for maximum benefit. ▪ Tell patient to report dyspnea or aggravation of preexisting dyspnea immediately.
nisoldipine Sular	*Hypertension* — **Adults:** 20 mg (10 mg if patient > 65 or has liver dysfunction) P.O. q.d.;	▪ Monitor carefully. Some patients experience increased frequency, duration, or

Antihypertensive Pregnancy Risk Category: C	increased by 10 mg/wk or at longer intervals, p.r.n. Usual maintenance dosage 20 to 40 mg/day. Maximum 60 mg/day.	severity of angina or even acute MI after starting drug or when dosage increased. ▪ Monitor BP regularly.
nitrofurantoin macrocrystals Macrobid, Macrodantin **nitrofurantoin microcrystals** Furadantin, Mac *Urinary tract anti-infective* Pregnancy Risk Category: B	*UTIs caused by susceptible organisms* — **Adults and children > 12 yr:** 50 to 100 mg P.O. q.i.d. with meals and h.s. **Children 1 mo to 12 yr:** 5 to 7 mg/kg P.O. q.d. divided q.i.d. *Long-term suppression therapy* — **Adults:** 50 to 100 mg P.O. q.d. h.s. **Children:** 1 mg/kg P.O. q.d. in single dose h.s. or divided into 2 doses.	▪ Obtain urine specimen for culture and sensitivity tests before therapy. ▪ May cause growth of nonsusceptible organisms. ▪ Give with food or milk to minimize GI distress and improve absorption. ▪ Monitor I&O carefully. ▪ Drug may darken urine.
nitrofurazone Furacin *Topical antibacterial* Pregnancy Risk Category: C	*Adjunct treatment of 2nd- and 3rd-degree burns; prevention of skin allograft rejection* — **Adults and children:** Apply directly to lesion daily or q few days, depending on burn severity. May also apply to dressings used to cover affected area.	▪ Clean wound before reapplying dressings. ▪ When using wet dressing, protect skin around wound with zinc oxide ointment. ▪ Report irritation, sensitization, or infection.
nitroglycerin (glyceryl trinitrate) Anginine‡, Deponit, Minitran, Nitro-Bid, Nitrocine, Nitrodisc, Nitro-Dur, Nitrogard, Nitroglyn, Nitrol, Nitrolingual, Nitrostat, Transderm-Nitro, Transiderm-Nitro‡, Tridil *Antianginal, vasodilator*	*To prevent chronic anginal attacks* — **Adults:** 2.5 mg or 2.6 mg sustained-release capsule q 8 to 12 hr. Or, use 2% ointment range ½″ to 5″. Or, transdermal disc or pad 0.2 to 0.4 mg/hr q.d. *Acute angina pectoris; to prevent or minimize anginal attacks* — **Adults:** 1 S.L. tablet. Repeat q 5 min, p.r.n., for 15 min. Or, using Nitrolingual, 1 or 2 sprays into mouth. Repeat q 3 to 5 min, p.r.n., to maximum 3 doses in 15-min. Or, 1 to 3 mg transmu-	▪ Advise patient that stopping drug abruptly can cause coronary vasospasms. ▪ ***ALERT*** Closely monitor vital signs during infusion. Excessive hypotension may worsen MI. ▪ Measure prescribed amount on application paper; then place on nonhairy area. Don't rub in. Cover with plastic film. If using Tape-Surrounded Appli-Ruler (TSAR) system, keep TSAR on skin to protect clothing.

(continued)

DRUG & CLASS	INDICATIONS & DOSAGES	NURSING CONSIDERATIONS
nitroglycerin *(continued)* Pregnancy Risk Category: C	cosally q 3 to 5 hr while awake. *Hypertension; heart failure; acute angina pectoris; to control hypotension during surgery (by I.V. infusion)* — **Adults:** 5 mcg/min, increased p.r.n. by 5 mcg/min q 3 to 5 min until response.	▪ Remove transdermal patch before defibrillation. ▪ Keep S.L. tablets capped in original container. Protect from heat and moisture.
nitroprusside sodium Nitropress *Antihypertensive* Pregnancy Risk Category: C	*Hypertensive emergencies* — **Adults and children:** 50-mg vial diluted with 2 to 3 ml of D_5W and added to 250, 500, or 1,000 ml of D_5W; infuse I.V. at 0.3 to 10 mcg/kg/min titrated to BP. Maximum rate 10 mcg/kg/min. *Acute heart failure* — **Adults and children:** I.V. infusion titrated to cardiac output and systemic BP. Same dosage range as for hypertensive emergencies.	▪ ***I.V. use:*** Obtain vital signs and parameters before giving. Check BP q 5 min at start and then q 15 min. If severe hypotension occurs, stop infusion and notify doctor. Check serum thiocyanate levels q 72 hr. Levels > 100 mcg/ml associated with toxicity. ▪ Sensitive to light; wrap I.V. solution in foil. Fresh solution should be faintly brownish. ▪ Don't piggyback with other drugs.
nizatidine Axid, Axid AR, Tazac‡ *Antiulcer agent* Pregnancy Risk Category: C	*Active duodenal ulcer* — **Adults:** 300 mg P.O. q.d. h.s. Or, 150 mg P.O. b.i.d. *Maintenance therapy for duodenal ulcer* — **Adults:** 150 mg P.O. q.d. h.s. *Benign gastric ulcer* — **Adults:** 150 mg P.O. b.i.d. or 300 mg h.s. for 8 wk. *Gastroesophageal reflux disease* — **Adults:** 150 mg P.O. b.i.d.	▪ Tell patient with trouble swallowing capsules that contents may be mixed with apple juice but not with tomato-based juices. ▪ Encourage patient to avoid cigarette smoking; may increase gastric acid secretion and worsen disease. ▪ Increases serum salicylate levels when used with high doses of aspirin.
norepinephrine bitartrate Levophed *Vasopressor*	*To maintain BP in acute hypotensive states* — **Adults:** initially, 8 to 12 mcg/min I.V. infusion, then adjust to maintain normal BP. Average maintenance2 to 4 mcg/min.	▪ Check BP q 2 min until stabilized; then q 5 min. Frequently monitor ECG, cardiac output, CVP, PAWP, pulse rate, urine output, and color and temperature of extremities.

Pregnancy Risk Category: C	**Children:** 2 mcg/m²/min I.V. infusion. Adjust dose per response.	▪ Phentolamine is antidote for extravasation. ▪ When stopping, gradually slow rate.
norethindrone Micronor, Nor-Q.D. **norethindrone acetate** Aygestin, Norlu *Contraceptive* Pregnancy Risk Category: X	*Amenorrhea; abnormal uterine bleeding* — **Adults:** 2.5 to 20 mg norethindrone acetate P.O. q.d. on days 5 to 25 of menstrual cycle. *Endometriosis* — **Adults:** 5 to 10 mg norethindrone acetate P.O. q.d. for 2 wk; increase by 2.5 to 5 mg q.d. for 2 wk, up to 15 mg q.d. *Contraception* — **Women:** 0.35 mg norethindrone P.O. q.d., starting on 1st day of cycle.	▪ Norethindrone acetate is twice as potent as norethindrone. Don't use acetate for contraception. ▪ Watch carefully for signs of edema. ▪ Tell patient to report unusual symptoms immediately and to stop drug and call doctor if visual disturbance or migraine occurs.
norfloxacin *Broad-spectrum antibiotic* Pregnancy Risk Category: C	*UTIs caused by susceptible organisms* — **Adults:** for uncomplicated infections, 400 mg P.O. q 12 hr for 7 to 10 days. For complicated infections, 400 mg P.O. q 12 hr for 10 to 21 days. *Acute uncomplicated urethral, cervical gonorrhea* — **Adults:** 800 mg P.O. as single dose.	▪ Advise patient to take 1 hr before or 2 hr after meals. ▪ Tell patient to drink several glasses of water throughout day. ▪ Caution patient to avoid hazardous tasks that require alertness until CNS effects known.
norgestrel Ovrette *Contraceptive* Pregnancy Risk Category: X	*Contraception in women* — **Adults:** 0.075 mg P.O. q.d.	▪ Instruct patient to take every day at same time, even if menstruating.
nortriptyline hydrochloride Allegron‡, Aventyl, Pamelor *Antidepressant* Pregnancy Risk Category: NR	*Depression* — **Adults:** 25 mg P.O. t.i.d. or q.i.d., gradually increased to maximum 150 mg q.d. Entire dosage may be given h.s. Monitor plasma levels when giving doses > 100 mg/day. **Elderly:** 30 to 50 mg P.O. q.d. in single or divided doses.	▪ Adverse anticholinergic effects can occur rapidly. ▪ Warn patient to avoid activities that require alertness until CNS effects known. ▪ Tell patient to consult doctor before taking other prescription or OTC drugs.

†Canadian ‡Australian

DRUG & CLASS	INDICATIONS & DOSAGES	NURSING CONSIDERATIONS
nystatin Mycostatin, Nadostine†, Nilstat, Nystex *Antifungal* Pregnancy Risk Category: C	*Intestinal candidiasis* — **Adults:** 500,000 to 1 million U as oral tablets t.i.d. *Oral infections* — **Adults and children:** 400,000 to 600,000 U oral suspension q.i.d. **Infants:** 200,000 U oral suspension q.i.d. **Neonates and premature infants:** 100,000 U oral suspension q.i.d. *Vaginal infections* — **Adults:** 100,000 U (tablets) high into vagina q.d. for 14 days.	▪ Not effective against systemic infections. ▪ Pregnant patients can use vaginal tablets up to 6 wk before term. ▪ For treatment of oral candidiasis (thrush): After mouth cleaned of food debris, instruct patient to hold suspension in mouth for several min before swallowing. When treating infants, swab medication on oral mucosa.
octreotide acetate Sandostatin, Sandostatin LAR *Somatotropic hormone* Pregnancy Risk Category: B	*Flushing and diarrhea caused by carcinoid tumors* — **Adults:** 100 to 600 mcg q.d. S.C. in 2 to 4 divided doses for first 2 wk of therapy, then dose per response. *Watery diarrhea caused by vasoactive intestinal polypeptide–secreting tumors* — **Adults:** 200 to 300 mcg q.d. S.C. in 2 to 4 divided doses for first 2 wk of therapy. *Acromegaly* — **Adults:** initially, 50 mcg S.C. t.i.d., then adjusted according to somatomedin C levels q 2 wk. May switch patients currently receiving Sandostatin injection directly to depot. Give 20 mg I.M. intragluteally q 4 wk for 3 mo, then adjust dose according to growth hormone levels.	▪ LAR preparation for intragluteal use only. ▪ Monitor somatomedin C levels q 2 wk. ▪ Monitor urine 5-hydroxin-doleacetic acid, plasma serotonin, and substance P levels and thyroid function test results. ▪ May be linked to development of cholelithiasis. ▪ Monitor patient closely for symptoms of glucose imbalance.
ofloxacin Floxin, Floxin I.V. *Antibiotic*	*Lower respiratory tract infections* — **Adults:** 400 mg I.V. or P.O. q 12 hr for 10 days. *Cervicitis; urethritis* — **Adults:** 300 mg I.V.	▪ Use cautiously and with dosage adjustment in renal failure. ▪ Give serologic test for syphilis to patient

or P.O. q 12 hr for 7 days.

Acute, uncomplicated gonorrhea — **Adults:** 400 mg I.V. or P.O. as single dose with doxycycline.

Mild to moderate skin infections — **Adults:** 400 mg I.V. or P.O. q 12 hr for 10 days.

Cystitis; UTI — **Adults:** 200 mg I.V. or P.O. q 12 hr for 3 to 10 days.

Prostatitis — **Adults:** 300 mg I.V. or P.O. q 12 hr for 6 wk.

Pelvic inflammatory disease (outpatient) — **Adults:** 400 mg P.O. q 12 hr for 14 days.

Adjust-a-dose: Decrease dose or interval in patients with renal failure.

treated for gonorrhea. Drug not effective against syphilis; gonorrhea treatment may mask or delay symptoms of syphilis.

- Advise patient to take with plenty of fluids but not with meals.
- Instruct patient to stop drug and notify doctor if rash or other hypersensitivity signs occur.
- Advise patient to use sunscreen and wear protective clothing.

---

olanzapine
Zyprexa, Zyprexa Zydis
Antipsychotic
Pregnancy Risk Category: C

Short-term treatment of acute manic episodes from bipolar I disorder — **Adults:** Initially, 10 to 15 mg P.O. q.d. Adjust dose p.r.n. by increments of 5 mg q.d. at intervals of 24 hr or more. Maximum daily dose is 20 P.O. Duration of treatment is 3 to 4 wk.

Schizophrenia — **Adults:** Initially, 5 to 10 mg P.O. q.d. Target dose is 10 mg P.O. q.d. within several days of starting therapy. Dosage may be increased q wk in increments of 5 mg q.d. to a maximum daily dose of 20 mg P.O. Doses > 10 mg q.d. only after clinical assessment.

Adjust-a-dose: For debilitated and elderly patients, start therapy at low end of dosage range.

- Monitor patient for signs of neuroleptic malignant syndrome. Stop drug immediately.
- Monitor patient for tardive dyskinesia.
- Obtain baseline and periodic LFTs.

†Canadian ‡Australian

DRUG & CLASS	INDICATIONS & DOSAGES	NURSING CONSIDERATIONS
olsalazine sodium Dipentum *Anti-inflammatory* Pregnancy Risk Category: C	*Maintenance of remission of ulcerative colitis in patients who can't tolerate sulfasalazine* — **Adults:** 500 mg P.O. b.i.d. with meals.	▪ Regularly monitor BUN, creatinine, and urinalysis in preexisting renal disease. ▪ Give in divided doses and with food to minimize adverse GI reactions.
omeprazole Losec†‡, Prilosec *Gastric acid suppressant* Pregnancy Risk Category: C	Helicobacter pylori *eradication to reduce risk of duodenal ulcer recurrence; triple therapy consisting of omeprazole, clarithromycin, and amoxicillin* — **Adults:** 20 mg P.O. with clarithromycin 500 mg P.O. and amoxicillin 1 g P.O., each given b.i.d. for 10 days. *Patients with an ulcer present at initiation of therapy* — **Adults:** Additional 18 days of omeprazole 20 mg P.O. once daily. *Severe erosive esophagitis; gastroesophageal reflux disease* — **Adults:** 20 mg P.O. q.d. for 4 to 8 wk. *Hypersecretory conditions* — **Adults:** 60 mg P.O. q.d.; adjust to response. If dose > 80 mg, give in divided doses. *Duodenal ulcer* — **Adults:** 20 mg P.O. q.d. for 4 to 8 wk. *Active benign gastric ulcer* — **Adults:** 40 mg P.O. q.d. for 4 to 8 wk. H. pylori — **Adults:** 40 mg P.O. q morning with clarithromycin 500 mg t.i.d. for 14 days, then 20 mg q.d. for 14 days. Or, 20 mg P.O. with clarithromycin 500 mg P.O. and amoxicillin 1,000 mg P.O., each given for	▪ Increases its own bioavailability with repeated doses. ▪ Caution patient not to perform hazardous activities if dizziness occurs. ▪ Instruct patient to swallow capsules whole. ▪ Advise patient to report signs and symptoms of overdose: confusion, drowsiness, blurred vision, tachycardia, nausea and vomiting, diaphoresis, dry mouth, and headache.

	10 days, then 20 mg omeprazole for additional 18 days.	
ondansetron hydrochloride Zofran, Zofran ODT *Antiemetic* Pregnancy Risk Category: B	*Prevention of nausea and vomiting from chemotherapy* — **Adults and children ≥ 12 yr:** 8 mg P.O. 30 min before chemotherapy. Then 8 mg P.O. 8 hr after 1st dose, then 8 mg q 12 hr for 1 to 2 days. Or, single dose of 32 mg by I.V. infusion over 15 min, given 30 min before chemotherapy; or 3 divided doses of 0.15 mg/kg I.V. given over 15 min, 4 and 8 hr after 1st dose (30 min before chemotherapy). **Children 4 to 12 yr:** 4 mg P.O. 30 min before chemotherapy. Then 4 mg P.O. 4 and 8 hr after 1st dose, then 4 mg q 8 hr for 1 to 2 days. Or, 3 doses of 0.15 mg/kg I.V., given as for adults. *Prevention of nausea and vomiting from radiotherapy* — **Adults:** 8 mg P.O. t.i.d.	▪ Dilute I.V. form in 50 ml 5% dextrose or 0.9% NaCl before giving. ▪ Tell patient to alert nurse immediately for difficulty breathing after use. ▪ Tell patient receiving I.V. form to report discomfort at insertion site promptly. ▪ Watch for common adverse reactions, including headache, malaise, dizziness, sedation, diarrhea or constipation, and musculoskeletal pain. ▪ Don't remove orally disintegrating tablet until immediately before use.
opium tincture; opium tincture, camphorated (paregoric) *Antidiarrheal* Pregnancy Risk Category: NR Controlled Substance Schedule: II (tincture) or III (camphorated)	*Acute diarrhea* — ***Tincture*** — **Adults:** 0.6 ml (range 0.3 to 1 ml) P.O. q.i.d. Maximum 6 ml/day. ***Camphorated tincture*** — **Adults:** 5 to 10 ml P.O. once daily, b.i.d., t.i.d., or q.i.d. until diarrhea subsides. **Children:** 0.25 to 0.5 ml/kg camphorated tincture P.O. once daily, b.i.d., t.i.d., or q.i.d. until diarrhea subsides.	▪ Mix with enough water to ensure passage to stomach. ▪ For overdose, use narcotic antagonist naloxone to reverse respiratory depression. ▪ Opium content of tincture 25 times greater than that of camphorated tincture. Don't confuse the two. ▪ Risk of physical dependence; don't use for longer than 2 days.
oprelvekin Neumega *Platelet production stimulator*	*Prevention of severe thrombocytopenia and reduction of need for platelet transfusions after myelosuppressive chemotherapy with*	▪ Start 6 to 24 hr after chemotherapy ends, and stop at least 2 days before starting next cycle.

(continued)

†Canadian ‡Australian

DRUG & CLASS	INDICATIONS & DOSAGES	NURSING CONSIDERATIONS
oprelvekin *(continued)* Pregnancy Risk Category: C	*nonmyeloid malignancies* — **Adults:** 50 mcg/kg S.C. q.d.	▪ Use reconstituted drug within 3 hr. ▪ Refrigerate drug and diluent. ▪ Monitor fluid and electrolyte status in patients receiving diuretics.
orlistat Xenical *Antihyperlipidemic* Pregnancy Risk Category: B	*Obesity management when used with reduced-calorie diet; risk reduction for regaining weight after weight loss; for obese patients with initial body mass index ≥ 30 kg (66 lb)/m² or ≥ 27 kg (60 lb)/m² with other risk factors* — **Adult:** 120 mg P.O. t.i.d. with each main meal containing fat.	▪ Patient should take vitamin supplement q day at least 2 hr before or after use. ▪ Advise patient to distribute fat, carbohydrate, and protein intake over 3 main meals. ▪ If patient occasionally misses meal or eats meal without fat, dose can be omitted.
oseltamivir phosphate Tamiflu *Antiviral* Pregnancy Risk Category: C	*Uncomplicated, acute influenza infection in patients symptomatic for ≤ 2 days* — **Adults:** 75 mg P.O. b.i.d. for 5 days. ***Adjust-a-dose:*** For patients with CrCl < 30 ml/min, reduce dose to 75 mg P.O. q.d. for 5 days. *Prevention of influenza after close contact with infected person* — **Adults and adolescents ≥ 13 yr:** 75 mg P.O. q.d. beginning ≤ 2 days of exposure, for ≥ 1 wk. *Prevention of influenza during community outbreak* — **Adults and adolescents ≥ 13 yr:** 75 mg P.O. q.d. for < 6 wk.	▪ Use cautiously in patients with chronic cardiac or respiratory diseases, or any medical condition that may require imminent hospitalization. Also use cautiously in patients with renal failure, especially if CrCl < 10 ml/min. ▪ Drug treats influenza virus types A and B only. ▪ Give drug ≤ 2 days of symptom onset. ▪ Drug isn't a replacement for annual flu vaccine. Patients for whom vaccine is indicated should continue annual vaccine. ▪ Give drug with meals to decrease GI adverse effects.
oxacillin sodium Bactocill *Antibiotic*	*Infections from penicillinase-producing staphylococci* — **Adults and children > 40 kg (88 lb):** 500 mg to 1 g P.O. q 4 to 6	▪ Obtain specimen for culture and sensitivity tests before 1st dose. ▪ Watch for superinfection.

Pregnancy Risk Category: B	hr; or 1 to 2 g I.M. or I.V. q 4 to 6 hr. **Children ≤ 40 kg:** 50 to 100 mg/kg P.O. q.d. in divided doses q 6 hr; or 50 to 200 mg/kg I.M. or I.V. q.d. in divided doses q 4 to 6 hr.	▪ When given P.O., give 1 to 2 hr before or 2 to 3 hr after meals. ▪ Give at least 1 hr before bacteriostatic antibiotics.
oxaprozin Daypro *Anti-inflammatory* Pregnancy Risk Category: C	*Osteoarthritis; rheumatoid arthritis* — **Adults:** initially, 600 to 1,200 mg P.O. q.d. Then individualized to smallest effective dose. Maximum 1,800 mg or 26 mg/kg.	▪ May cause renal toxicity in susceptible patients. Closely monitor renal function. ▪ Elevated LFT results can occur after long-term use. ▪ May mask signs of infection.
oxazepam Alepam‡, Serax, Zapex† *Anxiolytic, sedative-hypnotic* Pregnancy Risk Category: NR Controlled Substance Schedule: IV	*Alcohol withdrawal; severe anxiety* — **Adults:** 15 to 30 mg P.O. t.i.d. or q.i.d. *Mild to moderate anxiety* — **Adults:** 10 to 15 mg P.O. t.i.d. or q.i.d. **Elderly:** initially, 10 mg t.i.d., increased to 15 mg t.i.d. to q.i.d., p.r.n.	▪ Use cautiously in elderly patients or in those with history of drug abuse. ▪ Monitor liver, renal, and hematopoietic function studies periodically. ▪ Possibility of abuse and addiction exists. Don't stop drug abruptly; withdrawal symptoms may occur.
oxcarbazepine Trileptal *Antiepileptic* Pregnancy Risk Category: C	*Adjunct treatment for partial seizures* — **Adults:** 300 mg P.O. b.i.d. Increase by ≤ 600 mg q wk, to 1,200 mg q.d., divided b.i.d. **Children 4 to 16 yr:** 8 to 10 mg/kg/day P.O., divided b.i.d., not to exceed 600 mg daily. Target maintenance dose (TMD) depends on patient weight and should be divided b.i.d. and achieved over 2 wk. If patient weighs 20 to 29 kg, TMD is 900 mg q.d.; if 29.1 to 39 kg, TMD is 1,200 mg q.d.; if > 39 kg, TMD is 1,800 mg q.d. *Conversion to monotherapy for partial seizures* — **Adults:** 300 mg P.O. b.i.d, while	▪ ***ALERT*** Ask patient if he is hypersensitive to carbamazepine; 25% to 30% of patients hypersensitive to carbamazepine are hypersensitive to oxcarbazepine. Gradually withdraw oxcarbazepine immediately if signs and symptoms of hypersensitivity occur. Gradual withdrawal minimizes potential for increased seizure frequency. ▪ Monitor for signs and symptoms of hyponatremia, including nausea, malaise, headache, lethargy, confusion, and decreased sensation. ▪ Monitor serum sodium *(continued)*

†Canadian ‡Australian

DRUG & CLASS	INDICATIONS & DOSAGES	NURSING CONSIDERATIONS
oxcarbazepine *(continued)*	gradually withdrawing concomitant antiepileptic dose (over 3 to 6 wk). Increase oxcarbazepine by ≤ 600 mg q wk over 2 to 4 wk to 2,400 mg q.d., divided b.i.d. *Monotherapy for partial seizures* — **Adults:** 300 mg P.O. b.i.d. Increase by 300 mg/day q 3rd day to 1,200 mg, divided b.i.d. ***Adjust-a-dose:*** For adults with CrCl < 30 ml/min, initiate therapy at 150 mg P.O. b.i.d. and increase slowly to achieve desired response.	levels in patients receiving oxcarbazepine for maintenance treatment, especially patients who are receiving other therapies that may decrease serum sodium levels. ▪ Use may cause CNS-related adverse effects, including psychomotor slowing; difficulty with concentration, speech, and language; fatigue and somnolence; and coordination abnormalities, including ataxia and gait disturbances.
oxycodone hydrochloride M-Oxy, Oxyfast, OxyContin, Oxy IR, Percolone, Roxicodone, Roxicodone Intensol, Supeudol† **oxycodone pectinate** *Analgesic* Pregnancy Risk Category: C Controlled Substance Schedule: II	*Moderate to severe pain for patients who need an around-the-clock analgesic for an extended time*— **Adults:** 5 mg P.O. q 6 hr.	▪ ***ALERT*** OxyContin tablets are to be swallowed whole. Breaking, crushing, or chewing them leads to rapid release of potentially fatal dose. ▪ Use single-agent solution or tablets in patients who shouldn't take aspirin or acetaminophen. ▪ Monitor circulatory and respiratory status. Withhold dose and notify doctor if respirations are shallow or if rate < 12 breaths per minute.
oxymetazoline hydrochloride (nasal) Afrin, Allerest 12 Hr Nasal Spray, Duramist Plus, Cheracol Nasal, Dristan 12 Hr Nasal, Genasol, Nostrilla	*Nasal congestion* — **Adults and children ≥ 6 yr:** 2 to 3 drops or sprays of 0.05% solution in each nostril b.i.d. **Children 2 to 6 yr:** 2 to 3 drops of 0.025% solution in each nostril b.i.d. Don't use > 3 to 5 days.	▪ Tell patient to hold head upright to avoid swallowing drug, and to sniff spray briskly. ▪ Tell patient not to exceed dosage and to use only p.r.n. ▪ Excessive use may cause bradycardia, hypotension, dizziness, and weakness.

Long-Acting Spray, Neo-Synephrine 12 Hr Nasal Spray *Decongestant, vasoconstrictor* Pregnancy Risk Category: NR		▪ Should be used by only 1 person.
oxytocin, synthetic injection Pitocin, Syntocinon *Oxytocic, lactation stimulant* Pregnancy Risk Category: NR	*Induction, stimulation of labor* — **Adults:** 1-ml (10 U) ampule in 1,000 ml dextrose 5% injection or 0.9% NaCl I.V. infused at 1 to 2 milliunits/min. Increase in increments of $\leq$ 1 to 2 milliunits/min q 15 to 30 min. Dose rarely exceeds 9 to 10 milliunits/min. *Reduction of postpartum bleeding after placenta expulsion* — **Adults:** 10 to 40 U added to 1 L D_5W or 0.9% NaCl infused at 20 to 40 milliunits/min. Also, 1 ml (10 U) can be given I.M. after placenta delivery. *Incomplete or inevitable abortion* — **Adults:** 10 U I.V. in 500 ml 0.9% NaCl or dextrose 5% in 0.9% NaCl at 10 to 20 milliunits/min.	▪ ***I.V. use:*** Don't give by bolus injection. Give by piggyback infusion only, so drug may be stopped without interrupting I.V. line. Use infusion pump. ▪ Monitor I&O. Antidiuretic effect may lead to fluid overload, seizures, and coma. ▪ Monitor and record uterine contractions, HR, BP, intrauterine pressure, fetal HR, and character of blood loss q 15 min. ▪ ***ALERT*** If contractions are < 2 min apart and if contractions > 50 mm Hg are recorded, or if contractions last $\geq$ 90 sec, stop infusion, turn patient on side, and notify doctor.
paclitaxel Taxol *Antineoplastic* Pregnancy Risk Category: D	*Metastatic ovarian cancer* — **Adults:** 135 or 175 mg/m² I.V. over 3 hr q 3 wk (monotherapy). *Breast cancer* — **Adults:** 175 mg/m² I.V. over 3 hr q 3 wk (monotherapy). *Adjuvant treatment of node-positive breast cancer* — **Adults:** 175 mg/m² I.V. over 3 hr q 3 wk for 4 courses given sequentially to doxorubicin-containing combination chemotherapy.	▪ Closely monitor patient throughout infusion. ▪ Monitor blood counts during therapy. ▪ Watch for signs of infection and bleeding.
pamidronate disodium Aredia	*Moderate to severe hypercalcemia from cancer* — **Patients with albumin corrected serum calcium (CCa) levels 12 to 13.5**	▪ Use after patient hydrated. ▪ Monitor serum electrolytes, especially calcium, phosphate, and *(continued)*

DRUG & CLASS	INDICATIONS & DOSAGES	NURSING CONSIDERATIONS
pamidronate disodium *(continued)* *Antihypercalcemic* Pregnancy Risk Category: C	**mg/dl:** 60 to 90 mg by I.V. infusion over 4 hr for 60-mg dose and over 24 hr for 90-mg dose. **Patients with CCa levels > 13.5 mg/dl:** 90 mg by I.V. infusion over 24 hr. Minimum of 7 days before retreatment. *Moderate to severe Paget's disease* — **Adults:** 30 mg I.V. as 4-hr infusion on 3 days for total dose of 90 mg. Repeat, p.r.n. *Osteolytic bone lesions of multiple myeloma* — **Adults:** 90 mg I.V. as 4-hr infusion q 4 wk.	magnesium levels. Also monitor creatinine, CBC and differential, Hct, and Hgb. ▪ Carefully monitor patients with preexisting anemia, leukopenia, or thrombocytopenia during first 2 wk of therapy. ▪ ***I.V. use:*** Reconstitute vial with 10 ml sterile water for injection. After completely dissolved, add to 1,000 ml 0.45% or 0.9% NaCl for injection or D_5W. Don't mix with infusion solutions that contain calcium.
pantoprazole Protonix *Gastric acid suppressant* Pregnancy Risk Category: B	*Erosive esophagitis from gastroesophageal reflux disorder (GERD)* — **Adults:** 40 mg P.O. q.d. for ≤ 8 wk. If not healed after 8 wk of treatment, give additional 8-wk course. *Maintenance of healing of erosive esophagitis* — **Adults:** 40 mg P.O. q.d.	▪ Drug not for maintenance therapy > 16 wk. ▪ Symptomatic response to therapy doesn't preclude presence of gastric malignancy. ▪ Tell patient to take exactly as prescribed and at about the same time q.d., without regard to meals. ▪ Advise patient to swallow tablet whole and not crush, split, or chew.
paricalcitol Zemplar *Antihyperparathyroid agent* Pregnancy Risk Category: C	*Prevention and treatment of secondary hyperparathyroidism from chronic renal failure* — **Adults:** 0.04 to 0.1 mcg/kg (2.8 to 7 mcg) I.V. every other day during dialysis. Maximum 0.24 mcg/kg (16.8 mcg). Dose may be increased by 2 to 4 mcg at 2- to 4-wk intervals.	▪ Patients taking digoxin are at greater risk for digitalis toxicity because of potential for hypercalcemia. ▪ Monitor serum calcium and phosphorus twice/wk when dose adjusted, then q mo. Check parathyroid hormone level q 3 mo. ▪ Give as I.V. bolus only.

paroxetine hydrochloride
Paxil
Antidepressant
Pregnancy Risk Category: B

Depression — **Adults:** 20 mg P.O. q morning. If no response, increase by 10 mg/day at least weekly to maximum 50 mg q.d. Give 25 mg/day (extended-release), initially; then increase to maximum of 62.5 mg/day. *Panic disorder* — **Adults:** 10 mg/day. Increase by 10 mg/wk, p.r.n. Maximum dose $\leq$ 60 mg/day. *Social anxiety disorder* — **Adults:** initially, 20 mg P.O. daily, usually in the morning. Dosing range is 20 to 60 mg daily. Maintain patient on the lowest effective dosage and periodically assess patient to determine need for continued treatment.
Obsessive-compulsive disorder — **Adults:** 20 mg P.O. daily. Increase by 10 mg/day at least weekly to target dose of 40 mg/day. Maximum dose is 60 mg/day.
Adjust-a-dose: Start elderly or debilitated patients or patients with severe hepatic or renal disease on 10 mg P.O. q.d. Increase dosage p.r.n., up to 40 mg q.d.

- If psychosis occurs or increases, expect to reduce dosage.
- Warn patient to avoid hazardous activities until CNS effects known.
- Inform patient that orthostatic hypotension may occur. Tell patient to get out of bed slowly. Supervise patient's walking.

---

pegaspargase (PEG-L-asparaginase)
Oncaspar
Antineoplastic
Pregnancy Risk Category: C

Acute lymphoblastic leukemia in patients who need L-asparaginase but are hypersensitive to native forms — **Adults and children with body surface area (BSA) $\geq$ 0.6 m²:** 2,500 IU/m² I.M. or I.V. q 14 days. **Children with BSA < 0.6 m²:** 82.5 IU/kg I.M. or I.V. q 14 days.

- When giving I.M., limit volume given at single injection site to 2 ml.
- ***I.V. use:*** Give over 1 to 2 hr in 100 ml 0.9% NaCl or D_5W through infusion already running.
- Handle with care. Use gloves and don't inhale vapor or let contact skin or mucous membranes.

DRUG & CLASS	INDICATIONS & DOSAGES	NURSING CONSIDERATIONS
pemoline Cylert, Cylert Chewable *Analeptic* Pregnancy Risk Category: B Controlled Substance Schedule: IV	*Attention deficit hyperactivity disorder* — **Children ≥ 6 yr:** initially, 37.5 mg P.O. in morning with daily dose raised by 18.75 mg weekly, p.r.n. Effective dose range 56.25 to 75 mg q.d.; maximum 112.5 mg/day.	▪ ***ALERT*** Perform LFTs before and during therapy. Give drug only to patients without liver dysfunction and with normal baseline LFT results. ▪ May induce Tourette syndrome in children. ▪ Advise patient to take ≥ 6 hr before bedtime to avoid sleep interference.
penicillamine Cuprimine, Depen, D-Penamine‡ *Anti-inflammatory* Pregnancy Risk Category: NR	*Wilson's disease* — **Adults and children:** 250 mg P.O. q.i.d. 30 to 60 min before meals. Adjust dosage to achieve urinary copper excretion of 0.5 to 1 mg q.d. *Cystinuria* — **Adults:** 250 mg to 1 g P.O. q.i.d. before meals. Adjust dosage to urinary cystine excretion < 100 mg q.d. with calculi present or 100 to 200 mg q.d. when no calculi present. Maximum 4 g q.d. **Children:** 30 mg/kg P.O. q.d., divided q.i.d. before meals. Dose adjusted to achieve urinary cystine excretion < 100 mg q.d. when renal calculi present, or 100 to 200 mg q.d. with no calculi. *Rheumatoid arthritis* — **Adults:** initially, 125 to 250 mg P.O. q.d., with increases of 125 to 250 mg q 1 to 3 mo, if necessary. Maximum 1.5 g/day.	▪ Give dose on empty stomach, preferably 1 hr before or 3 hr after meals. ▪ If patient has skin reaction, give antihistamines, as prescribed. ▪ Report rash and fever to doctor immediately. ▪ Monitor CBC and renal and hepatic function q 2 wk for first 6 mo, then q mo. Monitor urinalysis regularly for protein loss. ▪ Withhold drug and notify doctor if WBC count < 3,500/mm³ or platelet count < 100,000/mm³. Progressive decline in platelet or WBC count in three successive blood tests may necessitate temporary discontinuation. ▪ Give supplemental pyridoxine daily.
penicillin G benzathine (benzylpenicillin	*Congenital syphilis* — **Children < 2 yr:** 50,000 U/kg I.M. once. *Group A streptococcal upper respiratory tract*	▪ Obtain specimen for culture and sensitivity tests before 1st dose. ▪ Never give I.V. Inject deeply into upper

benzathine) Bicillin L-A, Permapen *Antibiotic* Pregnancy Risk Category: B	*infections* — **Adults:** 1.2 million U I.M. once. **Children > 27 kg (60 lb):** 900,000 U I.M. once. **Children < 27 kg:** 300,000 to 600,000 U I.M. once. *Prophylaxis of poststreptococcal rheumatic fever* — **Adults and children:** 1.2 million U I.M. q mo or 600,000 U twice monthly. *Syphilis* — **Adults:** 2.4 million U I.M. once (< 1-yr duration); or, q wk for 3 wk (> 1-yr duration).	outer quadrant of buttocks in adults; in midlateral thigh in infants and small children. Avoid injection into or near major nerves or blood vessels. ▪ With large doses and prolonged therapy, superinfection may occur. ▪ Shake syringe before giving.
penicillin G potassium (benzylpenicillin potassium) Megacillin†, Pfizerpen *Antibiotic* Pregnancy Risk Category: B	*Moderate to severe systemic infection* — **Adults and children ≥ 12 yr:** individualized; 1.6 to 3.2 million U P.O. q.d. in divided doses q 6 hr; 1.2 to 24 million U I.M. or I.V. q.d. in divided doses q 4 hr. **Children < 12 yr:** 25,000 to 100,000 U/kg P.O. q.d. in divided doses q 6 hr; or 25,000 to 400,000 U/kg I.M. or I.V. q.d. in divided doses q 4 hr.	▪ Obtain specimen for culture and sensitivity tests before 1st dose. ▪ Monitor renal function closely. ▪ Give 1 to 2 hr before or 2 to 3 hr after meals. Food may interfere with absorption. ▪ Give at least 1 hr before bacteriostatic antibiotics.
penicillin G procaine (benzylpenicillin procaine) Ayercillin†, Crysticillin 300 A.S., Wycillin *Antibiotic* Pregnancy Risk Category: B	*Moderate to severe systemic infection* — **Adults:** 600,000 to 1.2 million U I.M. q.d. in single dose. **Children > 1 mo:** 25,000 to 50,000 U/kg I.M. q.d. in single dose. *Uncomplicated gonorrhea* — **Adults and children > 12 yr:** 1 g probenecid P.O.; after 30 min, 4.8 million U I.M., divided between 2 sites. *Pneumococcal pneumonia* — **Adults and children > 12 yr:** 600,000 to 1.2 million U I.M. q.d. for 7 to 10 days.	▪ Obtain specimen for culture and sensitivity tests before 1st dose. ▪ Never give I.V. ▪ Give deep I.M. in upper outer quadrant of buttocks in adults; in midlateral thigh in small children. Don't give S.C. or massage injection site. Avoid injection near major nerves or blood vessels.

†Canadian ‡Australian

DRUG & CLASS	INDICATIONS & DOSAGES	NURSING CONSIDERATIONS
penicillin G sodium (benzylpenicillin sodium) Crystapen† *Antibiotic* Pregnancy Risk Category: B	*Moderate to severe systemic infection* — **Adults and children ≥ 12 yr:** 1.2 to 24 million U q.d. I.M. or I.V. in divided doses q 4 to 6 hr. **Children < 12 yr:** 25,000 to 400,000 U/kg q.d. I.M. or I.V. in divided doses q 4 to 6 hr.	▪ For patients receiving ≥ 10 million U q.d., dilute in 1 to 2 L of compatible solution and give over 24 hr. Otherwise, give by intermittent I.V. infusion: Dilute drug in 50 to 100 ml, and give over 1 to 2 hr. ▪ Give ≥ 1 hr before bacteriostatic antibiotics.
pentamidine isethionate NebuPent, Pentacarinat, Pentam 300 *Antiprotozoal* Pregnancy Risk Category: C	P. carinii *pneumonia* — **Adults and children:** 3 to 4 mg/kg I.V. or I.M. q.d. for 2 to 3 wk. *Prevention of* P. carinii *pneumonia in high-risk individuals* — **Adults:** 300 mg by inhalation q 4 wk.	▪ Give aerosol form only by Respirgard II nebulizer. ▪ Don't mix with other drugs. ▪ Monitor serum glucose, serum calcium, serum creatinine, and BUN levels daily.
pentazocine hydrochloride Fortral‡, Talwin† **pentazocine hydrochloride and naloxone hydrochloride** Talwin-Nx **pentazocine lactate** Fortral‡, Talwin *Analgesic, adjunct to anesthesia* Pregnancy Risk Category: C Controlled Substance Schedule: IV	*Moderate to severe pain* — **Adults:** 50 to 100 mg P.O. q 3 to 4 hr, p.r.n. Maximum P.O. dose 600 mg/day. Or, 30 mg I.M., I.V., or S.C. q 3 to 4 hr, p.r.n. Maximum parenteral dose 360 mg/day. Single doses > 30 mg I.V. or 60 mg I.M. or S.C. not recommended. *Labor* — **Adults:** 30 mg I.M. or 20 mg I.V. q 2 to 3 hr with regular contractions.	▪ Have naloxone available. ▪ ***ALERT*** May trigger withdrawal syndrome in narcotic-dependent patients. ▪ May cause psychological and physical dependence with prolonged use. ▪ Talwin-Nx contains naloxone. This prevents illicit I.V. use.

pentobarbital Nembutal **pentobarbital sodium** Nembutal Sodium, Nova Rectal† *Anticonvulsant, sedative-hypnotic* Pregnancy Risk Category: D (suppositories C) Controlled Substance Schedule: II (suppositories III)	*Sedation* — **Adults:** 20 to 40 mg P.O. b.i.d., t.i.d., or q.i.d. **Children:** 2 to 6 mg/kg/day P.O. in 3 divided doses. Maximum 100 mg/day. *Insomnia* — **Adults:** 100 to 200 mg P.O. h.s. or 150 to 200 mg deep I.M.; 100 mg I.V., then doses $\leq$ 500 mg; 120 or 200 mg P.R. **Children:** 2 to 6 mg/kg or 125 mg/m^2 I.M. Maximum 100 mg. **Children 2 mo to 1 yr:** 30 mg P.R. **Children 1 to 4 yr:** 30 or 60 mg P.R. **Children 5 to 11 yr:** 60 mg P.R. **Children 12 to 14 yr:** 60 or 120 mg P.R. *Preoperative sedation* — **Adults:** 150 to 200 mg I.M. **Children:** 5 mg/kg P.O. or I.M. $\geq$ 10 yr; 5 mg/kg I.M. or P.R. if < 10 yr.	▪ ***I.V. use:*** May cause severe respiratory depression, laryngospasm, or hypotension. Have emergency resuscitation equipment available. ▪ Watch for signs of barbiturate toxicity. ▪ Assess mental status before starting therapy. Elderly patients more sensitive to adverse CNS effects. ▪ Inspect skin. If skin reactions occur, discontinue drug and call doctor. In some patients, high fever, stomatitis, headache, or rhinitis may precede skin reactions.
pentoxifylline Trental *Hemorheologic agent* Pregnancy Risk Category: C	*Intermittent claudication caused by chronic occlusive vascular disease* — **Adults:** 400 mg P.O. t.i.d. with meals. May decrease to 400 mg b.i.d. if adverse GI and CNS effects occur.	▪ Elderly patients may be more sensitive to effects. ▪ Instruct patient to swallow medication whole.
pergolide mesylate Permax *Antiparkinsonian* Pregnancy Risk Category: B	*Adjunctive treatment of Parkinson's disease* — **Adults:** 0.05 mg P.O. q.d. for first 2 days, then increase to 0.1 to 0.15 mg q 3rd day over 12 days. Then increase by 0.25 mg q 3rd day, p.r.n., until best response seen. Give in divided doses t.i.d.	▪ Monitor BP. Symptomatic orthostatic or sustained hypotension may occur. ▪ Advise patient of potential adverse reactions, especially hallucinations and confusion.
perindopril erbumine Aceon *Antihypertensive*	*Essential hypertension* — **Adults:** 4 mg P.O. q.d. Increase dosage until BP controlled or up to 16 mg q.d.; usual maintenance, 4 to 8 mg P.O., divided b.i.d.	▪ ***ALERT*** If angioedema of face, hands or feet, lips, tongue, glottis, or larynx occurs, stop drug and observe patient until swelling disappears. Angioedema *(continued)*

†Canadian ‡Australian

DRUG & CLASS	INDICATIONS & DOSAGES	NURSING CONSIDERATIONS
perindopril erbumine *(continued)* Pregnancy Risk Category: C (1st trimester) and D (2nd and 3rd trimesters)	***Adjust-a-dose:*** **Elderly (> 65 yr):** 4 mg P.O. q.d. or divided b.i.d. Dosage increases > 8 mg q.d. only under close medical supervision. **For renally impaired patients (CrCl > 30 ml/min):** 2 mg P.O. q.d.; maximum maintenance, 8 mg/day. **For patients taking diuretics:** 2 to 4 mg P.O. q.d. or divided b.i.d., with close medical supervision for several hours, until BP stabilizes. Adjust dosage based on patient's BP response.	of tongue, glottis, or larynx may fatally obstruct airway. ▪ Patients with history of angioedema unrelated to therapy may be at increased risk for angioedema. ▪ Excessive hypotension can occur when drug is given with diuretics. ▪ Closely monitor patients at risk for hypotension at start of therapy, for first 2 wk of therapy, and when increasing dose of perindopril or concomitant diuretic. ▪ Monitor serum potassium levels closely.
perphenazine Apo-Perphenazine†, PMS Perphenazine†, Trilafon, Trilafon Concentrate *Antipsychotic, antiemetic* Pregnancy Risk Category: NR	*Psychosis in nonhospitalized patients* — **Adults:** 4 to 8 mg P.O. t.i.d., reduced as soon as possible to minimum effective dosage. **Children > 12 yr:** lowest adult dose. *Psychosis in hospitalized patients* — **Adults:** 8 to 16 mg P.O. b.i.d., t.i.d., or q.i.d., increased to 64 mg/day, p.r.n. Or, 5 to 10 mg I.M. q 6 hr, p.r.n. Maximum 30 mg. **Children > 12 yr:** lowest adult dose. *Severe nausea and vomiting* — **Adults:** 8 to 16 mg P.O. q.d. in divided doses to maximum 24 mg. Or, 5 to 10 mg I.M., p.r.n. May give I.V., diluted to 0.5 mg/ml with 0.9% NaCl. Maximum 5 mg.	▪ Obtain baseline BP before therapy and monitor regularly. Watch for orthostatic hypotension. Keep patient supine for 1 hr after giving; tell him to change positions slowly. ▪ Monitor for tardive dyskinesia. ▪ Assess for neuroleptic malignant syndrome. ▪ Monitor weekly bilirubin tests during 1st mo; periodic CBC, LFTs, and ophthalmic tests (long-term use). ▪ Wear gloves to prepare liquid forms.

phenazopyridine hydrochloride (phenylazo diamino pyridine hydrochloride) Azo-Standard, Baridium, Phenazo†, Prodium, Pyridiate, Pyridium, Urogesic, UTI Relief *Urinary analgesic* Pregnancy Risk Category: B	*Pain with urinary tract irritation or infection* — **Adults:** 200 mg P.O. t.i.d. after meals for 2 days. **Children:** 12 mg/kg P.O. q.d. in 3 equal doses after meals for 2 days.	▪ Caution patient to stop taking drug and notify doctor if skin or sclerae yellow-tinged. ▪ When used with antibacterial agent, therapy shouldn't last longer than 2 days. ▪ Advise patient to take with meals. ▪ Tell diabetic patient to use Clinitest for accurate urine glucose results. Also inform him that drug may interfere with Acetest or Ketostix. ▪ Tell patient that drug turns urine red or orange; may stain fabrics or contact lenses.
phenobarbital (phenobarbitone) Ancalixir†, Barbita, Solfoton **phenobarbital sodium (phenobarbitone sodium)** Luminal Sodium *Anticonvulsant, sedative-hypnotic* Pregnancy Risk Category: D Controlled Substance Schedule: IV	*All forms of epilepsy, febrile seizures* — **Adults:** 60 to 200 mg P.O. q.d. in divided doses t.i.d. or as single dose h.s. **Children:** 3 to 6 mg/kg P.O. q.d., divided q 12 hr. *Status epilepticus* — **Adults:** 200 to 600 mg I.V. **Children:** 100 to 400 mg I.V. *Sedation* — **Adults:** 30 to 120 mg P.O. q.d. in 2 or 3 divided doses. **Children:** 3 to 5 mg/kg P.O. q.d. in divided doses t.i.d. *Preoperative sedation* — **Adults:** 100 to 200 mg I.M. 60 to 90 min before surgery. **Children:** 16 to 100 mg I.M. or 1 to 3 mg/kg I.V., I.M., or P.O. 60 to 90 min before surgery.	▪ ***I.V. use:*** I.V. injection for emergencies only. Give slowly under close supervision. Monitor respirations closely. Don't give > 60 mg/min. Have resuscitation equipment available. ▪ Watch for signs of barbiturate toxicity; overdose can be fatal. ▪ Don't stop abruptly; seizures may worsen. Call doctor if adverse reactions develop. ▪ Therapeutic blood levels 10 to 25 mcg/ml.
phentermine hydrochloride Fastin, Adipex-P, Obe-Nix, Phentercot, Phentride *Anorexigenic, indirect-*	*Short-term adjunct in exogenous obesity* — **Adults:** 8 mg P.O. t.i.d. ½ hr before meals. Or, 15 to 30 mg (resin complex) or 15 to 37.5 mg (hydrochloride) P.O. q.d. as single dose in morning.	▪ Use in conjunction with weight-reduction program. ▪ Monitor patient for tolerance or dependence.

(continued)

†Canadian ‡Australian

DRUG & CLASS	INDICATIONS & DOSAGES	NURSING CONSIDERATIONS
phentermine hydrochloride *(continued)* *acting sympathomimetic amine* Pregnancy Risk Category: X Controlled Substance Schedule: IV		▪ Tell patient to take ≥ 6 hr before bedtime to avoid sleep interference. ▪ Use cautiously in patient with mild hypertension.
phentolamine mesylate Regitine, Rogitine† *Antihypertensive for pheochromocytoma, cutaneous vasodilator* Pregnancy Risk Category: C	*To aid pheochromocytoma diagnosis; to control or prevent hypertension before or during pheochromocytomectomy* — **Adults:** I.V. diagnostic dose 2.5 mg. Before tumor removal, 5 mg I.M. or I.V. During surgery, may give 5 mg I.V. **Children:** I.V. diagnostic dose 1 mg. Before tumor removal, 1 mg I.V. or I.M. During surgery, may give 1 mg I.V. *Dermal necrosis and sloughing after I.V. extravasation of norepinephrine* — **Adults and children:** infiltrate with 5 to 10 mg in 10 ml 0.9% NaCl, or half through infiltrated I.V. and other half around site.	▪ When given to diagnose pheochromocytoma, take BP first; monitor BP frequently during use. Positive for pheochromocytoma if I.V. test dose causes severe hypotension. ▪ Don't give epinephrine to treat hypotension induced by phentolamine. Use norepinephrine instead. ▪ Tell patient to report adverse reactions. ▪ Must perform treatment for infiltration within 12 hr.
phenylephrine hydrochloride (systemic) Neo-Synephrine *Vasoconstrictor* Pregnancy Risk Category: C	*Mild to moderate hypotension* — **Adults:** 2 to 5 mg S.C. or I.M.; repeat in 1 to 2 hr, p.r.n. Or, 0.1 to 0.5 mg by slow I.V.; repeat 10 to 15 min. **Children:** 0.1 mg/kg I.M. or S.C.; repeat in 1 to 2 hr, p.r.n. *Severe hypotension and shock* — **Adults:** 10 mg in 250 to 500 ml D_5W or 0.9% NaCl.	▪ Use CV catheter or large vein to minimize extravasation. Use continuous infusion pump to regulate infusion flow rate. ▪ Frequently monitor ECG, BP, HR, cardiac output, CVP, PAWP, urine output, and color and temperature of extremities. ▪ To treat extravasation, infiltrate site

	Start infusion at 100 to 180 mcg/min; decrease to 40 to 60 mcg/min when BP stable.	promptly with phentolamine.
phenylephrine hydrochloride (ophthalmic) AK-Dilate, AK-Nefrin Ophthalmic, Isopto Frin, Mydfrin, Neo-Synephrine, Prefrin Liquifilm Relief *Vasoconstrictor* Pregnancy Risk Category: C	*Mydriasis without cycloplegia* — **Adults and children:** 1 drop of 2.5% or 10% solution instilled before examination. May repeat in 1 hr. *Mydriasis and vasoconstriction* — **Adults and adolescents:** 1 drop 2.5% or 10% solution. **Children:** 1 drop 2.5% solution. *Chronic mydriasis* — **Adults and adolescents:** 1 drop 2.5% or 10% solution b.i.d. or t.i.d. **Children:** 1 drop 2.5% solution b.i.d. or t.i.d.	▪ Wash hands before and after instilling. Apply light pressure on lacrimal sac for 1 min after drops instilled. ▪ Tell patient not to use brown solutions or solutions that contain precipitate. ▪ Monitor BP and pulse rate. ▪ Advise patient to contact doctor if condition persists > 12 hr after drug stopped.
phenylephrine hydrochloride (nasal) Alconefrin, Neo-Synephrine, Sinex *Vasoconstrictor* Pregnancy Risk Category: NR	*Nasal congestion* — **Adults and children ≥ 12 yr:** 1 to 2 sprays in nostril or small amount of jelly to nasal mucosa q 4 hr. Don't use > 3 to 5 days. **Children 6 to 12 yr:** 1 to 2 sprays of 0.25% solution in nostril q 4 hr. **Children < 6 yr:** 2 to 3 drops of 0.125% solution q 4 hr.	▪ Tell patient to hold head upright to avoid swallowing medication, then sniff spray briskly. After use, rinse tip of spray with hot water and dry. ▪ Tell patient not to exceed recommended dosage.
phenytoin (diphenylhydantoin) Dilantin, Dilantin Infatabs **phenytoin sodium** Dilantin, Phenytex **phenytoin sodium (extended)** Dilantin Kapseals *Anticonvulsant* Pregnancy Risk Category: NR	*Control of tonic-clonic and complex partial seizures* — **Adults:** 100 mg P.O. t.i.d., increased in increments of 100 mg P.O. q 2 to 4 wk until desired response. **Children:** 5 mg/kg or 250 mg/m^2 P.O. divided b.i.d. or t.i.d. Maximum 300 mg/day. *For patients requiring loading dose* — **Adults:** 1 g P.O. divided into 3 doses given at 2-hr intervals. Or, 10 to 15 mg/kg I.V. at rate ≤ 50 mg/min. **Children:** 5 mg/kg/day P.O. in 2 or 3 equally divided doses with later dose	▪ Extravasation has caused severe local tissue damage. Avoid administering by I.V. push into veins on back of hand. Inject into larger veins or central venous catheter, if available. ▪ Check vital signs, BP, and ECG during I.V. administration. Monitor blood levels. Therapeutic level 10 to 20 mcg/ml. Monitor CBC and serum calcium level q 6 mo, and periodically monitor hepatic function. ▪ Advise patient to avoid *(continued)*

DRUG & CLASS	INDICATIONS & DOSAGES	NURSING CONSIDERATIONS
phenytoin *(continued)*	individualized to maximum 300 mg/day. *Status epilepticus* — **Adults:** loading dose 10 to 15 mg/kg I.V. at rate ≤ 50 mg/min, then maintenance doses of 100 mg P.O. or I.V. q 6 to 8 hr. **Children:** loading dose 15 to 20 mg/kg I.V., at rate ≤ 1 to 3 mg/kg/min, then individualized maintenance doses.	hazardous activities until CNS effects known. ▪ Inform patient that drug may color urine pink, red, or reddish brown. ▪ After loading dose, start normal maintenance dose in 24 hr.
phytonadione (vitamin K_1) AquaMEPHYTON, Mephyton *Blood coagulation modifier* Pregnancy Risk Category: C	*Hypoprothrombinemia from vitamin K malabsorption, drug therapy, excessive vitamin A dosage* — **Adults:** 2.5 to 10 mg P.O., S.C., or I.M.; repeat and increase up to 50 mg. **Infants:** 2 mg P.O., I.M., or S.C. **Children:** 5 to 10 mg P.O., I.M., or S.C. *Hypoprothrombinemia from oral anticoagulants* — **Adults:** 2.5 to 10 mg P.O., S.C., or I.M. based on PT and INR. In emergency, 10 to 50 mg slow I.V., rate ≤ 1 mg/min, repeated q 4 hr, p.r.n.	▪ ***I.V. use:*** Give I.V. by slow infusion over 2 to 3 hr. Rate ≤ 1 mg/min in adults. ▪ For I.M. use in adults and older children, inject in upper outer quadrant of buttocks; for infants, inject in anterolateral aspect of thigh or deltoid region. ▪ Monitor PT and INR. ▪ Watch for flushing, weakness, tachycardia, and hypotension. ▪ Protect parenteral products from light.
pilocarpine Ocusert Pilo **pilocarpine hydrochloride** Adsorbocarpine, Akarpine, Isopto Carpine, Miocarpine†, Pilocar, Pilopt‡ **pilocarpine nitrate** Pilagan, P.V. Carpine	*Primary open-angle glaucoma* — **Adults and children:** 1 to 2 drops up to q.i.d., or 1-cm ribbon of 4% gel q h.s. Or, 1 Ocusert Pilo system (20 or 40 mcg/hr) q 7 days. *Emergency treatment of acute angle-closure glaucoma* — **Adults and children:** 1 drop 2% solution q 5 to 10 min for 3 to 6 doses, then 1 drop q 1 to 3 hr until pressure controlled.	▪ Instruct patient to apply gel h.s. Warn him to avoid hazardous activities until temporary blurring subsides. ▪ Apply light finger pressure on lacrimal sac for 1 min afterward. ▪ If Ocusert Pilo system falls out of eye during sleep, tell patient to wash hands, rinse insert in cool tap water, and reposition in eye.

pilocarpine *(continued)* Liquifilm *Miotic* Pregnancy Risk Category: C	*Mydriasis caused by mydriatic or cycloplegic agents* — **Adults and children:** 1 drop 1% solution.	▪ Inform patient that transient brow pain and myopia usually subside within 2 wk.
pimozide Orap *Antipsychotic* Pregnancy Risk Category: C	*Suppression of motor and phonic tics in Tourette syndrome* — **Adults and children > 12 yr:** 1 to 2 mg P.O. q.d. in divided doses; increase every other day, p.r.n. Maintenance dose < 0.2 mg/kg/day or 10 mg/day, whichever less. Maximum 10 mg/day.	▪ Monitor for prolonged QT interval before and during treatment. ▪ Monitor for tardive dyskinesia. May treat acute dystonic reactions with diphenhydramine. ▪ May lower seizure threshold.
pindolol Apo-Pindol†, Visken *Antihypertensive* Pregnancy Risk Category: B	*Hypertension* — **Adults:** initially, 5 mg P.O. b.i.d. Increase q 3 to 4 hr p.r.n. and as tolerated, to maximum of 60 mg/day.	▪ Check apical pulse before giving. If extreme, withhold dose and call doctor. ▪ Monitor BP frequently. ▪ Withdraw over 1 to 2 wk after long-term therapy.
pioglitazone hydrochloride Actos *Antidiabetic* Pregnancy Risk Category: C	*Monotherapy for type 2 diabetes mellitus, or combination therapy with a sulfonylurea, metformin, or insulin* — **Adults:** 15 or 30 mg P.O. q.d. Dose may be increased in increments, p.r.n.; maximum, 45 mg/day. If used in combination therapy, maximum dose 30 mg/day.	▪ ***ALERT*** Measure liver enzyme levels at the start of therapy, every 2 mo for the 1st year of therapy, and periodically thereafter. Obtain LFT results in patients who develop signs and symptoms of liver dysfunction. Stop drug if patient develops jaundice or if LFTs show ALT elevations > 3 times the upper limit of normal. ▪ Because ovulation may resume in premenopausal, anovulatory women with insulin resistance, tell patient to use contraception. ▪ Use in pregnancy only if benefit justifies risk to fetus. Insulin is *(continued)*

†Canadian ‡Australian

DRUG & CLASS	INDICATIONS & DOSAGES	NURSING CONSIDERATIONS
pioglitazone hydrochloride *(continued)*		preferred during pregnancy. ▪ Monitor heart failure patients for increased edema. ▪ Hgb and Hct fall, usually during the first 4 to 12 wk of therapy.
piperacillin sodium Pipracil, Pipril‡ *Antibiotic* Pregnancy Risk Category: B	*Systemic infections from susceptible strains of gram-positive and gram-negative organisms* — **Adults and children > 12 yr:** 100 to 300 mg/kg I.V. or I.M. q.d. in divided doses q 4 to 6 hr. Maximum 24 g/day. *Prophylaxis of surgical infections* — **Adults:** 2 g I.V. 30 to 60 min before surgery.	▪ Obtain specimen for culture and sensitivity tests before 1st dose. ▪ Monitor patient for superinfection. ▪ Give ≥ 1 hr before bacteriostatic antibiotics. ▪ Monitor serum potassium level. ▪ Alter dosage in impaired renal function.
piperacillin sodium and tazobactam sodium Zosyn *Antibiotic* Pregnancy Risk Category: B	*Appendicitis; skin, skin-structure infections; postpartum endometritis; pelvic inflammatory disease; moderately severe community-acquired pneumonia* — **Adults:** 3 g piperacillin and 0.375 g tazobactam I.V. q 6 hr. *Renal impairment* — **Adults:** if CrCl 20 to 40 ml/min, 2 g piperacillin and 0.25 g tazobactam I.V. q 6 hr; if < 20 ml/min, 2 g piperacillin and 0.25 g tazobactam I.V. q 8 hr. *Moderate to severe nosocomial pneumonia* — **Adults:** initially, 3.375 g I.V. over 30 min q 4 hr. Give with aminoglycoside. ***Adjust-a-dose:*** If CrCl 20 to 40 ml/min, give 2 g piperacillin and 0.25 g tazobactam I.V. q 6 hr; if < 20 ml/min, 2 g piperacillin and 0.25 g tazobactam I.V. q 8 hr.	▪ Obtain specimen for culture and sensitivity tests before 1st dose. ▪ Superinfection may occur, especially in elderly, debilitated, or immunosuppressed patients. Observe closely. ▪ Infuse over ≥ 30 min. Don't mix with other drugs. Discard unused drug after 24 hr if stored at room temperature; after 48 hr if refrigerated. Once diluted, drug stable in I.V. bags for 24 hr at room temperature or 1 wk if refrigerated.

pirbuterol acetate Maxair, Maxair Autohaler *Bronchodilator* Pregnancy Risk Category: C	*Prevention and reversal of bronchospasm, asthma* — **Adults and children ≥ 12 yr:** 1 or 2 inhalations (0.2 to 0.4 mg) repeated q 4 to 6 hr. Maximum 12 inhalations daily.	▪ Tell patient to wait ≥ 2 min before repeating. ▪ If patient also using steroid inhaler, instruct to use bronchodilator first, then wait 5 min before using steroid.
piroxicam Apo-Piroxicam†, Feldene, Novo-Pirocam† *Nonnarcotic analgesic, antipyretic, anti-inflammatory* Pregnancy Risk Category: NR	*Osteoarthritis; rheumatoid arthritis* — **Adults:** 20 mg P.O. q.d. May divide dosage b.i.d.	▪ May lead to reversible renal impairment. ▪ Check renal, hepatic, and auditory function and CBC during prolonged therapy. ▪ May mask infection.
plicamycin (mithramycin) Mithracin *Antineoplastic, hypocalcemic agent* Pregnancy Risk Category: X	Dosage and indications vary. *Hypercalcemia and hypercalciuria associated with advanced malignant disease* — **Adults:** 25 mcg/kg/day I.V. for 3 to 4 days. Repeat dosage weekly until patient responds. *Testicular cancer* — **Adults:** 25 to 30 mcg/kg/day I.V. for 8 to 10 days or until toxicity occurs.	▪ To reduce nausea, give antiemetic before using drug. Infuse over 4 to 6 hr. ▪ If solution extravasates, stop immediately, notify doctor, and use ice packs. ▪ Monitor CBC, platelets, and PT. ▪ Monitor for tetany, carpopedal spasm, Chvostek's sign, and muscle cramps.
pneumococcal 7-valent conjugate vaccine (diphtheria CRM_{197} protein) Prevnar *Bacterial vaccine* Pregnancy Risk Category: C	*Immunization against invasive disease from* Streptococcus pneumoniae *capsular serotypes 4, 6B, 9V, 14, 18C, 19F, and 23F* — **Infants and toddlers:** Four 0.5-ml doses, given I.M. at 2, 4, 6, and 12 to 15 mo. **Previously unvaccinated older infants and children:** 0.5 ml I.M., according to the following schedule based on age at 1st dose: **Children ages 7 to 11 mo:** Two doses ≥ 4 wk apart, then 3rd dose after the 1st birthday and ≥ 2 mo after	▪ Take thorough allergy history, including reactions to immunizations. ▪ Shake well to produce a uniform suspension. A nodule may form at injection site if vaccine isn't shaken. ▪ ***ALERT*** Don't inject I.V. Give I.M. only, using the deltoid muscle or, in infants, the anterolateral thigh. Don't inject into or near a nerve or blood vessel. ▪ Delay giving the vaccine

(continued)

†Canadian ‡Australian

DRUG & CLASS	INDICATIONS & DOSAGES	NURSING CONSIDERATIONS
pneumococcal 7-valent conjugate vaccine *(continued)*	2nd dose. **Children ages 12 to 23 mo:** Two doses ≥ 2 mo apart. **Children ages 2 to 9 yr:** One dose.	if the patient has recently had moderate to severe febrile illness; this may impair development of immunity.
polymyxin B sulfate *Ophthalmic antibiotic* Pregnancy Risk Category: C	*Alone or with other agents to treat superficial eye infections from* Pseudomonas *or other gram-negative organisms* — **Adults and children:** 1 to 3 drops of 0.1% to 0.25% (10,000 to 25,000 U/ml) q hr. Increase interval according to response; or up to 10,000 U injected subconjunctivally q.d.	▪ Don't touch dropper tip to eye or surrounding tissue. ▪ Apply light pressure on tear duct for 1 min after drops instilled. ▪ Tell patient not to share drug, washcloths, or towels and to notify doctor if anyone in household develops same symptoms.
potassium bicarbonate K + Care ET, K-Ide, Klor-Con/EF, K-Lyte *Therapeutic agent for electrolyte balance* Pregnancy Risk Category: NR	*Hypokalemia* — **Adults:** 25 to 50 mEq dissolved in half to full glass of water (120 to 240 ml) once daily to q.i.d.	▪ Dissolve tablets in 6 to 8 oz (180 to 240 ml) cold water. ▪ Monitor BUN, serum potassium and creatinine, and I&O. ▪ Tell patient to take with meals and sip slowly. ▪ Warn patient not to use salt substitutes, except with doctor's permission.
potassium chloride K+10, Kaochlor 10%, K-Dur, K-Lyte/Cl, K-Tab, Slow-K *Therapeutic agent for electrolyte balance* Pregnancy Risk Category: C	*Hypokalemia* — **Adults:** 40 to 100 mEq P.O. q.d. in 3 or 4 divided doses or 10 to 20 mEq for prevention. **Children:** 3 mEq/kg q.d. Maximum daily dose 40 mEq/m^2. If potassium < 2 mEq/ml, maximum infusion rate 40 mEq/hr; maximum infusion concentration 80 mEq/L; maximum 24-hr dose 400 mEq. If potassium > 2 mEq/ml, maximum infusion rate 10 mEq/hr; maximum infusion concentration 40 mEq/L; maximum 24-hr dose 200 mEq.	▪ Never switch potassium products without doctor's order. ▪ ***I.V. use:*** Give by infusion only. Give slowly as dilute solution. ▪ Make sure powder is completely dissolved before giving. ▪ Monitor ECG and serum electrolytes.

potassium gluconate
Glu-K, Kaon Liquid
Therapeutic agent for electrolyte balance
Pregnancy Risk Category: C

Hypokalemia — **Adults:** 40 to 100 mEq P.O. q.d. in 3 or 4 divided doses for treatment; 10 to 20 mEq q.d. for prevention. Further dosage adjustments based on serum potassium levels.

- Don't give potassium supplements postoperatively until urine flow established.
- Instruct patient to take with meals with full glass of water or juice.
- Caution patient not to use salt substitutes, unless medically advised.

---

potassium iodide
Pima, Thyro-Block
potassium iodide, saturated solution (SSKI), strong iodine solution
Antihyperthyroid agent
Pregnancy Risk Category: D

Preparation for thyroidectomy — **Adults and children:** strong iodine solution (USP), 0.1 to 0.3 ml P.O. t.i.d., or SSKI, 1 to 5 drops in water P.O. t.i.d. after meals for 10 to 14 days before surgery.
Thyrotoxic crisis — **Adults and children:** 500 mg P.O. q 4 hr (SSKI) or 1 ml strong iodine solution t.i.d.
Radiation protectant for thyroid gland — **Adults and children ≥ 1 yr:** 130 mg P.O. q.d. for 7 to 14 days after radiation exposure. **Children < 1 yr:** 65 mg P.O. q.d. for 7 to 14 days after exposure.

- Doctor may avoid prescribing enteric-coated tablets, which can lead to perforation, hemorrhage, or obstruction.
- Dilute oral solutions in water, milk, or fruit juice; give after meals to prevent gastric irritation, hydrate patient, and mask salty taste.
- Give iodides through straw to avoid tooth discoloration.
- Irritation and swollen eyelids are earliest signs of delayed hypersensitivity reactions to iodides.

---

pramipexole dihydrochloride
Mirapex
Antiparkinsonian
Pregnancy Risk Category: C

Signs and symptoms of idiopathic Parkinson's disease — **Adults:** 0.375 mg P.O. q.d. in divided doses t.i.d.; increase q 5 to 7 days. Maintenance range 1.5 to 4.5 mg/day in 3 divided doses.
Adjust-a-dose: In patients with CrCl ≥ 60 ml/min, give 0.125 mg P.O. t.i.d., up to 1.5 mg t.i.d.; in those with CrCl 35 to 59 ml/min, give 1.25 mg P.O. b.i.d., up to 1.5 mg b.i.d.; in those with CrCl 15 to 34 ml/min, give 0.125 mg P.O. q.d., up to 1.5 mg/day.

- If drug needs to be stopped, withdraw over 1-wk period.
- Drug may cause orthostatic hypotension, especially when dose is increased. Monitor patient carefully.
- Adjust dose gradually to achieve maximum therapeutic effect, balanced against dyskinesia, hallucinations, somnolence, and dry mouth.

DRUG & CLASS	INDICATIONS & DOSAGES	NURSING CONSIDERATIONS
pravastatin sodium (eptastatin) Pravachol *Antilipemic* Pregnancy Risk Category: X	*Reduction of LDL and total cholesterol levels in primary hypercholesterolemia (types IIa and IIb); reduction of risk of stroke or transient ischemic attacks in post-MI patients with normal cholesterol levels* — **Adults:** 10 or 20 mg P.O. q.d. h.s. Adjust q 4 wk per response; maximum 40 mg/day. *Increasing HDL-C in patients with primary hypercholesterolemia and mixed dyslipidemia (Frederickson types IIa and IIb)* — **Adults:** 10 mg, 20 mg, or 40 mg P.O. q.d. ***Adjust-a-dose:*** Most elderly patients and patients on immunosuppressant therapy respond to ≤ 20 mg q.d.	▪ Initiate only after other nonpharmacologic therapies prove ineffective. ▪ Obtain LFT results at start of therapy and periodically thereafter. ▪ Instruct patient to take in evening.
prazosin hydrochloride Minipress *Antihypertensive* Pregnancy Risk Category: C	*Mild to moderate hypertension* — **Adults:** P.O. test dose 1 mg h.s. Initial dose 1 mg P.O. b.i.d. or t.i.d. Increase slowly. Maximum 20 mg q.d. Maintenance 6 to 15 mg q.d. in 3 divided doses.	▪ Monitor BP and HR frequently. Elderly patients may be more sensitive to hypotensive effects. ▪ Give 1st dose of each increment h.s. to reduce episodes of syncope.
prednisolone Delta-Cortef **prednisolone sodium phosphate** Hydeltrasol, Key-Pred-SP **prednisolone tebutate** Hydeltra-T.B.A., Nor-Pred	*Severe inflammation or immunosuppression* — **Adults:** 2.5 to 15 mg P.O. b.i.d., t.i.d., or q.i.d.; 2 to 30 mg I.M. (phosphate) or I.V. (phosphate) q 12 hr; or 2 to 30 mg (phosphate) into joints (depending on joint size), lesions, or soft tissue; or 4 to 40 mg (tebutate) into joints (depending on joint size) and lesions, p.r.n.	▪ Give P.O. dose with food to reduce GI irritation. ▪ Give I.M. injection deeply into gluteal muscle. Rotate injection sites to prevent muscle atrophy. Avoid S.C. injection. ▪ Monitor weight, BP, and serum electrolytes.

T.B.A. *Anti-inflammatory, immunosuppressant* Pregnancy Risk Category: C		
prednisolone acetate (suspension) Econopred Plus, Pred-Forte **prednisolone sodium phosphate** AK-Pred, Inflamase Forte *Ophthalmic anti-inflammatory* Pregnancy Risk Category: C	*Inflammation* — **Adults and children:** 1 to 2 drops instilled into eye. In severe conditions, may use q hr, tapering to discontinuation as inflammation subsides. In mild conditions, may use b.i.d. to q.i.d.	▪ Wash hands before and after use. Don't touch dropper tip to eye or surrounding area. ▪ Apply light pressure on lacrimal sac for 1 min after instillation. ▪ Instruct patient to notify doctor if anyone in household develops same symptoms. ▪ Shake suspension. Store in tightly covered container.
prednisone Liquid Pred, Meticorten, Panasol, Prednicen-M, Prednisone Intensol *Anti-inflammatory, immunosuppressant* Pregnancy Risk Category: C	*Severe inflammation or immunosuppression* — **Adults:** 5 to 60 mg P.O. q.d. in 2 to 4 divided doses. Give maintenance dose daily or every other day. Dosage individualized. **Children:** 0.14 to 2 mg/kg or 4 to 60 mg/m^2 P.O. q.d. in 4 divided doses.	▪ Monitor BP, sleep patterns, daily weight, and serum potassium. Report sudden weight gain. ▪ Watch for depression or psychotic episodes, especially with high-dose therapy. ▪ Diabetic patients may need more insulin. ▪ May mask or exacerbate infections, including latent amebiasis.
primaquine phosphate *Antimalarial* Pregnancy Risk Category: C	*Radical cure for treatment or prevention of* P. vivax *malaria* — **Adults:** 15 mg (base) P.O. q.d. for 2 wk. (26.3-mg tablet provides 15 mg of base.) **Children:** 0.5 mg/kg/day (0.3 mg base/kg/day; maximum 15 mg base/dose) P.O. for 2 wk.	▪ Give with fast-acting antimalarial to reduce risk of drug-resistant strains. ▪ Monitor for sudden fall in Hgb, erythrocyte, or leukocyte count and for marked urine darkening. Discontinue immediately and notify doctor.

DRUG & CLASS	INDICATIONS & DOSAGES	NURSING CONSIDERATIONS
primidone Apo-Primidone†, Mysoline, PMS Primidone†, Sertan† *Anticonvulsant* Pregnancy Risk Category: NR	*Tonic-clonic, complex partial, and simple partial seizures* — **Adults and children ≥ 8 yr:** initially, 100 to 125 mg P.O. h.s. on days 1 to 3, 100 to 125 mg P.O. b.i.d. on days 4 to 6, 100 to 125 mg P.O. t.i.d. on days 7 to 9, then 250 mg P.O. t.i.d. Increase to 250 mg q.i.d., p.r.n. Maximum 2 g/day in divided doses. **Children < 8 yr:** 50 mg P.O. h.s. on days 1 to 3, then 50 mg P.O. b.i.d. on days 4 to 6, 100 mg P.O. b.i.d. on days 7 to 9, then 125 to 250 mg P.O. t.i.d.	▪ Don't withdraw suddenly; seizures may worsen. Call doctor if adverse reactions develop. ▪ Therapeutic primidone blood level 5 to 12 mcg/ml; therapeutic phenobarbital level 15 to 40 mcg/ml. ▪ Monitor CBC and routine blood chemistry q 6 mo.
probenecid Benuryl† *Uricosuric* Pregnancy Risk Category: NR	*Gonorrhea* — **Adults:** 3.5 g ampicillin P.O. with 1 g probenecid P.O. given together; or 1 g probenecid P.O. 30 min before dose of 4.8 million U of aqueous penicillin G procaine I.M., injected at 2 different sites. *Hyperuricemia of gout, gouty arthritis* — **Adults:** 250 mg P.O. b.i.d. for 1st wk, then 500 mg b.i.d., up to 2 g/day. *Prevention of renal failure caused by cidofovir* — **Adults:** 2 g P.O. 3 hr before cidofovir infusion, then 1 g P.O. 2 and 8 hr after infusion.	▪ Give with milk, food, or antacids. ▪ Monitor periodic BUN and renal function with long-term therapy. ▪ Force fluids to maintain ≥ 2 to 3 L/day output. ▪ May increase frequency, severity, and length of gout attacks during first 6 to 12 mo.
procainamide hydrochloride Procanbid, Pronestyl, Pronestyl-SR *Ventricular antiarrhythmic,*	*Life-threatening ventricular arrhythmias* — **Adults:** 100 mg slow I.V. push q 5 min, until arrhythmias disappear, adverse reactions develop, or 1 g given. Then give continuous infusion of 1 to 6 mg/min. If arrhythmias recur,	▪ ***I.V. use:*** Monitor BP and ECG continuously. If prolonged QT intervals and QRS complexes, heart block, or increased arrhythmias occur, withhold drug and notify doctor. ▪ To suppress ventricular arrhythmias, drug

supraventricular anti-arrhythmic Pregnancy Risk Category: C	repeat bolus and increase infusion rate. Or, 0.5 to 1 g I.M. q 4 to 8 hr until P.O. therapy begins. P.O.: 50 mg/kg/day in divided doses q 3 hr. May divide sustained-release P.O. forms q 6 or 12 hr, depending on product.	levels 4 to 8 mcg/ml; N-acetyl procainamide (NAPA) levels 10 to 30 mcg/ml.
procarbazine hydrochloride Matulane, Natulan† *Antineoplastic* Pregnancy Risk Category: D	*Adjunct treatment of Hodgkin's disease* — **Adults:** 2 to 4 mg/kg P.O. q.d. for 1st wk. Then, 4 to 6 mg/kg/day until WBC count < 4,000/mm^3 or platelet count < 100,000/mm^3. After bone marrow recovers, resume maintenance of 1 to 2 mg/kg/day. For MOPP regimen, 100 mg/m^2/day P.O. for 14 days. **Children:** 50 mg/m^2/day P.O. for 1st wk; then 100 mg/m^2 until response or toxicity occurs. Maintenance dosage 50 mg/m^2/day P.O. after bone marrow recovery.	▪ Monitor CBC and platelet count. ▪ If confusion, paresthesia, or other neuropathies develop, stop drug and notify doctor. ▪ Give h.s. and in divided doses. ▪ Watch for signs of infection and bleeding. Take temperature daily. ▪ Warn patient to avoid alcohol. Urge him to stop drug and call doctor immediately if disulfiram-like reaction occurs.
prochlorperazine Compazine, PMS Prochlorperazine†, Prorazin†, **prochlorperazine edisylate** Compa-Z, Compazine, Cotranzine, Ultrazine-10 **prochlorperazine maleate** Compazine, PMS Prochlorperazine†, Prorazin†, Stemetil† *Antipsychotic, antiemetic,*	*Preoperative nausea control* — **Adults:** 5 to 10 mg I.M. 1 to 2 hr before anesthesia; repeat once in 30 min, p.r.n. Or, 5 to 10 mg I.V. 15 to 30 min before anesthesia; repeat once, p.r.n. *Severe nausea and vomiting* — **Adults:** 5 to 10 mg P.O., t.i.d. or q.i.d.; 25 mg P.R., b.i.d.; 5 to 10 mg I.M. repeated q 3 to 4 hr, p.r.n. Or, 2.5 to 10 mg I.V. at maximum rate 5 mg/min. **Children 9 to 13 kg (20 to 29 lb):** 2.5 mg P.O. or P.R. once daily or b.i.d. Or 0.132 mg/kg by I.M. injection. **Children 14 to 17 kg (31 to 38 lb):** 2.5 mg P.O. or P.R.,	▪ Dilute P.O. solution with tomato or fruit juice, milk, coffee, carbonated beverage, tea, water, or soup or mix with pudding. ▪ ***I.V. use:*** 15 to 30 min before induction, add 20 mg prochlorperazine/L D_5W and 0.9% NaCl. Infusion rate ≤ 5 mg/min. Parenteral dose ≤ 40 mg daily. Infuse slowly, never as bolus. ▪ Don't get concentrate or injection solution on hands or clothing. ▪ Watch for orthostatic hypotension, especially when giving I.V. ▪ For I.M. use, inject deeply *(continued)*

†Canadian ‡Australian

DRUG & CLASS	INDICATIONS & DOSAGES	NURSING CONSIDERATIONS
prochlorperazine *(continued)* *anxiolytic* Pregnancy Risk Category: NR	b.i.d. or t.i.d. Or 0.132 mg/kg by deep I.M. injection. **Children 18 to 39 kg (40 to 86 lb):** 2.5 mg P.O. or P.R., t.i.d.; or 5 mg P.O. or P.R., b.i.d. Or 0.132 mg/kg by deep I.M. injection. *Psychotic disorders* — **Adults:** 5 to 10 mg P.O., t.i.d. or q.i.d. **Children 2 to 12 yr:** 2.5 mg P.O. or P.R., b.i.d. or t.i.d. Maximum 10 mg on day 1. Increase dose gradually, p.r.n. In children 2 to 10 yr, maximum 25 mg daily. *Nonpsychotic anxiety* — **Adults:** 5 to 10 mg by deep I.M. injection q 3 to 4 hr, not to exceed 20 mg daily or to be given for longer than 12 wk. Or, 5 to 10 mg P.O., t.i.d. or q.i.d. Or, 15 mg extended-release capsules daily or 10 mg extended-release capsules q 12 hr.	into upper outer quadrant of gluteal region. ▪ Don't give S.C. or mix in syringe with other drug. ▪ Use only when vomiting can't be controlled by other measures. Notify doctor if > 4 doses needed q 24 hr. ▪ Advise patient to wear protective clothing when exposed to sunlight. ▪ Store in light-resistant container. Slight yellowing doesn't affect potency, but discard extremely discolored solutions.
progesterone Prometrium *Progestin, contraceptive* Pregnancy Risk Category: X	*Amenorrhea* — **Adults:** 5 to 10 mg I.M. q.d. for 6 to 8 days, beginning 8 to 10 days before anticipated start of menstruation. *Dysfunctional uterine bleeding* — **Adults:** 5 to 10 mg I.M. q.d. for 6 doses.	▪ Give oil solutions (peanut oil or sesame oil) via deep I.M. injection. Check sites frequently for irritation. ▪ Rotate injection sites.
promethazine hydrochloride Anergan, Histantil†, Phenazine, Phencen, Phenergan, Phenergan Fortis, Phenergan Syrup Plain, Phenoject,	*Motion sickness* — **Adults:** 25 mg P.O. b.i.d. **Children:** 12.5 to 25 mg P.O., I.M., or P.R. b.i.d. *Nausea* — **Adults:** 12.5 to 25 mg P.O., I.M., or P.R. q 4 to 6 hr, p.r.n. **Children:** 12.5 to 25 mg I.M. or P.R. q 4 to 6 hr, p.r.n.	▪ Used as adjunct to analgesics; has no analgesic activity. ▪ Don't give S.C. ▪ In patients scheduled for myelogram, discontinue drug 48 hr before procedure and don't resume until 24 hr after procedure.

PMS-Promethazine†, Prothazine†, V-Gan-25 **promethazine theoclate** Avomine‡ *Antiemetic; antivertigo agent; antihistamine; preoperative, postoperative, or obstetric sedative and adjunct to analgesics* Pregnancy Risk Category: C	*Rhinitis, allergy symptoms* — **Adults:** 12.5 mg P.O. q.i.d.; or 25 mg P.O. h.s. **Children:** 6.25 to 12.5 mg P.O. t.i.d. or 25 mg P.O. or P.R. h.s. *Sedation* — **Adults:** 25 to 50 mg P.O. or I.M. h.s. or p.r.n. **Children:** 12.5 to 25 mg P.O., I.M., or P.R. h.s. *Routine preoperative or postoperative sedation; adjunct to analgesics* — **Adults:** 25 to 50 mg I.M., I.V., or P.O. **Children:** 12.5 to 25 mg I.M., I.V., or P.O.	▪ ***I.V. use:*** Don't give concentration > 25 mg/ml or > 25 mg/min. ▪ May cause sedation. Warn patient to avoid alcohol and activities requiring alertness until CNS effects known.
propofol Diprivan *Anesthetic* Pregnancy Risk Category: B	*Initiation and maintenance of intensive care unit sedation in intubated, mechanically ventilated patients* — **Adults:** usually, 5 mcg/kg/min for 5 min. Increase rate at 5- to 10-min intervals in increments of 5 to 10 mcg/kg/min until desired response. Rates of 5 to 50 mcg/kg/min or higher may be required.	▪ Use cautiously in patients with seizures. ▪ Allow adequate interval between dosage adjustments to assess effects. ▪ Titrate drug daily to achieve only minimum effective drug concentration. ▪ Don't give in same I.V. line with blood or plasma. ▪ Consult references for anesthesia dosages.
propoxyphene hydrochloride Darvon, 692† **propoxyphene napsylate** Darvon-N, Doloxene‡ *Opioid analgesic* Pregnancy Risk Category: C Controlled Substance Schedule: IV	*Mild to moderate pain* — **Adults:** 65 mg (hydrochloride) P.O. q 4 hr, p.r.n. Maximum 390 mg/day. Or, 100 mg (napsylate) P.O. q 4 hr, p.r.n. Maximum 600 mg/day.	▪ Mild narcotic analgesic. ▪ ***ALERT*** Warn patient not to exceed dosage or use with other CNS depressant; respiratory depression, hypotension, profound sedation, and coma may result. ▪ Advise patient to avoid alcohol or other CNS depressants.

†Canadian ‡Australian

DRUG & CLASS	INDICATIONS & DOSAGES	NURSING CONSIDERATIONS
propranolol hydrochloride Deralin‡, Detensol†, Inderal, Inderal LA, Novopranol† *Antihypertensive, antianginal, antiarrhythmic, adjunctive therapy for MI* Pregnancy Risk Category: C	*Angina pectoris* — **Adults:** total daily dose, 80 to 320 mg P.O. b.i.d., t.i.d., or q.i.d.; or one 80-mg extended-release capsule q.d. Increase dose at 7- to 10-day intervals. *Mortality reduction after MI* — **Adults:** 180 to 240 mg P.O. t.i.d. or q.i.d. 5 to 21 days after MI. *Supraventricular and ventricular arrhythmias; tachyarrhythmias from excessive catecholamine action during anesthesia or in hyperthyroidism or pheochromocytoma* — **Adults:** 0.5 to 3 mg by slow I.V. push ($\leq$ 1 mg/min). After 3 mg, give next dose in 2 min; other doses > q 4 hr. Maintenance 10 to 30 mg P.O. t.i.d. or q.i.d. *Hypertension* — **Adults:** 80 mg P.O. daily in 2 to 4 divided doses or extended-release once a day. Increase at 3- to 7-day intervals. Maintenance 160 to 480 mg daily. Maximum 640 mg daily. *Essential tremor* — **Adults:** 40 mg P.O. b.i.d. Maintenance 120 to 320 mg daily in 3 divided doses. *Hypertrophic subaortic stenosis* — **Adults:** 20 to 40 mg P.O. t.i.d. or q.i.d., or 80 to 160 mg extended-release capsules q.d. *Adjunct therapy in pheochromocytoma* — **Adults:** 60 mg P.O. daily in divided doses with an alpha blocker 3 days before surgery.	▪ Check apical pulse before giving drug. If extremes detected, stop drug and call doctor. ▪ Double-check dose and route. ▪ ***I.V. use:*** Give by direct injection into a large vessel or into the tubing of a free-flowing, compatible I.V. solution; don't give by continuous I.V. infusion. Or, dilute drug with 0.9% NaCl and give by intermittent infusion over 10 to 15 min in 0.1- to 0.2-mg increments. Drug is compatible with D_5W and 0.45% and 0.9% NaCl and lactated Ringer's. ▪ Give drug with meals. ▪ If severe hypotension occurs, notify doctor. ▪ Drug masks common signs of shock and hypoglycemia.

propylthiouracil (PTU) Propyl-Thyracil† *Antihyperthyroid agent* Pregnancy Risk Category: D	*Hyperthyroidism* — **Adults:** 100 to 150 mg P.O. t.i.d.; up to 1,200 mg/day. Maintenance 100 to 150 mg q.d. in divided doses t.i.d. **Children ≥ 10 yr:** 150 to 300 mg P.O. q.d. in divided doses t.i.d. **Children 6 to 10 yr:** 50 to 150 mg P.O. q.d. in divided doses t.i.d. *Thyrotoxic crisis* — **Adults and children:** 200 mg P.O. q 4 to 6 hr on first day. Reduce dose gradually to maintenance level.	▪ Watch for hypothyroidism (depression; cold intolerance; hard, nonpitting edema); adjust dosage as ordered. ▪ Discontinue drug if patient develops severe rash or enlarged lymph nodes. ▪ Best response occurs when drug is given around the clock at the same time q.d. with respect to meals.
protamine sulfate *Heparin antagonist* Pregnancy Risk Category: C	*Heparin overdose* — **Adults:** dosage based on blood coagulation studies, usually 1 mg for each 90 to 115 U heparin. Maximum 50 mg.	▪ ***I.V. use:*** Give slowly over 10 min. Have emergency equipment available. ▪ May act as anticoagulant in high doses.
pseudoephedrine hydrochloride Children's Sudafed, Drixoral, Efidac/24, Genaphed, Pedia Care Infant's Decongestant, Sudafed **pseudoephedrine sulfate** Afrin, Drixoral *Decongestant* Pregnancy Risk Category: C	*Nasal and eustachian tube decongestion* — **Adults:** 60 mg P.O. q 4 hr. Maximum 240 mg/day. Or, 120 mg extended-release form P.O. q 12 hr or 240 mg extended-release form once daily. **Children ≥ 12 yr:** 120 mg P.O. q 12 hr, or 240 mg P.O. q.d. **Children 6 to 12 yr:** 30 mg P.O. regular-release form q 4 to 6 hr. Maximum 120 mg/day. **Children 2 to 6 yr:** 15 mg P.O. regular-release form q 4 to 6 hr. Maximum 60 mg/day. **Children 1 to 2 yr:** 7 drops (0.2 ml)/kg q 4 to 6 hr. Maximum 4 doses/day. **Children 3 to 12 mo:** 3 drops/kg q 4 to 6 hr. Maximum 4 doses/day.	▪ Elderly patients more sensitive to drug effects. ▪ Warn patient against using OTC products containing other sympathomimetics. ▪ Tell patient not to take within 2 hr of bedtime. ▪ Don't use with MAO inhibitors. ▪ Tell patient not to crush or break forms. ▪ Instruct patient to stop drug and notify doctor if unusual restlessness occurs.
psyllium Fiberall, GenFiver, Hydrocil, Konsyl, Metamucil, Modane	*Constipation; bowel management* — **Adults:** 1 to 2 tsp (rounded) P.O. in full glass liquid once daily, b.i.d., or t.i.d.; or 1 packet dis-	▪ Mix with ≥ 8 oz (240 ml) of cold, pleasant-tasting liquid to mask grittiness; stir only few sec. Have patient *(continued)*

†Canadian ‡Australian

DRUG & CLASS	INDICATIONS & DOSAGES	NURSING CONSIDERATIONS
psyllium *(continued)* Bulk, Reguloid, Serutan Concentrated Powder *Bulk laxative* Pregnancy Risk Category: NR	solved in water once daily, b.i.d., or t.i.d. **Children > 6 yr:** 1 tsp (level) P.O. in half glass liquid h.s.	drink immediately. Follow with additional glass of liquid.
pyrazinamide Pyrazinamide†, Tebrazid† *Antituberculotic* Pregnancy Risk Category: C	*Adjunctive treatment of TB* — **Adults:** 15 to 30 mg/kg P.O. q.d. Maximum 2 g/day. Or, if patient noncompliant, 50 to 70 mg/kg P.O. twice weekly.	▪ Given for initial 2 mo of ≥ 6-mo regimen. Patients with HIV may require longer course. ▪ Watch for signs of gout and liver impairment.
pyridostigmine bromide Mestinon, Mestinon-SR, Mestinon Timespans, Regonol *Muscle stimulant* Pregnancy Risk Category: NR	*Antidote for nondepolarizing neuromuscular blockers* — **Adults:** 10 to 20 mg I.V., following atropine sulfate 0.6 to 1.2 mg I.V. *Myasthenia gravis* — **Adults:** 60 to 120 mg P.O. q 3 or 4 hr. Usual dose, 600 mg q.d.; higher dose p.r.n. For I.M. or I.V. use, give 1⁄30 of P.O. dose. Or, 180 to 540 mg extended-release tablets (1 to 3 tablets) P.O. b.i.d., with ≥ 6 hr between doses. **Children:** 7 mg/kg P.O. or 200 mg/m^2 P.O. daily in 5 or 6 divided doses. *Supportive treatment of neonates born to myasthenic mothers* — **Neonates:** 0.05 to 0.15 mg/kg I.M. q 4 to 6 hr. Decrease dose q.d. until drug can be stopped.	▪ Stop other cholinergics before giving drug. ▪ ***I.V. use:*** Give I.V. injection no faster than 1 mg/min. Monitor vital signs. Position patient to ease breathing. Be ready to give atropine injection; provide respiratory support, p.r.n. ▪ Don't crush extended-release (Timespans) tablets. ▪ Test dose of edrophonium I.V. aggravates drug-induced weakness but temporarily relieves weakness caused by disease. ▪ Regonol (U.S. only) contains benzyl ethanol; can cause toxicity in neonates in high doses.

pyridoxine hydrochloride (vitamin B_6) Nestrex, Rodex *Nutritional supplement* Pregnancy Risk Category: A	*Dietary vitamin B_6 deficiency* — **Adults:** 10 to 20 mg P.O., I.M., or I.V. q.d. for 3 wk; then 2 to 5 mg q.d. as supplement to proper diet. *Seizures related to vitamin B_6 deficiency or dependency* — **Adults and children:** 100 mg I.M. or I.V. in single dose. *Isoniazid poisoning (> 10 g)* — **Adults:** give equal amount of pyridoxine: 4 g I.V., followed by 1 g I.M. q 30 min.	▪ Protect from light. Don't use solution if it contains precipitate, although slight darkening acceptable. ▪ High doses (2 to 6 g/day) may cause difficulty walking. ▪ Monitor diet. Excessive protein intake increases daily pyridoxine requirements.
pyrimethamine Daraprim **pyrimethamine with sulfadoxine** Fansidar *Antimalarial* Pregnancy Risk Category: C	*Malaria prophylaxis and transmission control (pyrimethamine)* — **Adults and children ≥ 10 yr:** 25 mg P.O. q wk. **Children 4 to 10 yr:** 12.5 mg P.O. q wk **Children < 4 yr:** 6.25 mg P.O. q wk. Continue 6 to 10 wk after leaving endemic areas. *Acute attacks of malaria (Fansidar)* — **Adults and children ≥ 14 yr:** 2 to 3 tablets as single dose. **Children 9 to 14 yr:** 2 tablets/wk. **Children 4 to 8 yr:** 1 tablet/wk. **Children < 4 yr:** ¾ tablet/wk. *Malaria prophylaxis (Fansidar)* — **Adults and children ≥ 14 yr:** 1 tablet/wk. **Children 9 to 14 yr:** ¾ tablet/wk. **Children 4 to 8 yr:** ½ tablet/wk. **Children < 4 yr:** ¼ tablet/wk. *Acute attacks of malaria (pyrimethamine)* — **Adults and children ≥ 15 yr:** 25 mg P.O. q.d. for 2 days. **Children < 15 yr:** 12.5 mg P.O. q.d. for 2 days. *Toxoplasmosis (pyrimethamine)* — **Adults:**	▪ Obtain twice-weekly blood counts, including platelets, for toxoplasmosis patient. ▪ Fansidar should be used in areas where chloroquine-resistant malaria are prevalent and if traveler stays > 3 wk. ▪ Tell patient to take with meals. ▪ Instruct patient to stop drug and notify doctor at 1st sign of rash. ▪ Use with faster-acting antimalarials for 2 days to initiate transmission control and suppressive cure. Don't use alone. ▪ Give sulfadiazine with pyrimethamine to treat toxoplasmosis.

(continued)

DRUG & CLASS	INDICATIONS & DOSAGES	NURSING CONSIDERATIONS
pyrimethamine *(continued)*	50 to 75 mg P.O. q.d. for 1 to 3 wk, then reduce dose by 50% and continue for additional 4 to 5 wk. **Children:** 1 mg/kg P.O. (< 100 mg) in 2 equally divided doses for 2 to 4 days, then 0.5 mg/kg/day for 4 wk.	
quetiapine fumarate Seroquel *Antipsychotic* Pregnancy Risk Category: C	*Psychotic disorders* — **Adults:** 25 mg P.O. b.i.d. Increase by 25 to 50 mg P.O. b.i.d. or t.i.d. on days 2 and 3, as tolerated. Target dose of 300 to 400 mg P.O. q.d., divided b.i.d. or t.i.d., by day 4. Further dose adjustments should occur at intervals of ≥ 2 days, p.r.n. **Elderly:** give lower doses, slow titration, and carefully monitor in the initial dosing period. ***Adjust-a-dose:*** In patients with hepatic impairment or hypotension or in debilitated patients, use lower doses and slower titration.	▪ Use cautiously in patients with CV or cerebrovascular disease, hypotension, seizures, or low seizure threshold. ▪ Use cautiously in patients who may experience elevated core body temperature. ▪ Watch for symptoms of neuroleptic malignant syndrome (extrapyramidal effects, hyperthermia, autonomic disturbance). ▪ Monitor patient for tardive dyskinesia.
quinapril hydrochloride Accupril, Asig‡ *Antihypertensive* Pregnancy Risk Category: C (1st trimester); D (2nd and 3rd trimesters)	*Hypertension* — **Adults:** initially, 10 mg P.O. q.d. or 5 mg q.d. if patient takes diuretic. Adjust based on response at 2-wk intervals. Maintenance dose is 20 to 80 mg once daily or b.i.d. *Heart failure* — **Adults:** 5 mg P.O. b.i.d. Increase q wk to 20 to 40 mg/day in 2 equally divided doses b.i.d. ***Adjust-a-dose:*** Patients with impaired renal function require dosage adjustments.	▪ Advise patient to report angioedema (including laryngeal edema). ▪ Monitor BP for effectiveness. ▪ Observe for light-headedness and syncope. ▪ Monitor serum potassium level.

quinidine gluconate Quinaglute Dura-Tabs, Quinalan, Quinate† **quinidine sulfate** Apo-Quinidine†, Cin-Quin, Quinidex Extentabs *Antitachyarrhythmic* Pregnancy Risk Category: C	*Atrial flutter or fibrillation* — **Adults:** 200 mg P.O. q 2 to 3 hr for 5 to 8 doses, then increase q.d. Maximum 3 to 4 g/day. *Paroxysmal supraventricular tachycardia* — **Adults:** 400 to 600 mg I.M. or P.O. q 2 to 3 hr. *Premature atrial contractions; PVCs; paroxysmal atrial tachycardia; paroxysmal ventricular tachycardia; maintenance after cardioversion of atrial fibrillation* — **Adults:** test dose 200 mg P.O. or I.M. Then 200 to 400 mg (sulfate or equivalent base) P.O. q 4 to 6 hr; or 600 mg (gluconate) I.M., then 400 mg q 2 hr, p.r.n.; or 800 mg (gluconate) in 40 ml D_5W I.V. infusion at 16 mg/min. **Children:** test dose 2 mg/kg P.O.; then 30 mg/kg/24 hr P.O. or 900 mg/m^2/24 hr P.O. in 5 divided doses.	▪ Use cautiously in impaired renal or hepatic function, asthma, muscle weakness, or infection with fever. ▪ Check apical pulse and BP before therapy. ▪ Adverse GI reactions signal toxicity. Check blood drug levels; > 8 mcg/ml toxic. ▪ Give with meals to prevent GI symptoms. ▪ Give sulfate or equivalent base for atrial flutter or fibrillation only if AV node has been blocked by another agent to prevent increased AV conduction.
quinupristin/ dalfopristin Synercid *Antibiotic* Pregnancy Risk Category: B	*Serious or life-threatening infections from vancomycin-resistant* Enterococcus faecium *(VREF) bacteremia* — **Adults and adolescents ≥ 16 yr**: 7.5 mg/kg I.V. infusion over 1 hr, q 8 hr. Treatment duration determined by infection site and severity. *Complicated skin and skin-structure infections from* Staphylococcus aureus *(methicillin susceptible) or* Streptococcus pyogenes — **Adults and adolescents ≥ 16 yr:** 7.5 mg/kg by I.V. infusion over 1 hr, q 12 hr for ≥ 1 wk.	▪ Drug isn't active against *Enterococcus faecalis*. Appropriate blood cultures are needed to avoid misidentifyiing *E. faecalis* or *E. faecium.* ▪ ***I.V. use:*** Reconstitute powder for injection: Add 5 ml of sterile water for injection or D_5W, then gently swirl vial by manual rotation to ensure dissolution; avoid shaking, to limit foaming. Further dilute reconstituted solutions within 30 min. ▪ Because this drug may cause mild to life-threatening *(continued)*

†Canadian ‡Australian

DRUG & CLASS	INDICATIONS & DOSAGES	NURSING CONSIDERATIONS
quinupristin/ dalfopristin *(continued)*		pseudomembranous colitis, consider this diagnosis in patients who develop diarrhea during or after drug therapy. ▪ The appropriate dose of reconstituted solution, based on patient's weight, should be added to 250 ml D_5W to make final concentration of ≤ 2 mg/ml. This diluted solution is stable for 5 hr at room temperature or 54 hr refrigerated. ▪ Give by I.V. infusion over 1 hr, using infusion pump to control rate of infusion. ▪ Drug is incompatible with saline and heparin solutions. Don't dilute drug with solutions that contain saline or infuse into lines that contain saline or heparin. Flush line with D_5W before and after each dose.
rabeprazole sodium Aciphex *Antiulcerative* Pregnancy Risk Category: B	*Healing of erosive or ulcerative gastroesophageal reflux disease (GERD)* — **Adults:** 20 mg P.O. q.d. for 4 to 8 wk. May give additional 8-week course p.r.n. *Maintenance of healing of erosive or ulcerative GERD* — **Adults:** 20 mg P.O. q.d. *Healing of duodenal ulcers* — **Adults:** 20 mg P.O. q.d. after morning meal for ≤ 4 wk. *Pathological hypersecretory conditions including Zollinger-Ellison syndrome* — **Adults:** 60 mg P.O. q.d.; increase, p.r.n., to 100 mg P.O. once daily or 60 mg P.O. b.i.d.	▪ Use cautiously in patients with severe hepatic impairment. ▪ May give additional courses of therapy when duodenal ulcers or GERD doesn't heal after 1st course. ▪ Symptomatic response to therapy doesn't preclude gastric malignancy. ▪ Delayed-release tablets should be swallowed whole. Tell patient not to crush, chew, or split.

raloxifene hydrochloride Evista *Antiosteoporotic* Pregnancy Risk Category: X	*Prevention and treatment of osteoporosis in postmenopausal women* — **Adults:** 60 mg P.O. q.d.	▪ Use cautiously in those with liver disease. ▪ Greatest risk for thromboembolic events occurs during first 4 mo of treatment. ▪ Stop ≥ 72 hr before prolonged immobilization and resume after patient fully mobilized. ▪ Report unexplained uterine bleeding.
ramipril Altace, Ramace‡, Tritace‡ *Antihypertensive* Pregnancy Risk Category: C (1st trimester); D (2nd and 3rd trimesters)	*Hypertension* — **Adults:** initially, 2.5 mg P.O. q.d. for patient not taking diuretic; 1.25 mg P.O. q.d. for patient taking diuretic. Increase, p.r.n., based on response. Maintenance 2.5 to 20 mg q.d. as single or divided doses. *Heart failure* — **Adults:** 2.5 mg P.O. b.i.d. If hypotension, decrease to 1.25 mg P.O. b.i.d. May increase slowly to maximum 5 mg P.O. b.i.d., p.r.n. *Reduction in risk of MI, stroke, and death from CV causes* — **Adults ≥ 55:** 2.5 mg P.O. q.d. for 1 wk, then 5 mg P.O. q.d. for 3 wk. Increase as tolerated up to 10 mg P.O. q.d. ***Adjust-a-dose:*** In patients with CrCl < 40 ml/min, give 1.25 mg P.O. q.d. Adjust gradually according to response.	▪ Advise patient to report angioedema (including laryngeal edema). ▪ Monitor BP regularly. ▪ Watch for light-headedness and syncope. ▪ Monitor serum potassium level.
ranitidine bismuth citrate Tritec *Antiulcerative* Pregnancy Risk Category: C	*Combined with clarithromycin for active duodenal ulcer from* H. pylori *infection* — **Adults:** 400 mg P.O. b.i.d. for 28 days with clarithromycin.	▪ Don't use with clarithromycin in patients with history of acute porphyria. ▪ Don't use alone to treat active duodenal ulcers. ▪ May cause temporary and harmless darkening of the tongue or stool.

DRUG & CLASS	INDICATIONS & DOSAGES	NURSING CONSIDERATIONS
ranitidine hydrochloride Apo-Ranitidine†, Zantac, Zantac-C†, Zantac 75, Zantac EFFERdose, Zantac GELdose *Antiulcerative* Pregnancy Risk Category: B	*Duodenal and gastric ulcer (short-term treatment); pathologic hypersecretory conditions, such as Zollinger-Ellison syndrome* — **Adults:** 150 mg P.O. b.i.d. or 300 mg q.d. h.s. Or, 50 mg I.V. or I.M. q 6 to 8 hr. Patients with Zollinger-Ellison syndrome may need up to 6 g P.O. q.d. *Maintenance therapy for duodenal or gastric ulcer* — **Adults:** 150 mg P.O. h.s. *Gastroesophageal reflux disease* — **Adults:** 150 mg P.O. b.i.d. *Erosive esophagitis* — **Adults:** 150 mg P.O. q.i.d. Maintenance is 150 mg P.O. b.i.d. ***Adjust-a-dose:*** In patients with CrCl < 50 ml/min, give 150 mg P.O. q 24 hr or 50 mg I.V. q 18 to 24 hr.	▪ ***I.V. use:*** When giving I.V. push, dilute to total volume of 20 ml and inject over 5 min. ▪ For intermittent I.V. infusion, dilute 50 mg in 100 ml compatible solution, and infuse over 15 to 20 min. ▪ For continuous I.V. infusion: 150 mg in 250 ml compatible solution. Give at 6.25 mg/hr using infusion pump. ▪ Incompatible with aluminum. ▪ Dissolve EFFERdose tablets or granules in 6 to 8 oz of water before giving.
repaglinide Prandin *Antidiabetic* Pregnancy Risk Category: C	*Adjunct to diet and exercise in lowering blood glucose level in type 2 diabetes mellitus with hyperglycemia that can't be controlled by diet and exercise alone; combined with metformin to lower blood glucose level in hyperglycemia that can't be controlled by exercise, diet, and either repaglinide or metformin alone* — **Adults:** for patients not previously treated or whose glycosylated hemoglobin (HbA_{1c}) is < 8%, 0.5 mg P.O. taken up to 30 min before meals; for those previously treated with glucose-lowering drugs	▪ Use cautiously in elderly, debilitated, or malnourished patients and in those with adrenal or pituitary insufficiency because glucose-lowering drugs may make them hypoglycemic. ▪ Increase dosage carefully in patients with impaired renal function or renal failure requiring dialysis. ▪ Adjust dosage by blood glucose response. May double dose up to 4 mg with each meal until response satisfactory. Allow ≥ 1 wk between dosage adjustments.

	and whose HbA_{1c} is ≥ 8%, 1 to 2 mg P.O., taken up to 30 min before each meal. Dose range is 0.5 to 4 mg with meals, divided b.i.d., t.i.d., or q.i.d. Maximum 16 mg daily.	▪ Patients can lose glycemic control during stress. ▪ Hypoglycemia may be difficult to recognize in the elderly and in patients taking beta blockers.
respiratory syncytial virus immune globulin intravenous, human (RSV-IGIV) RespiGam *Immune serum* Pregnancy Risk Category: C	*Prevention of serious lower respiratory tract infections caused by RSV in children with bronchopulmonary dysplasia (BPD) or premature birth* — **Premature infants and children < 2 yr:** single infusion monthly. Give 1.5 ml/kg/hr I.V. for 15 min; then may increase to 3 ml/kg/hr for 15 min to maximum 6 ml/kg/hr until infusion ends. Maximum total per monthly infusion, 750 mg/kg.	▪ Assess cardiopulmonary status and vital signs before infusion, each rate increase, and q 30 min until 30 min after infusion. ▪ May use slower rate in critically ill children with BPD. ▪ Monitor for fluid overload. ▪ ***I.V. use:*** Use single-use vial only once; don't shake, avoid foaming. Begin infusion within 6 hr and complete by 12 hr.
reteplase, recombinant Retavase *Thrombolytic* Pregnancy Risk Category: C	*Management of acute MI* — **Adults:** double-bolus of 10 + 10 U. Give each bolus I.V. over 2 min. If no complications after 1st bolus, give 2nd bolus 30 min after start of 1st.	▪ Carefully monitor ECG during treatment. ▪ Monitor for bleeding and mental status changes. Avoid I.M. injections, invasive procedures, and nonessential patient handling. If bleeding or anaphylactoid reactions occur after 1st bolus, notify doctor. ▪ Don't give with other I.V. medications.
ribavirin Virazole *Antiviral* Pregnancy Risk Category: X	*Hospitalized infants and young children infected by RSV* — **Infants and young children:** solution in concentration of 20 mg/ml delivered via Viratek Small Particle Aerosol Generator (SPAG-2) and mechanical ventilation, or via oxygen mask, hood, or tent at	▪ Give aerosol form by SPAG-2 only. ▪ Use sterile USP water for injection only. ▪ Discard solutions placed in SPAG-2 unit ≥ q 24 hr before adding newly reconstituted solution. ▪ Health care personnel *(continued)*

DRUG & CLASS	INDICATIONS & DOSAGES	NURSING CONSIDERATIONS
ribavirin *(continued)*	flow rate of 12.5 L/min mist. Treat for 12 to 18 hr/day for 3 to 7 days, with flow rate of 12.5 L/min of mist.	exposed to aerosolized drug may have eye irritation and headache. ▪ Monitor ventilator function frequently.
riboflavin (vitamin B_2) *Vitamin B complex vitamin* Pregnancy Risk Category: A	*Riboflavin deficiency or adjunct to thiamine treatment for polyneuritis or cheilosis from pellagra* — **Adults:** 5 to 30 mg P.O. q.d., in divided doses, depending on severity. **Children:** 3 to 10 mg P.O. q.d., depending on severity.	▪ Deficiency often accompanies other vitamin B complex deficiencies; may require multivitamin therapy. ▪ Tell patient to take with meals; food increases absorption. ▪ Urine may appear bright yellow.
rifabutin Mycobutin *Antibiotic* Pregnancy Risk Category: B	*Prevention of disseminated MAC in advanced HIV infection* — **Adults:** 300 mg P.O. q.d. as single dose or divided b.i.d., with food.	▪ Use cautiously in preexisting neutropenia and thrombocytopenia. ▪ Perform baseline hematologic studies; repeat periodically. ▪ May stain soft contact lenses.
rifampin (rifampicin) Rifadin, Rifadin IV, Rimactane, Rimycin‡, Rofact† *Antituberculotic* Pregnancy Risk Category: C	*Pulmonary TB* — **Adults:** 10 mg/kg, up to 600 mg/day P.O. or I.V. in single dose 1 hr before or 2 hr after meals. **Children:** 10 to 20 mg/kg P.O. or I.V. q.d. in single dose 1 hr before or 2 hr after meals. Maximum 600 mg/day. *Meningococcal carriers* — **Adults:** 600 mg P.O. or I.V., b.i.d. for 2 days, or 600 mg/day P.O. or I.V. for 4 days. **Children 1 mo to 12 yr:** 10 mg/kg P.O. or I.V. b.i.d. for 2 days, ≤ 600 mg/day, or 10 to 20 mg/kg/day for 4 days. **Neonates:** 5 mg/kg P.O. or I.V. b.i.d. for 2 days.	▪ Give 1 hr before or 2 hr after meals. ▪ ***I.V. use:*** Reconstitute with 10 ml sterile water for injection to make solution containing 60 mg/ml. Add to 100 ml D_5W and infuse over 30 min, or add to 500 ml D_5W and infuse over 3 hr. ▪ Give with other antituberculotics. ▪ May stain urine, feces, saliva, sweat, sputum, and tears red-orange. ▪ May stain soft contact lenses.

	Prophylaxis of H. influenzae *type b* — **Adults and children:** 20 mg/kg/day P.O. for 4 days; maximum 600 mg/day.	
rifapentine Priftin *Antituberculotic* Pregnancy Risk Category: C	*Pulmonary TB, with ≥ 1 other antituberculotic* — **Adults:** during intensive phase of short-course therapy, 600 mg P.O. twice weekly for 2 mo, with an interval between doses of ≥ 3 days (≥ 72 hr). During continuation phase of short-course therapy, 600 mg P.O. q wk for 4 mo.	▪ Monitor LFTs before therapy. ▪ ***ALERT*** Must give with appropriate daily companion drugs. Compliance crucial for early sputum conversion and to prevent tuberculosis relapse. ▪ Giving during last 2 wk of pregnancy may lead to postnatal hemorrhage in mother or infant. ▪ Notify doctor of persistent or severe diarrhea.
riluzole Rilutek *Neuroprotector* Pregnancy Risk Category: C	*Amyotrophic lateral sclerosis* — **Adults:** 50 mg P.O. q 12 hr, on empty stomach.	▪ Tell patient to take at same time daily. ▪ Instruct patient to report fever. ▪ Caution patient to avoid hazardous activities. ▪ Obtain LFT results periodically.
rimantadine hydrochloride Flumadine *Antiviral* Pregnancy Risk Category: C	*Prevention of influenza A* — **Adults and children ≥ 10 yr:** 100 mg P.O. b.i.d. **Children < 10 yr:** 5 mg/kg (maximum 150 mg) P.O. q.d. **Elderly:** 100 mg P.O. q.d. *Influenza A* — **Adults:** 100 mg P.O. b.i.d., within 24 to 48 hr of symptom onset and for 24 to 48 hr after symptoms disappear. ***Adjust-a-dose:*** In patients with severe hepatic or renal dysfunction or with adverse effects at normal dosage, give 100 mg P.O. q.d.	▪ Use cautiously in renal or hepatic impairment and in history of seizures. Pregnant patients should compare risks versus benefits before starting. ▪ Tell patient to take several hr before h.s. ▪ Tell patient to take infection-control precautions. ▪ Resistant strains may emerge during therapy.
risperidone Risperdal	*Psychosis* — **Adults:** initially, 1 mg P.O. b.i.d., increased in 1-mg increments b.i.d.	▪ Obtain baseline BP; monitor often. ▪ Monitor patient for orthostatic *(continued)*

DRUG & CLASS	INDICATIONS & DOSAGES	NURSING CONSIDERATIONS
risperidone *(continued)* *Antipsychotic* Pregnancy Risk Category: C	on days 2 and 3 to 3 mg b.i.d. Wait ≥ 1 wk before adjusting dose. Safety of > 16 mg/day not known. ***Adjust-a-dose:*** In debilitated patients or those with hypotension or severe renal or hepatic impairment, give 0.5 mg P.O. b.i.d. Increase by 0.5-mg increments b.i.d. on days 2 and 3 to 1.5 mg P.O. b.i.d. Wait ≥ 1 wk before increasing.	hypotension and tardive dyskinesia. ▪ Assess for neuroleptic malignant syndrome. ▪ Use lower dose in elderly patients. ▪ Mix oral solution with 3 to 4 oz of coffee, orange juice, water, or low-fat milk. Don't mix with cola or tea.
ritonavir Norvir *Antiviral* Pregnancy Risk Category: B	*HIV infection, in combination with nucleoside analogues* — **Adults:** 600 mg P.O. b.i.d. before meals. If nausea occurs, adjust dosage: 300 mg b.i.d. for 1 day, 400 mg b.i.d. for 2 days, 500 mg b.i.d. for 1 day, and 600 mg b.i.d. thereafter.	▪ Give before meals to decrease nausea. ▪ Oral solution may be more palatable if mixed with chocolate milk, Ensure, or Advera. ▪ Adverse reactions may diminish as therapy continues.
rituximab Rituxan *Antineoplastic* Pregnancy Risk Factor: C	*B-cell malignant lymphoma with relapsed or refractory low-grade or follicular, CD20 positive disease* — **Adults:** 375 mg/m^2 as I.V. infusion q wk for 4 doses (days 1, 8, 15, and 22). Start initial infusion at 50 mg/hr. If no hypersensitivity or infusion-related events occur, increase to 50 mg/hr q 30 min, to maximum of 400 mg/hr. Can give subsequent infusions, initially, at 100 mg/hr and increase by 100 mg/hr at 30-min intervals, to maximum of 400 mg/hr, as tolerated.	▪ Monitor patient closely for signs and symptoms of hypersensitivity reaction. ▪ Give acetaminophen and diphenhydramine before each infusion. ▪ Obtain CBC at regular intervals. ▪ Don't give as I.V. push or bolus. ▪ ***ALERT*** Monitor BP closely during infusion. If hypotension, bronchospasm, or angioedema occurs, stop and restart at 50% rate reduction when symptoms resolve. Stop infusion if serious arrhythmias occur.

rivastigmine tartrate Exelon *Anti–Alzheimer's disease agent* Pregnancy Risk Category: B	*Alzheimer's disease* — **Adults:** 1.5 mg P.O. b.i.d. with food. If tolerated, dosage may be increased to 3 mg b.i.d. after 2 wk. Further increases to 4.5 mg b.i.d. and 6 mg b.i.d. may be implemented as tolerated after 2 wk on previous dose. Dosage ranges from 6 to maximum 12 mg/day.	▪ Expect GI adverse effects such as nausea, vomiting, anorexia, and weight loss; these occur less commonly during maintenance doses. ▪ Monitor for symptoms of active or occult GI bleeding. ▪ Dramatic memory improvement is unlikely. As disease progresses, drug benefits may decline. ▪ Monitor patient for severe nausea, vomiting, and diarrhea, which may lead to dehydration and weight loss. ▪ Carefully monitor patient for adverse effects if he has a history of GI bleeding, NSAID use, arrhythmias, seizures, or pulmonary conditions.
rizatriptan benzoate Maxalt, Maxalt-MLT *Antimigraine agent* Pregnancy Risk Category: C	*Acute migraine headaches with or without aura* — **Adults:** 5 or 10 mg P.O. If 1st dose ineffective, can give another dose 2 hr after first. Maximum dose is 30 mg/24 hr. For patients receiving propranolol, give 5 mg P.O. up to maximum of 3 doses (15 mg) in 24 hr.	▪ Use cautiously in patients with hepatic or renal impairment or risk of CAD. ▪ Don't use for prophylactic therapy or in patients with hemiplegic or basilar migraine or cluster headaches.
rofecoxib Vioxx *Nonnarcotic analgesic, anti-inflammatory* Pregnancy Risk Category: C	*Osteoarthritis* — **Adults:** 12.5 mg P.O. q.d., increased p.r.n. up to 25 mg P.O. q.d. *Acute pain; primary dysmenorrhea* — **Adults:** 50 mg P.O. q.d. p.r.n. for ≤ 5 days.	▪ ***ALERT*** Use cautiously in patients with asthma; they may suffer severe, potentially fatal bronchospasm after taking aspirin or other NSAIDs. ▪ Use cautiously in patients with renal disease. If drug therapy must be initiated, renal function should be *(continued)*

†Canadian ‡Australian

DRUG & CLASS	INDICATIONS & DOSAGES	NURSING CONSIDERATIONS
rofecoxib *(continued)*		closely monitored. Don't give to patients with advanced renal disease. ▪ NSAIDs may cause serious GI toxicity at any time without warning. ▪ Use cautiously in dehydrated patients. Rehydrate before starting therapy. ▪ In patients with fluid retention, hypertension, or heart failure, begin therapy at lowest dosage. Monitor BP and check patient for fluid retention or worsening heart failure.
ropinirole hydrochloride Requip *Antiparkinsonian* Pregnancy Risk Category: C	*Idiopathic Parkinson's disease* — **Adults:** 0.25 mg P.O. t.i.d. Adjust q wk. After wk 4, may increase by 1.5 mg/day q wk up to 9 mg/day, then increase q wk by up to 3 mg/day. Maximum 24 mg/day.	▪ ***ALERT*** Monitor patient carefully for orthostatic hypotension, especially during dose escalation. May cause syncope. ▪ Can increase adverse effects of levodopa and may cause or exacerbate dyskinesia. ▪ May cause hallucinations. ▪ Withdraw gradually over 7 days.
rosiglitazone maleate Avandia *Antidiabetic* Pregnancy Risk Category: C	*Type 2 diabetes mellitus, alone or combined with metformin* — **Adults:** 4 mg P.O. q.d. in morning or in divided doses b.i.d. morning and evening. Dosage may be increased to 8 mg P.O. q.d. or in divided doses b.i.d., p.r.n., after 12 wk of treatment. *Adjunct to sulfonylureas for type 2 diabetes mellitus* — **Adults:** 4 mg P.O. q.d. or in 2 divided doses.	▪ ***ALERT*** Check liver enzyme levels before therapy starts and monitor every 2 mo for the 1st 12 mo of treatment and periodically afterward. If ALT level is elevated, recheck as soon as possible. Stop drug if levels remain elevated. ▪ Because ovulation may resume in premenopausal, anovulatory women with insulin resistance, tell patient to use con-

	Adjunct to sulfonylureas, diet, and exercise in patients with type 2 diabetes mellitus — **Adults:** 4 mg P.O. q.d. or in 2 divided doses.	traceptives. ▪ Hgb and Hct may fall, usually in the 1st 4 to 8 wk of therapy. ▪ For patients whose blood glucose levels are inadequately controlled with metformin, drug should be added to — not substituted for — metformin.
salmeterol xinafoate Serevent, Serevent Diskus *Bronchodilator* Pregnancy Risk Category: C	*Long-term maintenance of asthma; prevention of bronchospasm for nocturnal asthma or reversible obstructive airway disease* — **Adults and children > 12 yr:** 2 inhalations q 12 hr, a.m. and p.m. **Adults and children ≥ 4 yr:** 1 inhalation q 12 hr, a.m. and p.m. *Prevention of exercise-induced bronchospasm* — **Adults and children ≥ 12 yr:** 2 inhalations 30 to 60 min before exercise. **Adults and children ≥ 4 yr**: 1 inhalation ≥ 30 min before exercise. *Maintenance of bronchospasm linked to COPD, including emphysema and chronic bronchitis* —**Adults:** 2 inhalations (42 mcg; inhalation aerosol) q 12 hr, a.m. and p.m.	▪ Use cautiously in patients with CV disorders, thyrotoxicosis, or seizure disorders and if overly responsive to sympathomimetics. ▪ Tell patient to take at 12-hr intervals. ▪ Instruct patient to use 30 to 60 min before exercise. ▪ ***ALERT*** Don't use for acute bronchospasm.
saquinavir Fortovase **saquinavir mesylate** Invirase *Antiviral* Pregnancy Risk Category: B	*Adjunct treatment of advanced HIV infection in selected patients* — **Adults:** 600 mg (Invirase) or 1,200 mg (Fortovase) P.O. t.i.d. within 2 hr after meals and with nucleoside analogue.	▪ Monitor hydration if adverse GI reactions occur. ▪ Adverse reactions include headache, nausea, and diarrhea.

DRUG & CLASS	INDICATIONS & DOSAGES	NURSING CONSIDERATIONS
sargramostim (granulocyte-macrophage colony-stimulating factor, GM-CSF) Leukine *Colony-stimulating factor* Pregnancy Risk Category: C	*Acceleration of hematopoietic reconstitution after autologous bone marrow transplantation (BMT)* — **Adults:** 250 mcg/m^2/day for 3 wk given as 2-hr I.V. infusion starting 2 to 4 hr after BMT. *BMT failure or engraftment delay* — **Adults**: 250 mcg/m^2/day for 2 wk as 2-hr I.V. infusion. May repeat dose after 1-wk rest period.	▪ Don't add other medications to infusion. ▪ Don't give within 24 hr of last chemotherapy dose or within 12 hr of last radiotherapy dose. ▪ Monitor CBC with differential. ▪ Transient rash and local reactions at injection site may occur. ▪ Duration of therapy based on indications and response.
scopolamine (hyoscine) Isopto Hyoscine, Scopace, Transderm-Scop, Transderm-V† **scopolamine butylbromide (hyoscine butylbromide)** Buscopan†‡ **scopolamine hydrobromide (hyoscine hydrobromide; systemic)** *Antimuscarinic, cycloplegic mydriatic* Pregnancy Risk Category: C	*Spastic states* — **Adults:** 10 to 20 mg P.O. t.i.d. or q.i.d. Adjust dosage, p.r.n. Or 10 to 20 mg (butylbromide) S.C., I.M., or I.V. t.i.d. or q.i.d. *Delirium; preanesthetic sedation and obstetric amnesia with analgesics* — **Adults:** 0.3 to 0.65 mg I.M., S.C., or I.V. **Children:** 0.006 mg/kg I.M., S.C., I.V.; maximum 0.3 mg. *Prevention of motion sickness* — **Adults:** 1 Transderm-Scop or Transderm-V patch applied to skin behind ear at least 4 hr before antiemetic required. One patch lasts 72 hr. Or 300 to 600 mcg (hydrobromide) S.C., I.M., or I.V. **Children:** 6 mcg/kg or 200 mcg/m^2 (hydrobromide) S.C., I.M., or I.V.	▪ Use cautiously in autonomic neuropathy, hyperthyroidism, CAD, arrhythmias, heart failure, hypertension, hiatal hernia with reflux esophagitis, hepatic or renal disease, or ulcerative colitis; in children < 6 yr; or in hot or humid environments. ▪ ***I.V. use:*** Avoid intermittent and continuous infusions. For direct I.V. use, dilute with sterile water. ▪ Protect I.V. solutions from freezing and light; store at room temperature. ▪ Tolerance may develop with long-term use.
scopolamine hydrobromide	*Cycloplegic refraction* — **Adults:** 1 to 2 drops 0.25% solution 1 hr before refraction.	▪ Warn patient to avoid hazardous activities until blurring subsides.

(ophthalmic) Isopto Hyoscine *Antimuscarinic, cycloplegic mydriatic* Pregnancy Risk Category: NR	**Children:** 1 drop 0.25% solution b.i.d. for 2 days before refraction. *Iritis; uveitis* — **Adults:** 1 to 2 drops 0.25% solution once daily to q.i.d. **Children:** 1 drop once daily to q.i.d.	▪ Observe for adverse CNS effects. ▪ Advise patient to wear dark glasses. ▪ May use in patients sensitive to atropine. ▪ Apply light pressure to lacrimal sac for 1 min after instillation.
secobarbital sodium Novosecobarb†, Seconal Sodium *Sedative-hypnotic, anticonvulsant* Pregnancy Risk Category: D Controlled Substance Schedule: II	*Preoperative sedation* — **Adults:** 200 to 300 mg P.O. 1 to 2 hr before surgery or 1 mg/kg I.M. 15 min before procedure. **Children:** 2 to 6 mg/kg P.O. Maximum single dose 100 mg. *Insomnia* — **Adults:** 100 to 200 mg P.O. or I.M. *Status epilepticus* — **Adults:** 250 to 350 mg I.M. or I.V. **Children:** 15 to 20 mg/kg I.V. over 15 min.	▪ ***I.V. use:*** I.V. injection for emergency use; give by direct injection. Give at rate $\leq$ 50 mg/15 sec. ▪ I.V. use may cause respiratory depression, laryngospasm, or hypotension; keep emergency resuscitation equipment available. ▪ Assess mental status before initiating.
selegiline hydrochloride Carbex, Eldepryl *Antiparkinsonian* Pregnancy Risk Category: C	*Adjunct treatment with levodopa-carbidopa to manage Parkinson's disease* — **Adults:** 10 mg/day P.O. (5 mg at breakfast, 5 mg at lunch). After 2 or 3 days, slowly decrease levodopa-carbidopa dose.	▪ Some patients may experience more adverse reactions with levodopa and need 10% to 30% reduction of levodopa-carbidopa dose. ▪ May cause dizziness at start of therapy.
senna Fletcher's Castoria, Senexon, Senokot *Stimulant laxative* Pregnancy Risk Category: C	*Acute constipation; preparation for bowel or rectal exam* — **Adults:** 1 to 8 tablets (Senokot) P.O.; ½ to 4 tsp granules added to liquid P.O.; 1 to 2 suppositories P.R. h.s.; or 1 to 4 tsp syrup P.O. h.s.	▪ Don't expose drug to excessive heat or light.
sertraline hydrochloride Zoloft	*Depression* — **Adults:** 50 mg/day P.O.; adjust as tolerated and p.r.n. at $\geq$ 1-wk intervals. *Obsessive-compulsive disorder* — **Adults:**	▪ Use cautiously in patients at risk for suicide and in seizure disorders, major affective disorder, or *(continued)*

†Canadian ‡Australian

DRUG & CLASS	INDICATIONS & DOSAGES	NURSING CONSIDERATIONS
sertraline hydrochloride *(continued)* *Antidepressant* Pregnancy Risk Category: B	50 mg/day P.O. Maximum 200 mg/day. Adjust at ≥ 1-wk intervals. *Posttraumatic stress disorder; panic disorder* — **Adults:** initially, 25 mg P.O. q.d. Increase to 50 mg P.O. q.d. 1 wk after therapy. Dosage may be increased at 1-wk intervals to a maximum of 200 mg/day. Maintain patient on lowest effective dosage.	conditions that affect metabolism or hemodynamic responses. ▪ Monitor for suicidal tendencies and allow minimum drug supply.
sibutramine hydrochloride monohydrate Meridia *Antiobesity agent* Pregnancy Risk Category: C Controlled Substance Schedule: IV	*Management of obesity* — **Adults:** 10 mg P.O. q.d. May increase to 15 mg P.O. q.d. after 4 wk, p.r.n. Reduce to 5 mg P.O. q.d. in patients intolerant of higher dose. Maximum 15 mg/day.	▪ Use cautiously in patients with history of seizures or narrow-angle glaucoma. ▪ Rule out organic causes of obesity before starting therapy. ▪ Measure BP and pulse before starting, with dose changes, and regularly during therapy. ▪ Allow 2 wk between MAO inhibitor and starting drug therapy.
sildenafil citrate Viagra *Erectile dysfunction therapy* Pregnancy Risk Category: B	*Erectile dysfunction* — **Adults < 65 yr:** 50 mg P.O., p.r.n., 1 hr before sexual activity. Dose range is 25 mg to 100 mg. Maximum 1 dose/day. **Elderly:** 25 mg P.O., p.r.n., 1 hr before sexual activity. Adjust p.r.n., based on patient response. Maximum 1 dose/day. ***Adjust-a-dose:*** In adults with hepatic or severe renal impairment, 25 mg P.O., 1 hr before sexual activity. Adjust p.r.n., based on patient response. Maximum 1 dose/day.	▪ Systemic vasodilatory effects cause transient decreases in supine BP and cardiac output (about 2 hr after ingestion). ▪ May cause serious CV events. ▪ Don't give with nitrates.

silver sulfadiazine Flamazine†, Flint SSD, Silvadene, Thermazene *Topical antibacterial* Pregnancy Risk Category: B	*Prevention and treatment of wound infection in 2nd- and 3rd-degree burns* — **Adults:** apply 1/16" thickness to clean, debrided burn once daily or b.i.d.	▪ Use sterile application technique. ▪ Use only on affected areas; keep medicated at all times. ▪ Inspect skin daily, noting changes. Notify doctor of burning or excessive pain. ▪ Discard darkened cream.
simethicone Flatulex, Gas-X, Mylanta Gas, Mylicon, Phazyme *Antiflatulent* Pregnancy Risk Category: NR	*Flatulence; functional gastric bloating* — **Adults and children > 12 yr:** 40 to 125 mg before meals and h.s.; **Children 2 to 12 yr:** 40 mg (drops) P.O. q.i.d.; **Children < 2 yr:** 20 mg (drops) P.O. q.i.d., up to 240 mg/day.	▪ Don't use for infant colic. ▪ Doesn't prevent gas formation.
simvastatin (syvinolin) Lipex‡, Zocor *Antilipemic* Pregnancy Risk Category: X	*Reduction of LDL, total cholesterol, apolipoprotein B, and triglycerides and increase of HDL in primary hypercholesterolemia and mixed dyslipidemia (types IIa and IIb); hypertriglyceridemia (type IV); primary dysbetalipoproteinemia (type III)* — **Adults:** initially, 20 mg P.O. q.d. h.s. Adjust dose q 4 wk based on tolerance and response. Dosage range is 5 to 80 mg/day. ***Adjust-a-dose:*** Give elderly patients ≤ 20 mg q.d.	▪ Use cautiously in patients who use alcohol excessively or have history of liver disease. ▪ Obtain LFT results before therapy and periodically thereafter; if liver enzyme levels stay elevated, may do liver biopsy. ▪ Used as an adjunct to diet.
sirolimus Rapamune *Immunosuppressant* Pregnancy Risk Category: C	*Prevention, with cyclosporine and corticosteroids, of renal organ rejection after transplant* — **Adults and adolescents ≥ 13 yr weighing ≥ 40 kg:** 6 mg P.O. as a 1-time loading dose immediately after transplant; then maintenance dose of 2 mg P.O. q.d.	▪ After transplant, give antimicrobials to prevent *Pneumocystis carinii* and *Cytomegalovirus* infections for 1 yr and 3 mo, respectively. ▪ Patients taking drug are more susceptible to infection and possible *(continued)*

†Canadian ‡Australian

DRUG & CLASS	INDICATIONS & DOSAGES	NURSING CONSIDERATIONS
sirolimus *(continued)*	**Adolescents ≥ 13 yr weighing < 40 kg**: 3 mg/m^2 P.O. as a 1-time loading dose after transplant; then maintenance dose of 1 mg/m^2 P.O. q.d. ***Adjust-a-dose:*** In patients with mild to moderate hepatic impairment, loading dose can stay the same, but reduce maintenance dose by about one-third.	development of lymphoma, which may result from immunosuppression. ▪ If patient is on sirolimus and cyclosporine is started as an HMG-CoA reductase inhibitor, monitor for development of rhabdomyolysis. ▪ When diluting drug, empty correct amount into glass or plastic container filled with ≥ 2 oz (60 ml) of water or orange juice only; don't use any other liquid. Stir vigorously and have patient drink immediately. Refill container with ≥ 4 oz (120 ml) of water or orange juice, stir, and have patient drink all contents. ▪ Store away from light, and refrigerate at 36° to 46° F (2° to 8° C). After opening bottle, use contents within 1 mo. If necessary, bottles and pouches can be stored at room temperature (up to 77° F [25° C]) for several days. Drug can be kept in oral dosing syringe for 24 hr at room temperature or refrigerated at 36° to 46° F (2° to 8° C).
sodium bicarbonate Bell/ans, Citrocarbonate, Soda Mint *Systemic and urinary*	*Cardiac arrest* — **Adults and children:** 1 mEq/kg I.V. of 7.5% or 8.4% solution, then 0.5 mEq/kg I.V. q 10 min, based on ABGs. If ABGs unavailable, use 0.5 mEq/kg I.V. q 10 min until spontaneous circula-	▪ ***I.V. use:*** Don't mix with I.V. norepinephrine, dopamine, or calcium. ▪ Obtain blood pH, Pao_2, $Paco_2$, and serum electrolytes; report results to doctor. ▪ Don't use in cardiac arrest or during early

Drug	Indications and dosages	Key considerations
alkalinizer Pregnancy Risk Category: C	tion returns. **Infants < 2 yr:** ≤ 8 mEq/kg/day I.V. of 4.2% solution. *Metabolic acidosis* — **Adults and children:** 2 to 5 mEq/kg I.V. over 4 to 8 hr. *Systemic or urinary alkalinization* — **Adults:** 4 g P.O., then 1 to 2 g q 4 hr. **Children:** 84 to 840 mg/kg/day P.O.	resuscitation stages unless preexisting acidosis exists. ▪ When used as urinary alkalinizer, monitor urine pH. ▪ Dosage based on blood CO_2 content, pH, and clinical condition.
sodium chloride *Sodium and chloride replacement* Pregnancy Risk Category: C	*Hyponatremia from electrolyte loss or in severe salt depletion* — **Adults:** Use 3% or 5% solution only with frequent electrolyte determination. With 0.45% solution: 3% to 8% of body weight, according to deficiencies, over 18 to 24 hr; with 0.9% solution: 2% to 6% of body weight, according to deficiencies, over 18 to 24 hr. *Heat cramp from excessive perspiration* — **Adults:** 1 g P.O. with water.	▪ Never give concentrated solutions (> 5%) without diluting. Read labels carefully. ▪ ***I.V. use:*** Infuse 3% and 5% solutions slowly and cautiously. Use only for critical situations. Observe patient continually. ▪ Monitor serum electrolytes, acid-base balance, and changes in fluid balance. ▪ Never use bacteriostatic NaCl injection with newborns.
sodium ferric gluconate complex Ferrlecit *Hematinic* Pregnancy Risk Category: B	*Iron deficiency anemia in patients undergoing chronic hemodialysis while receiving supplemental erythropoietin therapy* — **Adults:** Before starting therapeutic doses, give test dose of 2 ml (25 mg elemental iron) diluted in 50 ml normal saline and given I.V. over 1 hr. If test dose is tolerated, give therapeutic dose of 10 ml (125 mg elemental iron) diluted in 100 ml normal saline I.V. over 1 hr. Usual minimum cumulative dose is 1 g elemental iron at > 8 sequential dialysis treatments to achieve fa-	▪ Potentially life-threatening hypersensitivity reactions (characterized by CV collapse, cardiac arrest, bronchospasm, oral or pharyngeal edema, dyspnea, angioedema, urticaria, or pruritus sometimes with pain and muscle spasm of chest or back) may occur during infusion. Have adequate supportive measures readily available. Monitor patient closely during infusion. ▪ Ask patient about other sources of iron, such as nonprescription iron preparations and iron-containing *(continued)*

DRUG & CLASS	INDICATIONS & DOSAGES	NURSING CONSIDERATIONS
sodium ferric gluconate complex *(continued)*	vorable Hgb or Hct response.	multiple vitamins. ▪ ***I.V. use:*** Don't mix with other drugs or add to parenteral nutrition solutions for I.V. infusion. Use immediately after dilution in normal saline. ▪ Profound hypotension with flushing, lightheadedness, malaise, fatigue, weakness, or severe chest, back, flank, or groin pain may occur after too-rapid I.V. infusion of iron. These aren't hypersensitivity reactions. Don't exceed rate of 2.1 mg/min. Monitor patient closely during infusion.
sodium phosphates Fleet Enema *Saline laxative* Pregnancy Risk Category: C	*Constipation* — **Adults:** 20 ml solution mixed with 120 ml cold water P.O., or as enema, 120 ml P.R. **Children:** 5 to 10 ml solution mixed with 120 ml cold water P.O.; or as enema, 60 ml P.R.	▪ Use cautiously in patients with large hemorrhoids or anal excoriations. ▪ Before giving for constipation, assess for adequate fluid intake, exercise, and diet. ▪ Up to 10% of sodium content may be absorbed.
sodium polystyrene sulfonate Kayexalate, SPS *Potassium-removing resin* Pregnancy Risk Category: C	*Hyperkalemia* — **Adults:** 15 g P.O. once daily to q.i.d. in water or sorbitol (3 to 4 ml/g of resin). Or, mix powder with appropriate medium and instill through NG tube. Or, 30 to 50 g/100 ml of sorbitol q 6 hr as warm emulsion deep into sigmoid colon (20 cm). **Children:** 1 g/kg P.O. or P.R., q 6 hr p.r.n. P.O. route preferred (drug should be in intestine $\geq$ 30 min).	▪ Monitor serum potassium at least daily; stop drug when 4 or 5 mEq/L. Monitor serum calcium if receiving drug for > 3 days. ▪ Watch for signs of hypokalemia and digitalis toxicity in digitalized patients. ▪ Monitor for other electrolyte deficiencies. ▪ Prevent fecal impaction in elderly patients by giving resin P.R.

sotalol Betapace, Betapace AF, Sotacor†‡ *Antiarrhythmic* Pregnancy Risk Category: B	*Documented, life-threatening ventricular arrhythmias (Betapace)* — **Adults:** initially, 80 mg P.O. b.i.d. Increase q 2 to 3 days p.r.n. and as tolerated; most respond to 160 to 320 mg/day. *Maintenance of normal sinus rhythm or delay in time to recurrence of atrial fibrillation or atrial flutter, with symptomatic atrial fibrillation or atrial flutter, if currently in sinus rhythm (Betapace AF)* — **Adults:** 80 mg P.O. b.i.d. Increase p.r.n. to 120 mg P.O. b.i.d. after 3 days if QT interval < 500 msec. Maximum dose is 160 mg P.O. b.i.d. ***Adjust-a-dose:*** In patients with CrCl > 30 to 60 ml/min, increase dosage interval to q 24 hr; if between 10 and 30 ml/min, increase to q 36 to 48 hr; if < 10 ml/min, individualize dosage.	▪ Proarrhythmic events may occur at start of therapy and at dosage adjustments. Monitor cardiac rhythm. ▪ Withdraw other antiarrhythmics first. ▪ Monitor serum electrolytes regularly. ▪ ***ALERT*** Significant differences in dosing and warnings exist between Betapace and Betapace AF.
sparfloxacin Zagam *Anti-infective* Pregnancy Risk Category: C	*Community-acquired pneumonia and acute bacterial exacerbation of chronic bronchitis caused by susceptible organisms* — **Adults > 18 yr:** 400 mg P.O. on day 1 as loading dose, then 200 mg/day for 10 days. ***Adjust-a-dose:*** In patients with CrCl < 50 ml/min, 400 mg loading dose P.O.; then 200 mg P.O. q 48 hr for 9 days.	▪ Use cautiously in patients with renal impairment. ▪ If patient experiences excessive CNS stimulation, discontinue and notify doctor. Institute seizure precautions.
spironolactone Aldactone, Novo-Spiroton† *Diuretic, antihypertensive, antihypokalemic*	*Edema* — **Adults:** 25 to 200 mg P.O. once daily or in divided doses. **Children:** 3.3 mg/kg P.O. once daily or in divided doses. *Hypertension* — **Adults:** 50 to 100 mg P.O.	▪ Instruct patient to take with food in morning; if 2nd dose needed, tell him to take in early evening. ▪ Warn patient to avoid

(continued)

†Canadian ‡Australian

DRUG & CLASS	INDICATIONS & DOSAGES	NURSING CONSIDERATIONS
spironolactone *(continued)* Pregnancy Risk Category: NR	once daily or in divided doses. *Diuretic-induced hypokalemia* — **Adults:** 25 to 100 mg P.O. q.d.	excessive use of potassium-rich foods, salt substitutes, and potassium supplements. ▪ Notify doctor if breast enlargement occurs in men.
stavudine (d4T) Zerit *Antiviral* Pregnancy Risk Category: C	*HIV-infected patients on prolonged zidovudine therapy* — **Adults ≥ 60 kg (132 lb):** 40 mg P.O. q 12 hr. **Adults < 60 kg:** 30 mg P.O. q 12 hr.	▪ Monitor CBC, serum creatinine, AST, ALT, and alkaline phosphatase levels. ▪ Instruct patient not to take with other drugs for HIV or AIDS unless doctor orders. ▪ Instruct patient to tell doctor if peripheral neuropathy occurs.
streptokinase Streptase *Thrombolytic enzyme* Pregnancy Risk Category: C	*Arteriovenous cannula occlusion* — **Adults:** 250,000 IU in 2 ml I.V. solution by I.V. pump infusion into each occluded limb of cannula over 25 to 35 min. Clamp off cannula for 2 hr. Then aspirate, flush, and reconnect. *Venous thrombosis; pulmonary embolism (PE); arterial thrombosis and embolism* — **Adults:** loading dose 250,000 IU I.V. over 30 min. Sustaining dose 100,000 IU/hr I.V. for 72 hr for deep vein thrombosis and 100,000 IU/hr over 24 to 72 hr for PE and arterial thrombosis or embolism. *Lysis of coronary artery thrombi* — **Adults:** loading dose 20,000 IU bolus via coronary catheter; then 2,000 IU/min infusion over 60 min. Or, give as I.V. infusion. Usual adult dose 1.5 million IU I.V. over 60 min.	▪ Before initiating, draw blood for coagulation studies, Hct, platelet count, and type and crossmatching. Keep aminocaproic acid and corticosteroids available. ▪ Avoid I.M. injections and other invasive procedures during therapy. ▪ Check for hypersensitivity reactions. Monitor vital signs, particularly BP and pulse, and neurologic status often. ▪ Monitor patient closely for excessive bleeding. If bleeding occurs, stop therapy and notify doctor. ▪ Monitor pulses, color, and sensation of extremities q hr. ▪ Avoid unnecessary patient handling; pad side rails.

streptozocin Zanosar *Antineoplastic* Pregnancy Risk Category: C	*Metastatic islet cell carcinoma of pancreas* — **Adults and children:** 500 mg/m² I.V. for 5 consecutive days q 6 wk until maximum benefit or toxicity observed. Or, 1 g/m² q wk intervals for first 2 wk. Maximum single dose 1,500 mg/m². Infuse diluted solution over ≥ 15 min. Give with antiemetic.	• Monitor CBC and LFT at least weekly. • Check urine protein and glucose q shift. • If extravasation occurs, stop infusion; notify doctor. • Obtain urinalysis, BUN, creatinine, and electrolyte levels at least weekly and for 4 wk after each course.
sucralfate Carafate, SCF‡, Sulcrate† *Antiulcer agent* Pregnancy Risk Category: B	*Short-term (≤ 8 wk) treatment of duodenal ulcer* — **Adults:** 1 g P.O. q.i.d. 1 hr after meals and h.s. *Maintenance therapy for duodenal ulcer* — **Adults:** 1 g P.O. b.i.d.	• Monitor for severe, persistent constipation. • May be as effective as cimetidine in healing duodenal ulcers. • Avoid giving within 2 hr of quinolone antibiotics.
sulfamethoxazole Apo-Sulfamethoxazole†, Gantanol *Antibiotic* Pregnancy Risk Category: C (contraindicated at term)	*UTIs and systemic infections* — **Adults:** initially, 2 g P.O., then 1 g P.O. b.i.d. or t.i.d. for severe infections. C. trachomatis — **Adults:** 1 g P.O. b.i.d. for 21 days. **Children and infants > 2 mo:** initially, 50 to 60 mg/kg P.O., then 25 to 30 mg/kg b.i.d. Maximum dose 75 mg/kg/day.	• Monitor urine cultures, CBC, and urinalysis before and during therapy. • Monitor fluid I&O. Intake should be sufficient to produce output of 1,500 ml/day. If fluid intake not adequate, may give sodium bicarbonate. Monitor urine pH daily.
sulfasalazine (salazosulfapyridine, sulphasalazine) Azulfidine, Azulfidine EN-tab *Antibiotic* Pregnancy Risk Category: B	*Mild to moderate ulcerative colitis; adjunctive therapy in severe ulcerative colitis, Crohn's disease* — **Adults:** 3 to 4 g/day P.O. in evenly divided doses; usual maintenance: 2 g/day P.O. in divided doses q 6 hr. **Children > 2 yr:** 40 to 60 mg/kg/day P.O., divided into 3 to 6 doses; then 30 mg/kg/day in 4 doses. *Rheumatoid arthritis (Azulfidine EN-tab)* — **Adults:** 2 to 3 g q.d. in 2 divided doses.	• Give with food; space doses evenly. • May start at lower dose if GI intolerance occurs. • Advise patient to maintain adequate fluid intake. • Discontinue immediately and notify doctor if hypersensitivity occurs. • Warn patient to avoid ultraviolet light.

(continued)

†Canadian ‡Australian

DRUG & CLASS	INDICATIONS & DOSAGES	NURSING CONSIDERATIONS
sulfasalazine *(continued)*	*Juvenile rheumatoid arthritis* — **Children ≥ 6 yr:** 50 mg/kg (Azulfidine EN-tabs) P.O. q.d. in 2 divided doses. Maximum dose is 2 g/day. To reduce GI intolerance, start with ¼ to ⅓ of planned maintenance dose and increase q wk until maintenance dose is reached at 1 mo.	
sulfisoxazole Gantrisin, Novo-Soxazole† **sulfisoxazole acetyl** Gantrisin Pediatric *Antibiotic* Pregnancy Risk Category: C (contraindicated at term)	*UTIs; systemic infections* — **Adults:** initially, 2 to 4 g P.O., then 4 to 8 g/day divided into 4 to 6 doses. **Children > 2 mo:** initially, 75 mg/kg/day P.O. or 2 g/m^2 P.O., then 150 mg/kg or 4 g/m^2 P.O. q.d. in divided doses q 6 hr. Maximum total dose 6 g/day. ***Adjust-a-dose:*** Increase dosage interval if CrCl < 50 ml/min.	▪ Obtain specimen for culture and sensitivity tests before 1st dose. ▪ Monitor urine cultures, CBC, PT, and urinalyses before and during therapy. ▪ Watch for superinfection. ▪ Monitor fluid I&O. Intake should be sufficient to produce 1,500 ml/day output. If fluid intake not adequate, may give sodium bicarbonate. Monitor urine pH daily.
sulindac Aclin‡, Apo-Sulin†, Clinoril, Novo-Sundac† *Nonnarcotic analgesic, anti-inflammatory* Pregnancy Risk Category: NR	*Osteoarthritis; rheumatoid arthritis; ankylosing spondylitis* — **Adults:** initially, 150 mg P.O. b.i.d.; increase to 200 mg b.i.d., p.r.n. Maximum dose is 400 mg/day. *Acute subacromial bursitis or supraspinatus tendinitis; acute gouty arthritis* — **Adults:** 200 mg P.O. b.i.d. for 7 to 14 days. Reduce dose as symptoms subside.	▪ Give with food, milk, or antacids. ▪ May mask signs and symptoms of infection. ▪ May cause peptic ulceration and bleeding. ▪ Periodically monitor hepatic and renal function and CBC with long-term therapy.

sumatriptan succinate Imitrex *Antimigraine agent* Pregnancy Risk Category: C	*Acute migraine attacks (with or without aura)* — **Adults**: 6 mg S.C. Maximum dose two 6-mg injections q.d., ≥ 1 hr apart. Or, initial dose of 25 to 100 mg P.O. and 2nd dose of up to 100 mg in 2 hr, p.r.n. Further doses may be given q 2 hr, p.r.n., to maximum P.O. dose 300 mg/day. For intranasal solution, 5 or 20 mg given into1 nostril (for 10 mg, 5 mg each nostril). If headache returns, may repeat dose after 2 hr. Maximum dose 40 mg/day. ***Adjust-a-dose:*** Maximum P.O. dose in hepatic impairment is 50 mg/day.	▪ ***ALERT*** Tell patient to stop taking drug and call doctor if persistent or severe chest pain, tightness in throat, wheezing, heart throbbing, rash, lumps, hives, or swelling of eyelids, face, or lips develops.
tacrine hydrochloride Cognex *Psychotherapeutic agent* Pregnancy Risk Category: C	*Mild to moderate Alzheimer's dementia* — **Adults**: initially, 10 mg P.O. q.i.d. After 6 wk and if tolerated with no rise in transaminase, increase to 20 mg q.i.d. After 6 wk, adjust to 30 mg q.i.d. If still tolerated, increase to 40 mg q.i.d. after another 6 wk.	▪ Abruptly stopping or reducing daily dose (≥ 80 mg/day) may cause behavioral disturbances and loss of cognitive function. ▪ Monitor LFT results.
tacrolimus Prograf *Immunosuppressant* Pregnancy Risk Category: C	*Prophylaxis of organ rejection in allogenic liver transplant* — **Adults:** 0.05 to 0.1 mg/kg/day I.V. as controlled infusion ≥ 6 hr after transplant. Initial P.O. dosage 0.15 to 0.3 mg/kg/day in 2 divided doses q 12 hr. Start 8 to 12 hr after stopping I.V. Adjust per response. **Children:** 0.1 mg/kg/day I.V., then 0.3 mg/kg/day P.O. on schedule similar to adults, adjusted p.r.n.	▪ Monitor patient for anaphylaxis continuously during first 30 min and frequently thereafter. Keep epinephrine 1:1,000 available. ▪ Observe for hyperkalemia. ▪ Monitor for neurotoxicity and nephrotoxicity. ▪ Check blood glucose regularly. ▪ Increases risk for infections, lymphomas, and other malignant diseases.

DRUG & CLASS	INDICATIONS & DOSAGES	NURSING CONSIDERATIONS
tamoxifen citrate Nolvadex, Nolvadex-D†‡, *Antineoplastic* Pregnancy Risk Category: D	*Advanced premenopausal and postmenopausal breast cancers* — **Adults:** 10 to 20 mg P.O. b.i.d. *Reduction of breast cancer incidence in high-risk women* — **Adults:** 20 mg P.O. q.d. for 5 yr. *Adjunct treatment of breast cancer in women* — **Adults:** 10 mg P.O. b.i.d. for 5 yr.	▪ Monitor serum calcium. May compound hypercalcemia at start of therapy. ▪ Monitor CBC. ▪ Exacerbation of bone pain during therapy often indicates good response.
tamsulosin hydrochloride Flomax *Anti-BPH agent* Pregnancy Risk Category: B	*BPH* — **Adults:** 0.4 mg P.O. q.d. If no response after 2 to 4 wk, may increase to 0.8 mg P.O. q.d. If treatment interrupted for several days, restart therapy at 1 capsule daily.	▪ Tell patient to swallow capsules whole and to take 30 min after same meal daily. ▪ Monitor BP. ▪ Instruct patient not to perform hazardous tasks for 12 hr after dose changes.
telmisartan Micardis *Antihypertensive* Pregnancy Risk Category: C (D in 2nd and 3rd trimesters)	*Hypertension* — **Adults:** 40 mg P.O. q.d. BP response is dose-related over range of 20 to 80 mg q.d.	▪ Use cautiously in patients with biliary obstructive disorders, renal and hepatic insufficiency, or volume or salt depletion. ▪ Monitor for hypotension. ▪ Most antihypertensive effect occurs ≤ 2 wk. Maximal BP reduction may take 4 wk.
temazepam Restoril *Sedative-hypnotic* Pregnancy Risk Category: X Controlled Substance Schedule: IV	*Insomnia* — **Adults:** 7.5 to 30 mg P.O. h.s. **Elderly:** 7.5 mg P.O. h.s.	▪ Assess mental status before initiating therapy. Elderly patients more sensitive to adverse CNS effects. ▪ Prevent hoarding or self-overdosing by depressed, suicidal, or drug-dependent patients or those with drug abuse history.

temozolomide
Temodar
Antineoplastic
Pregnancy Risk Category: D

Refractory anaplastic astrocytoma that has relapsed after chemotherapy regimen containing nitrosourea and procarbazine — **Adults:** 150 mg/m^2 P.O. q.d. for first 5 days of initial 28-day treatment cycle; then, 100 to 200 mg/m^2 P.O. q.d. for first 5 days of subsequent 28-day treatment cycles.
Adjust-a-dose: Timing and dosage of subsequent cycles must be adjusted according to the absolute neutrophil count (ANC) and platelet count measured on cycle day 22 (expected nadir) and cycle day 29 (day 1 of next cycle).

- Use with caution in elderly patients and in patients with severe hepatic or renal impairment.
- A CBC should be drawn on days 22 and 29 of each treatment cycle. If the ANC falls to $< 1{,}500/mm^3$ or the platelet count falls to $< 100{,}000/mm^3$, a weekly CBC should be obtained until the counts have recovered.
- Women and elderly patients are at higher risk for developing myelosuppression.
- Nausea and vomiting, which may be self-limiting, are the most common side effects. Give drug on empty stomach or h.s. to lessen these effects. Antiemetics effectively control nausea and vomiting from drug.
- Avoid skin contact with, or inhalation of, capsule contents if capsule is accidentally opened or damaged. Follow procedures for safe handling and disposal of antineoplastics.

tenecteplase
TNKase
Thrombolytic agent
Pregnancy Risk Category: C

Reduction of death from acute myocardial infarction (MI) — **Adults weighing < 60 kg:** 30 mg (6 ml) I.V. bolus over 5 sec. **Adults weighing 60 to < 70 kg:** 35 mg (7 ml) I.V. bolus over 5 sec. **Adults weighing 70 to < 80 kg:** 40 mg (8 ml) I.V. bolus over 5 sec. **Adults weighing 80 to < 90 kg:** 45 mg (9 ml) I.V. bolus over 5 sec. **Adults weighing ≥ 90 kg:** 50 mg (10 ml) I.V. bolus over 5 sec. Maximum dose is 50 mg.

- Begin therapy as soon as possible after onset of MI symptoms.
- Give drug with aspirin and heparin.
- ***I.V. use:*** Remove shield assembly from supplied B-D 10-ml syringe with TwinPak dual cannula device. Withdraw 10 ml of supplied sterile water for injection, using the red hub cannula syringe-filling device. Inject entire contents into drug vial. Reconstituted solution *(continued)*

DRUG & CLASS	INDICATIONS & DOSAGES	NURSING CONSIDERATIONS
tenecteplase *(continued)*		concentration is 5 mg/ml. ▪ Don't give drug in the same I.V. line as dextrose. Flush dextrose-containing lines with normal saline before and after giving drug. ▪ Monitor patient for bleeding. If serious bleeding occurs, stop heparin and antiplatelet agents immediately.
terazosin hydrochloride Hytrin *Antihypertensive* Pregnancy Risk Category: C	*Hypertension* — **Adults:** initially, 1 mg P.O. h.s. Adjust dose gradually based on response. Usual range 1 to 5 mg/day; maximum, 20 mg/day. *Symptomatic BPH* — **Adults:** initially, 1 mg P.O. h.s. Increase stepwise to 2, 5, or 10 mg/day.	▪ Monitor BP frequently. ▪ If stopped for several days, restart using initial dosing regimen. ▪ Advise patient not to stop suddenly and to call doctor if adverse reactions occur. ▪ Caution patient to avoid hazardous activities for 12 hr after 1st dose.
terbinafine hydrochloride (oral) Lamisil *Antifungal* Pregnancy Risk Category: B	*Fingernail onychomycosis from dermatophytes (tinea unguium)* — **Adults:** 250 mg P.O. q.d. for 6 wk. *Toenail onychomycosis from dermatophytes (tinea unguium)* — **Adults:** 250 mg P.O. q.d. for 12 wk.	▪ Successful treatment may not be noticed for 4 wk for fingernails and 10 wk for toenails. ▪ Not recommended for pregnant or breast-feeding patients.
terbinafine hydrochloride (topical) Lamisil *Antifungal* Pregnancy Risk Category: B	*Interdigital tinea pedis; tinea cruris; tinea corporis* — **Adults:** cover affected and surrounding area with cream b.i.d. for 1 to 4 wk.	▪ Use as directed for full course, even if symptoms disappear. ▪ Don't apply near eyes, mouth, or mucous membranes or use occlusive dressings. ▪ Tell patient to stop use and contact doctor if irritation or sensitivity develops.

terbutaline sulfate Brethaire, Brethine, Bricanyl *Bronchodilator, premature labor inhibitor (tocolytic)* Pregnancy Risk Category: B	*Bronchospasm in patients with reversible obstructive airway disease* — **Adults and children ≥ 12 yr:** *Aerosol inhaler:* 2 inhalations separated by 60-sec interval; repeat q 4 to 6 hr. *Injection:* 0.25 mg S.C.; repeat in 15 to 30 min, p.r.n. Maximum 0.5 mg in 4 hr. *Tablets in adults:* 2.5 to 5 mg P.O. q 6 hr t.i.d. Maximum 15 mg/day. *Tablets in children 12 to 15 yr:* 2.5 mg P.O. q 6 hr t.i.d. while awake. Maximum 7.5 mg/day.	▪ Use cautiously in CV disorders, hyperthyroidism, diabetes, or seizure disorders. ▪ Give S.C. injections in lateral deltoid area. ▪ Protect injection from light; discard if discolored. ▪ May use tablets and aerosol together. ▪ Teach patient to perform inhalation correctly. ▪ Advise patient to stop drug and call doctor if paradoxical bronchospasm occurs.
terconazole Terazol 3 Vaginal Ovules, Terazol 7 Vaginal Ovules Cream *Antifungal* Pregnancy Risk Category: C	*Vulvovaginal candidiasis* — **Adults:** 1 applicatorful of cream or 1 suppository inserted into vagina h.s. Use 0.4% cream for 7 days; 0.8% cream or 80-mg suppository for 3 days. Repeat course, p.r.n., after reconfirmation by smear or culture.	▪ ***ALERT*** Stop drug and notify doctor if fever, chills, flulike symptoms, or sensitivity develops. ▪ Persistent infection may be caused by reinfection. Evaluate for possible sources. ▪ Continue treatment during menses. Avoid tampons.
testosterone Andro 100, Testamone 100 **testosterone cypionate** Depo-Testosterone, depAndro, Duratest, Depotest **testosterone propionate** **testosterone transdermal system** Androderm, Testoderm,	*Male hypogonadism* — **Adults:** 10 to 25 mg (testosterone or propionate) I.M. 2 to 3 times/wk or 50 to 400 mg (cypionate) I.M. q 2 to 4 wk, in divided doses. *Metastatic breast cancer in women 1 to 5 yr postmenopausal* — **Adults:** 100 mg I.M. 2 times/wk; 50 to 100 mg (propionate) I.M. 3 times/wk; or 200 to 400 mg (cypionate) I.M. q 2 to 4 wk, in divided doses. *Primary or hypogonadotropic hypogonadism in men* — **Adults:** (Testoderm) one 4- to 6-mg/day patch on scrotal area q.d.	▪ Use cautiously in elderly patients and in patients with renal, hepatic, or cardiac disease. ▪ Don't use in women of childbearing age until pregnancy ruled out. ▪ Assess LFTs, serum lipid profiles, Hgb and Hct, and prostate antigen levels.

(continued)

†Canadian ‡Australian

DRUG & CLASS	INDICATIONS & DOSAGES	NURSING CONSIDERATIONS
testosterone *(continued)* Testoderm TTS *Androgen replacement, antineoplastic* Pregnancy Risk Category: X Controlled Substance Schedule: III	Patch worn for 22 to 24 hr/day. **Adults:** (Androderm) 2 systems applied nightly. Apply to clean, dry skin on back, abdomen, upper arms, or thigh.	
tetracycline hydrochloride (oral) Achromycin V, Panmycin P‡, Robitet, Sumycin, Tetracyn† *Antibiotic* Pregnancy Risk Category: D	*Infections* — **Adults:** 250 to 500 mg P.O. q 6 hr. **Children > 8 yr:** 25 to 50 mg/kg/day P.O., in divided doses q 6 hr. C. trachomatis *infections* — **Adults:** 500 mg P.O. q.i.d. for 7 to 21 days. *Brucellosis* — **Adults:** 500 mg P.O. q 6 hr for 3 wk, with streptomycin I.M. *Gonorrhea* — **Adults:** initially, 1.5 g P.O., then 500 mg P.O. q 6 hr for 4 days. *Acne* — **Adults and adolescents:** 500 mg to 1 g P.O. q.d. in 4 equally divided doses for 2 weeks or until clinical improvement.	▪ Use with extreme caution (if at all) during last half of pregnancy, in children < 9 yr, and in patients with impaired renal or hepatic function. ▪ Check tongue for candidal infection. Emphasize good oral hygiene. ▪ Take medication 2 hours before or after dairy products, iron preparations, or antacids.
theophylline *Immediate-release tablets and capsules:* Bronkodyl, Slo-Phyllin, Theolair; *timed-release tablets:* Respid, Theo-Dur; *timed-release capsules:* Aerolate, Slo-bid	*Acute bronchospasm if not on drug* — For I.V., loading dose 4.7 mg/kg slowly; then maintenance. **Adults (nonsmokers):** 6 mg/kg P.O., then 2 to 3 mg/kg q 6 hr for 2 doses. Maintenance: 3 mg/kg q 8 hr. Or, 0.55 mg/kg/hr I.V. for 12 hr, then 0.39 mg/kg/hr. **Adults (healthy smokers):** 6 mg/kg P.O., then 3 mg/	▪ For acute bronchospasm in patient already on drug, adjust dose per current level. Each 0.5 mg/kg I.V. or P.O. (load) increases levels 1 mcg/ml. ▪ Don't use extended-release preparations to treat acute bronchospasm. ▪ Monitor vital signs; measure and record

Gyrocaps, Theo-24

theophylline sodium glycinate
Bronchodilator
Pregnancy Risk Category: C

kg q 4 hr for 3 doses. Maintenance: 3 mg/kg q 6 hr. Or, 0.79 mg/kg/hr I.V. for 12 hr; then 0.63 mg/kg/hr. **Adults with heart failure or liver disease:** 6 mg/kg P.O., then 2 mg/kg q 8 hr for 2 doses. Maintenance: 1 to 2 mg/kg q 12 hr. Or, 0.39 mg/kg/hr I.V. for 12 hr; then 0.08 to 0.16 mg/kg/hr. **Children 9 to 16 yr:** 6 mg/kg P.O., then 3 mg/kg q 4 hr for 3 doses. Maintenance: 3 mg/kg q 6 hr. Or, 0.79 mg/kg/hr I.V. for 12 hr; then 0.63 mg/kg/hr. **Children 6 mo to 9 yr:** 6 mg/kg P.O., then 4 mg/kg q 4 hr for 3 doses. Maintenance: 4 mg/kg q 6 hr. Or, 0.95 mg/kg/hr I.V. for 12 hr; then 0.79 mg/kg/hr.

Chronic bronchospasm — **Adults and children:** 16 mg/kg or 400 mg P.O. q.d. in 3 to 4 divided doses q 6 to 8 hr; or, 12 mg/kg or 400 mg P.O. q.d. in extended-release preparation in 2 to 3 divided doses q 8 or 12 hr. Increase as tolerated q 2 to 3 days to maximum. **Adolescents > 16 yr:** 13 mg/kg or 900 mg P.O. q.d. in divided doses. **Children 12 to 16 yr:** 18 mg/kg P.O. q.d. in divided doses. **Children 9 to 12 yr:** 20 mg/kg P.O. q.d. in divided doses. **Children < 9 yr:** 24 mg/kg/day P.O. q.d. in divided doses.

I&O. Clinical effects include improved pulse quality and respirations.

- Don't confuse extended-release and regular forms.
- ***I.V. use:*** Use commercially available infusion solution, or mix in D_5W. Use infusion pump for continuous infusion.
- Give around-the-clock, using extended-release product h.s.
- Xanthine metabolism varies; dose based on response, tolerance, pulmonary function, and theophylline levels (10 to 20 mcg/ml); toxicity reported with levels > 20 mcg/ml.
- Teach patient to swallow extended-release preparations whole. For children who can't swallow these preparations, sprinkle contents over soft food.
- Adjust dose in chronic bronchospasm and in elderly patients with cor pulmonale to minimum needed for response.

---

thiamine hydrochloride (vitamin B_1)
Betamin‡

Beriberi — **Adults:** 10 to 20 mg I.M. t.i.d. for 2 wk, then diet correction and multivitamin supplement containing 5 to 10 mg/day thiamine for 1 mo. **Children:** depending on

- ***I.V. use:*** Dilute before giving. Give large doses cautiously; give skin test before therapy in history of hypersensitivity reactions. Have epinephrine available. *(continued)*

†Canadian ‡Australian

DRUG & CLASS	INDICATIONS & DOSAGES	NURSING CONSIDERATIONS
thiamine hydrochloride *(continued)* *Nutritional supplement* Pregnancy Risk Category: A	severity, 10 to 50 mg/day I.M. for several wk with adequate diet. *Wernicke's encephalopathy* — **Adults:** initially, 100 mg I.V., followed by 50 to 100 mg/day I.V. or I.M. until patient eats balanced diet.	▪ Obtain an accurate dietary history. ▪ Significant deficiency can occur in 3 wk of thiamine-free diet. Thiamine deficiency usually requires concurrent treatment for multiple deficiencies.
thioridazine hydrochloride Aldazine‡, Apo-Thioridazine†, Mellaril, Mellaril-S, Mellaril Concentrate, Novo-Ridazine†, PMS Thioridazine† *Antipsychotic* Pregnancy Risk Category: NR	*Psychosis* — **Adults:** 50 to 100 mg P.O. t.i.d., with gradual increases to 800 mg/day in divided doses, p.r.n. Dosage varies. *Short-term treatment of moderate to marked depression with anxiety; multiple symptoms in geriatric patients* — **Adults:** 25 mg P.O. t.i.d. Maintenance 20 to 200 mg/day. Maximum 200 mg/day. **Children 2 to 12 yr:** 0.5 to 3 mg/kg P.O. q.d. in divided doses.	▪ Different liquid formulations have different concentrations. Check dosage carefully. ▪ Keep drug away from skin and clothes; wear gloves when preparing liquid forms. ▪ Monitor for tardive dyskinesia. ▪ Shake suspension well before use. ▪ Dilute liquid concentrate with water or fruit juice before use. ▪ Advise patient to rise slowly to avoid dizziness from orthostatic hypotension.
thiotepa (TESPA, triethylenethiophosphoramide, TSPA) Thioplex *Antineoplastic* Pregnancy Risk Category: D	*Breast and ovarian cancers; lymphoma; Hodgkin's disease* — **Adults and children > 12 yr:** 0.3 to 0.4 mg/kg I.V. q 1 to 4 wk or 0.2 mg/kg for 4 to 5 days at 2- to 4-wk intervals.	▪ If pain occurs at insertion site, dilute further or use local anesthetic. ▪ Monitor CBC weekly for 3 wk after last dose. Notify doctor if WBC count $< 3{,}000/mm^3$ or if platelet count $< 150{,}000/mm^3$. ▪ Monitor serum uric acid. ▪ Tell patient to watch for signs of infection and bleeding and take temperature daily.
thiothixene Navane **thiothixene hydrochloride**	*Mild to moderate psychosis* — **Adults:** 2 mg P.O. t.i.d. Increase gradually to 15 mg/day. *Severe psychosis* — **Adults:** initially, 5 mg P.O. b.i.d. Increase slowly to 20 to	▪ Watch for orthostatic hypotension. Keep patient supine for 1 hr after giving drug. ▪ Keep drug off skin and clothes. Wear gloves when preparing liquid forms.

Navane *Antipsychotic* Pregnancy Risk Category: NR	30 mg/day. Maximum 60 mg/day. Or, 4 mg I.M. b.i.d. or q.i.d. Maximum 30 mg/day I.M. P.O. should replace I.M. promptly.	▪ Dilute liquid concentrate with fruit juice, milk, or semisolid food before use. ▪ Monitor patient for tardive dyskinesia.
tiagabine hydrochloride Gabitril Filmtabs *Anticonvulsant* Pregnancy Risk Category: C	*Adjunctive therapy for partial seizures* — **Adults:** initially, 4 mg P.O. q.d. May increase total daily dose by 4 to 8 mg q wk until clinical response or up to 56 mg/day, in divided doses b.i.d. to q.i.d. **Children 12 to 18 yr:** 4 mg P.O. q.d. May increase total daily dose by 4 mg at start of wk 2, then by 4 to 8 mg/wk until clinical response or up to 32 mg/day, in divided doses b.i.d. to q.i.d. ***Adjust-a-dose:*** In patients with impaired liver function, reduce initial and maintenance doses or lengthen dosing intervals, p.r.n.	▪ Withdraw drug gradually unless safety concerns require a more rapid withdrawal. ▪ May cause status epilepticus and sudden unexpected death in epilepsy. ▪ Patients who aren't receiving an enzyme-inducing anticonvulsant when tiagabine is started may require lower dose or slower adjustment. ▪ May cause moderately severe to incapacitating generalized weakness. Usually, weakness resolves after reducing dosage or stopping drug.
ticarcillin disodium Ticar, Ticillin‡ *Antibiotic* Pregnancy Risk Category: B	*Severe systemic infections from susceptible organisms* — **Adults and children:** 200 to 300 mg/kg/day I.V. in divided doses. *Uncomplicated UTI* — **Adults and children ≥ 40 kg:** 1 g I.M. or I.V. q 6 hr. **Children < 40 kg:** 50 to 100 mg/kg/day I.M. or I.V. in divided doses q 6 to 8 hr. *Complicated UTI* — **Adults and children:** 150 to 200 mg/kg/day I.V. in divided doses q 4 to 6 hr. ***Adjust-a-dose:*** In patients with renal impairment, if CrCl 30 to 60 ml/min, give 2 g I.V. q 4 hr; 10 to 29 ml/min, give 2 g I.V. q 8 hr; < 10 ml/min, give 2 g I.V. q 12 hr, or 1 g I.M. q 6 hr.	▪ Before giving, ask about previous allergic reactions to penicillin. ▪ Avoid continuous infusion. Change site q 48 hr. ▪ For I.M., use 2 ml diluent per g of drug. Inject deep I.M. into large muscle. Don't exceed 2 g/injection.

DRUG & CLASS	INDICATIONS & DOSAGES	NURSING CONSIDERATIONS
ticarcillin disodium/ clavulanate potassium Timentin *Antibiotic* Pregnancy Risk Category: B	*Infections of lower respiratory tract, urinary tract, bone and joint, and skin and skin structure; septicemia from beta-lactamase–producing bacteria or ticarcillin-susceptible organisms* — **Adults and children ≥ 60 kg:** 3.1 g (3 g ticarcillin and 100 mg clavulanic acid) by I.V. infusion q 4 to 6 hr. **Adults and children < 60 kg:** 200 to 300 mg/kg/day by I.V. infusion in divided doses q 4 to 6 hr. ***Adjust-a-dose:*** In patients with renal impairment, if CrCl 30 to 60 ml/min, give 2 g I.V. q 4 hr; 10 to 29 ml/min, give 2 g I.V. q 8 hr; < 10 ml/min, give 2 g I.V. q 12 hr.	▪ Before giving, ask about previous allergic reactions to penicillin. ▪ Check CBC and platelet counts frequently. May cause thrombocytopenia. ▪ With large doses and prolonged therapy, bacterial or fungal superinfection may occur.
ticlopidine hydrochloride Ticlid *Antithrombotic* Pregnancy Risk Category: B	*To reduce risk of thrombotic stroke in patients with history of stroke or with stroke precursors* — **Adults:** 250 mg P.O. b.i.d. with meals.	▪ Instruct patient to avoid aspirin and aspirin-containing products unless ordered by doctor and to check with doctor or pharmacist before taking OTC products. ▪ Report unusual or prolonged bleeding. ▪ Report signs of infection immediately.
tiludronate disodium Skelid *Antihypercalcemic agent* Pregnancy Risk Category: C	*Paget's disease of bone in patients who have serum alkaline phosphatase at least twice the upper limit of normal, who are symptomatic, or who are at risk for future complications of their disease* — **Adults:** 400 mg P.O. q.d. for 3 mo.	▪ Use cautiously in upper GI disease. ▪ Correct hypocalcemia and mineral metabolism disturbances (such as vitamin D deficiency) before starting therapy. ▪ Tell patient to take with 6 to 8 oz water 2 hr before or after meals.

Drug	Indications and dosages	Key considerations
timolol maleate (systemic) Apo-Timol†, Blocadren *Antihypertensive, adjunct in MI therapy* Pregnancy Risk Category: C	*Hypertension* — **Adults:** 10 mg P.O. b.i.d. Maximum 60 mg/day. Increase q wk, p.r.n. *MI (long-term prophylaxis in patients who have survived acute phase)* — **Adults:** 10 mg P.O. b.i.d. *Migraine headache prophylaxis* — **Adults:** 20 mg P.O. q.d. in 1 or divided doses b.i.d. Increase, p.r.n., to maximum 30 mg/day.	▪ Use cautiously in compensated heart failure, diabetes, hyperthyroidism, and hepatic, renal, or respiratory disease. ▪ Check apical pulse before giving and monitor BP closely. ▪ May mask signs and symptoms of hypoglycemia. Monitor blood glucose in diabetic patients.
timolol maleate (ophthalmic) Betimol, Timoptic Solution, Timoptic-XE *Antiglaucoma agent* Pregnancy Risk Category: C	*Chronic open-angle, secondary, and aphakic glaucomas; ocular hypertension* — **Adults:** initially, 1 drop 0.25% solution in each affected eye b.i.d.; maintenance, 1 drop/day. If no response, 1 drop 0.5% solution b.i.d. If IOP controlled, reduce to 1 drop/day. Or, 1 drop gel q.d.	▪ Give other ophthalmic agents ≥ 10 min before drops. ▪ Can mask signs of hypoglycemia. ▪ Some patients may need a few wk of treatment to stabilize pressure-lowering response. Determine IOP after 4 wk.
tinzaparin sodium Innohep *Anticoagulant* Pregnancy Risk Category: B	*Symptomatic deep vein thrombosis with or without pulmonary embolism, in conjunction with warfarin sodium* — **Adults:** 175 anti-Xa IU/kg of body weight S.C. q.d. for ≥ 6 days and until the patient is adequately anticoagulated with warfarin (INR of at least 2.0) for 2 consecutive days. Start warfarin when appropriate, usually within 1 to 3 days of starting Innohep. Volume of dose to be given may be calculated as follows: Patient weight (kg) x 0.00875 ml/kg = Volume to be given (ml).	▪ Drug shouldn't be interchanged (unit for unit) with heparin or other low molecular weight heparins. ▪ When you give drug, the patient should be sitting or lying down. Give by deep S.C. injection into the abdominal wall. Introduce the whole length of the needle into skinfold held between thumb and forefinger. Make sure to hold skinfold throughout injection. Rotate injection sites between the right and left anterolateral and posterolateral abdominal wall. To minimize bruising, don't rub the injection site *(continued)*

†Canadian ‡Australian

DRUG & CLASS	INDICATIONS & DOSAGES	NURSING CONSIDERATIONS
tinzaparin sodium *(continued)*	***Adjust-a-dose:*** Give cautiously in elderly patients and patients with renal insufficiency.	after giving. ▪ Monitor platelet count during therapy. Stop drug if platelet count < 100,000/mm^3. ▪ Periodically during treatment, check CBC and results of stool tests for occult blood. ▪ Drug may affect PT and INR. Patients also receiving warfarin should have blood for PT and INR drawn just before the next scheduled dose of drug.
tioconazole Vagistat-1 *Antifungal* Pregnancy Risk Category: C	*Vulvovaginal candidiasis* — **Adults:** 1 applicatorful (about 4.6 g) inserted intravaginally h.s. once.	▪ Instruct patient on proper use of drug and tell her to insert drug high into vagina. ▪ Report irritation or sensitivity. ▪ Tell patient to open applicator just before use.
tirofiban hydrochloride Aggrastat *Platelet aggregation inhibitor* Pregnancy Risk Category: B	*Acute coronary syndrome, given with heparin, in patients managed medically and those having PTCA or atherectomy* — **Adults:** I.V. loading dose of 0.4 mcg/kg/min for 30 min, then continuous infusion of 0.1 mcg/kg/min. Continue infusion through angiography and for 12 to 24 hr after PTCA or atherectomy. ***Adjust-a-dose:*** In patients with CrCl < 30 ml/min, give loading dose of 0.2 mcg/kg/min for 30 min, then continuous infusion of 0.05 mcg/kg/min. Continue infusion as above.	▪ Use cautiously in patients with increased risk of bleeding, including those with hemorrhagic retinopathy or platelet count below 150,000/mm^3. ▪ Monitor Hct, Hgb, and platelet counts before starting therapy, 6 hr after loading dose, and at least q.d. during therapy. ▪ Give drug with aspirin and heparin. ▪ Minimize use of artieral and venous punctures and I.M. injections. ▪ Avoid use of noncompressible I.V. access sites.

tobramycin AKTob, Tobrex *Antibiotic* Pregnancy Risk Category: B	*External ocular infections from susceptible bacteria* — **Adults and children:** in mild to moderate infections, 1 or 2 drops into affected eye q 4 hr, or thin strip (1 cm long) of ointment q 8 to 12 hr. In severe infections, 2 drops in infected eye q 30 to 60 min until improvement; then reduce frequency. Or, thin strip of ointment q 3 to 4 hr until improvement; then reduce frequency.	▪ Clean eye area before application. ▪ Advise patient to stop drug and call doctor if he has itching lids, swelling, or constant burning. ▪ Instruct patient not to share drug, washcloths, or towels and to notify doctor if family member develops symptoms. ▪ Discontinue if keratitis, erythema, lacrimation, edema, or lid itching occurs.
tobramycin sulfate Nebcin, TOBI *Antibiotic* Pregnancy Risk Category: D	*Serious infections* — **Adults:** 3 mg/kg/day I.M. or I.V. divided q 8 hr. Up to 5 mg/kg/day divided q 6 to 8 hr for life-threatening infections; reduce to 3 mg/kg/day based on therapeutic response. **Children:** 6 to 7.5 mg/kg/day I.M. or I.V. in 3 or 4 equal doses. **Neonates < 1 wk or premature infants:** up to 4 mg/kg/day I.V. or I.M. in 2 equal doses q 12 hr. *Cystic fibrosis with* Pseudomonas aeruginosa *infection* — **Adults and children ≥ 6 yr:** 300 mg (nebulizer solution) b.i.d., alternating 28 days on and 28 days off. Give with PARI LC PLUS nebulizer.	▪ ***I.V. use:*** Infuse over 20 to 60 min. ▪ Notify doctor if tinnitus, vertigo, or hearing loss occurs. ▪ Obtain blood for peak level 1 hr after I.M. injection and ½ to 1 hr after infusion ends; trough level just before next dose. ▪ Monitor renal function.
tocainide hydrochloride Tonocard *Ventricular antiarrhythmic* Pregnancy Risk Category: C	*Suppression of symptomatic life-threatening ventricular arrhythmias* — **Adults:** initially, 400 mg P.O. q 8 hr. Usual dosage 1,200 to 1,800 mg/day in 3 divided doses; maximum 2,400 mg/day. May give patients with renal or hepatic impairment < 1,200 mg/day.	▪ May ease transition from I.V. lidocaine to P.O. antiarrhythmic. Monitor carefully. ▪ Correct potassium deficit. ▪ Observe for tremor. ▪ Monitor blood levels. Therapeutic range 4 to 10 mcg/ml.

DRUG & CLASS	INDICATIONS & DOSAGES	NURSING CONSIDERATIONS
tolcapone Tasmar *Antiparkinsonian* Pregnancy Risk Category: C	*Adjunct to levodopa-carbidopa for idiopathic Parkinson's disease* — **Adults:** 100 mg P.O. t.i.d. (with levodopa-carbidopa). Daily dose 100 mg P.O. t.i.d.; 200 mg P.O. t.i.d. if anticipated benefit justified. If giving 200 mg t.i.d. and dyskinesia occurs, may reduce levodopa dose. Maximum 600 mg/day. ***Adjust-a-dose:*** Don't exceed 100 mg t.i.d. in severe renal dysfunction.	▪ ***ALERT*** Be sure patient has signed informed consent before use. ▪ Monitor LFTs before starting; then q 2 wk for 1st yr of therapy; then q 4 wk for next 6 mo, and then q 8 wk. ▪ Give 1st dose of day with levodopa-carbidopa. ▪ Diarrhea is common and usually resolves when drug stops. ▪ Stop drug if no benefit in 3 wk.
tolterodine tartrate Detrol *Anticholinergic* Pregnancy Risk Category: C	*Overactive bladder with symptoms of urinary frequency, urgency, or urge incontinence* — **Adults:** 2 mg P.O. b.i.d. Decrease to 1 mg P.O. b.i.d. based on response and tolerance. ***Adjust-a-dose:*** In adults whose hepatic function is significantly reduced or who are taking drug that inhibits cytochrome P-450 3A4 isoenzyme system, give 1 mg P.O. b.i.d.	▪ Use cautiously in patients with significant bladder outflow obstruction, GI obstructive disorders (such as pyloric stenosis), or controlled narrow-angle glaucoma, and hepatic or renal impairment. ▪ Assess baseline bladder function and monitor therapeutic effects. ▪ Tell patient to avoid driving and other hazardous activities until visual effects of drug known.
topiramate Topamax *Antiepileptic* Pregnancy Risk Category: C	*Adjunct therapy for partial-onset seizures and for primary generalized tonic-clonic seizures:* **Adults:** up to daily dose of 400 mg P.O. in divided doses b.i.d. Schedule as follows: wk 1, 50 mg P.O. q afternoon; wk 2, 50 mg P.O. b.i.d.; wk 3, 50 mg P.O. q morning and 100 mg P.O. q afternoon; wk 4, 100 mg	▪ Use cautiously in breast-feeding or pregnant patients and in those with hepatic impairment. ▪ Withdraw gradually to minimize risk of increased seizure activity. ▪ Monitor liver enzyme levels. ▪ Drug rapidly cleared by dialysis. Prolonged

	P.O. b.i.d.; wk 5, 100 mg P.O. q morning and 150 mg P.O. q afternoon; wk 6, 150 mg P.O. b.i.d.; wk 7, 150 mg P.O. q morning and 200 mg P.O. q afternoon; wk 8, 200 mg P.O. b.i.d. **Children 2 to 16 yr:** 1 to 3 mg/kg P.O. q.d. in afternoon for 1st week. Increase dose based on clinical response q 1 to 2 wk by 1 to 3 mg/kg/day in 2 divided doses. Dosage range is 5 to 9 mg/kg q.d. P.O. in 2 divided doses. ***Adjust-a-dose:*** In patients with CrCl < 70 ml/min, reduce dose by 50%.	period of dialysis may cause low drug levels and seizures.
topotecan hydrochloride Hycamtin *Antineoplastic* Pregnancy Risk Category: D	*Metastatic carcinoma of ovary after failure of initial or subsequent chemotherapy* — **Adults:** 1.5 mg/m^2 I.V. infusion over 30 min q.d. for 5 days, starting on day 1 of 21-day cycle. Give minimum 4 cycles. Reduce dose for next course if severe neutropenia occurs. *Small cell lung cancer after failure of first-line chemotherapy* — **Adults:** 1.5 mg/m^2 I.V. infusion given over 30 min daily for 5 days, starting on day 1 of 21-day cycle. Minimum of 4 cycles should be given.	▪ Before 1st course, baseline neutrophil count > 1,500 cells/mm^3 and platelet count > 100,000 cells/mm^3 required. Monitor CBC. ▪ Use reconstituted product immediately.
toremifene citrate Fareston *Antineoplastic* Pregnancy Risk Category: D	*Metastatic breast cancer in postmenopausal women with estrogen-receptor positive or unknown tumors* — **Adults:** 60 mg P.O. q.d.	▪ Obtain periodic CBC, calcium levels, and LFT results. ▪ Monitor for hot flashes and vaginal bleeding. ▪ Monitor PT and INR closely.
torsemide Demadex *Diuretic, antihypertensive*	*Diuresis in patients with heart failure* — **Adults:** 10 to 20 mg/day P.O. or I.V. If response inadequate, double dose until re-	▪ ***I.V. use:*** May give by direct injection over ≥ 2 min. Rapid injection may cause ototoxicity. Don't give > 200 mg *(continued)*

†Canadian ‡Australian

DRUG & CLASS	INDICATIONS & DOSAGES	NURSING CONSIDERATIONS
torsemide *(continued)* Pregnancy Risk Category: B	sponse obtained. Maximum 200 mg/day. *Diuresis in patients with chronic renal failure* — **Adults:** 20 mg/day P.O. or I.V. If response inadequate, double dose until response obtained. Maximum 200 mg/day. *Hypertension* — **Adults:** 5 mg/day P.O. Maximum to 10 mg, p.r.n.	at a time. Immediately report ringing in ears. ▪ Monitor I&O, serum electrolytes, BP, weight, and HR. ▪ Watch for hypokalemia. ▪ Tell patient to take in morning to prevent nocturia.
tramadol hydrochloride Ultram *Analgesic* Pregnancy Risk Category: C	*Moderate to moderately severe pain* — **Adults:** 50 to 100 mg P.O. q 4 to 6 hr, p.r.n. Maximum 400 mg/day. **Elderly:** in patients > 75 yr, maximum 300 mg/day in divided doses. ***Adjust-a-dose:*** In patients with CrCl < 30 ml/min, give 50 to 100 mg P.O. q 12 hr. In patients with cirrhosis, give 50 mg q 12 hr.	▪ Monitor CV and respiratory status. Withhold dose and notify doctor if respirations fall or respiratory rate < 12. ▪ Monitor bowel and bladder function. ▪ Give before onset of intense pain. ▪ Monitor patients at risk for seizures.
trandolapril Mavik *Antihypertensive* Pregnancy Risk Category: C (D in 2nd and 3rd trimesters)	*Hypertension* — **Adults:** for patients not receiving diuretics, initially 1 mg for nonblack patient and 2 mg for black patient P.O. q.d. If control not adequate, can increase dosage at ≥ 1-wk intervals. Maintenance dose 2 to 4 mg/day. May give 4-mg/day dose b.i.d. For patient receiving diuretic, give initial dose of 0.5 mg/day P.O. Dosage per BP response. *Heart failure post-MI or left-sided heart failure post-MI* — **Adults:** initially, 1 mg/day P.O., adjusted to 4 mg/day, as tolerated.	▪ Angioedema involving tongue, glottis, or larynx may be fatal. ▪ Monitor serum potassium level closely. ▪ Monitor patient for hypotension. If possible, discontinue diuretics 2 to 3 days before starting trandolapril. If drug doesn't control BP, diuretics may be reinstituted cautiously. ▪ Assess renal function before and during therapy.

trastuzumab Herceptin *Antineoplastic* Pregnancy Risk Category: B	*Metastatic breast cancer in patients whose tumors overexpress human epidermal growth factor receptor 2 (HER2) protein and who have received chemotherapy regimens for metastatic disease; combined with paclitaxel for metastatic breast cancer in patients whose tumors overexpress HER2 protein and who haven't received chemotherapy for metastatic disease* — **Adults:** initial loading dose 4 mg/kg I.V. over 90 min. Maintenance dose 2 mg/kg q wk as a 30-min I.V. infusion if initial loading dose well tolerated.	▪ Assess for cardiac dysfunction, especially if patient is receiving drug with anthracyclines and cyclophosphamide. ▪ Monitor patient for dyspnea, increased cough, paroxysmal nocturnal dyspnea, peripheral edema, or S_3 gallop. May stop drug if left ventricular function falls significantly. ▪ Watch for 1st-infusion symptom complex (chills or fever, nausea, vomiting, pain, rigors, headache, dizziness, dyspnea, hypotension, rash, and asthenia).
trazodone hydrochloride Desyrel, Desyrel Dividose *Antidepressant* Pregnancy Risk Category: C	*Depression* — **Adults:** initially, 150 mg P.O. q.d. in divided doses; increased by 50 mg/day q 3 to 4 days, p.r.n. Average dose 150 to 400 mg/day. Maximum daily dose for inpatients 600 mg; for outpatients, 400 mg.	▪ Give before meals or with light snack. ▪ Monitor for suicidal tendencies and allow only minimum drug supply. ▪ Report presence of priapism immediately. ▪ Warn patient to avoid hazardous activities until CNS effects known.
tretinoin (retinoic acid, vitamin A acid; topical) Avita, Renova, Retin-A, StieVA-A† *Antiacne agent* Pregnancy Risk Category: C	*Acne vulgaris* — **Adults and children:** clean affected area and lightly apply q.d. h.s. *Adjunct therapy to skin care and sun avoidance program; to improve fine facial wrinkles in patients on program* — **Adults:** Cover affected area lightly with small, pearl-sized amount (¼-inch or 5-mm diameter) q.d., h.s.	▪ Clean area thoroughly before application. Avoid getting in eyes, mouth, or mucous membranes. Instruct to wash face with mild soap no more than b.i.d. or t.i.d. ▪ Instruct patient to minimize exposure to sun, ultraviolet rays, wind, and cold.

†Canadian ‡Australian

DRUG & CLASS	INDICATIONS & DOSAGES	NURSING CONSIDERATIONS
tretinoin (oral) Vesanoid *Antineoplastic* Pregnancy Risk Category: D	*Induction of remission in patients with acute promyelocytic leukemia, French-American-British classification M3 (including M3 variant), when anthracycline chemotherapy contraindicated or unsuccessful* — **Adults and children ≥ 1 yr:** 45 mg/m^2/day P.O. in 2 even doses. Discontinue 30 days after complete remission or after 90 days of treatment, whichever is first.	▪ Notify doctor if fever, dyspnea, or weight gain occurs. ▪ Monitor CBC and platelet counts regularly. ▪ Maintain infection control and bleeding precautions. ▪ Watch for infection or bleeding.
triamcinolone acetonide (systemic) Azmacort, Kenalog-10, Triamonide 40, Trilog *Anti-inflammatory, antiasthmatic* Pregnancy Risk Category: C	*Severe inflammation or immunosuppression* — **Adults:** 4 to 48 mg/day P.O. in divided doses; 40 mg I.M. weekly; 1 mg into lesions; 2.5 to 40 mg into joints or soft tissue. *Persistent asthma* — **Adults:** Azmacort 2 inhalations t.i.d. or q.i.d. Maximum 16 inhalations daily. Total daily dose may be given b.i.d. for maintenance. **Children 6 to 12 yr:** Azmacort 1 to 2 inhalations t.i.d. or q.i.d. Maximum 12 inhalations daily.	▪ For better results and less toxicity, give daily dose in morning with food. ▪ Don't use diluents with preservatives. ▪ Monitor weight, BP, and serum electrolytes.
triamcinolone acetonide (topical) Aristocort, Flutex, Kenalog, Kenalone‡, Triacet *Anti-inflammatory* Pregnancy Risk Category: C	*Inflammation from corticosteroid-responsive dermatoses* — **Adults and children:** apply sparingly b.i.d. to q.i.d. *Inflammation from oral lesions* — **Adults and children:** apply paste h.s. and, if needed, b.i.d. or t.i.d., preferably after meals.	▪ Wash skin before applying. Rub in gently, leaving thin coat. Apply directly to lesions. ▪ Stop drug if infection, striae, or atrophy occurs. ▪ Don't leave occlusive dressing in place > 16 hr each day or use on infected or exudative lesions.

triamcinolone acetonide (nasal) Nasacort *Anti-inflammatory* Pregnancy Risk Category: C	*Symptoms of seasonal or perennial allergic rhinitis* — **Adults and children ≥ 12 yr:** 2 sprays (110 mcg) in each nostril q.d. Increase, p.r.n., to 440 mcg/day as daily dose or in divided doses ≤ q.i.d. Then decrease, if possible, to 1 spray in each nostril q.d.	▪ Instruct patient to instill properly. ▪ Stress importance of using regularly. Warn patient not to exceed dosage prescribed. ▪ Instruct patient to report nasal infection. ▪ Tell patient to notify doctor if symptoms worsen or don't diminish within 2 to 3 wk. ▪ Discard canister after 100 actuations.
triamterene Dyrenium *Diuretic* Pregnancy Risk Category: B	*Edema* — **Adults:** initially, 100 mg P.O. b.i.d. after meals. Maximum total dose 300 mg/day.	▪ Monitor BP, uric acid, CBC, serum glucose, BUN, and serum electrolytes. ▪ Warn patient to avoid potassium-rich foods and potassium supplements. ▪ Inform patient that urine may turn blue.
triazolam Apo-Triazo†, Halcion *Sedative-hypnotic* Pregnancy Risk Category: X Controlled Substance Schedule: IV	*Insomnia* — **Adults:** 0.125 to 0.5 mg P.O. h.s. **Adults > 65 yr:** 0.125 mg P.O. h.s.; increased, p.r.n., to 0.25 mg P.O. h.s.	▪ Assess mental status before initiating therapy. Elderly patients more sensitive to CNS effects. ▪ ***ALERT*** Prevent hoarding or overdosing if patient is depressed, suicidal, or drug-dependent or has drug abuse history.
trifluoperazine hydrochloride Apo-Trifluoperazine†, Solazine†, Stelazine, Terfluzine† *Antipsychotic, antiemetic* Pregnancy Risk Category: NR	*Anxiety states* — **Adults:** 1 to 2 mg P.O. b.i.d. Maximum 6 mg/day. Don't give > 12 wk. *Schizophrenia; other psychotic disorders* — **Adults:** 2 to 5 mg P.O. b.i.d., gradually increased until response. Or 1 to 2 mg deep I.M. q 4 to 6 hr, p.r.n. More than 6 mg I.M. in 24 hr rarely required. **Children 6 to 12 yr (hospitalized or under close supervision):** 1 mg P.O. once daily or b.i.d.; may increase gradually to 15 mg daily.	▪ Wear gloves when preparing liquid forms. ▪ Watch for orthostatic hypotension. Keep patient supine for 1 hr after giving. ▪ Dilute liquid concentration with 60 ml liquid or semisolid food. ▪ Protect from light. Slight yellowing of injection or concentration common. Discard markedly discolored solutions.

†Canadian ‡Australian

DRUG & CLASS	INDICATIONS & DOSAGES	NURSING CONSIDERATIONS
trihexyphenidyl hydrochloride Aparkane†, Apo-Trihex†, Artane, Novohexidyl†, Trihexane *Antiparkinsonian* Pregnancy Risk Category: NR	*Parkinsonism, drug-induced parkinsonism; adjunct treatment to levodopa for parkinsonism* — **Adults:** 1 mg P.O. 1st day, 2 mg 2nd day; then increased in 2-mg increments q 3 to 5 days until total of 6 to 10 mg/day. Usually given t.i.d. with meals or q.i.d. or switched to extended-release form b.i.d. Postencephalitic parkinsonism may require 12- to 15-mg total daily dose.	▪ Dose may need to be increased if tolerance develops. ▪ Adverse reactions are dose-related and transient. Monitor patient. ▪ May cause nausea if given after meals. ▪ Gonioscopic evaluation and IOP monitoring required, especially in patients > 40 yr.
trimethoprim Proloprim, Trimpex, Triprim‡ *Antibiotic* Pregnancy Risk Category: C	*Uncomplicated UTIs caused by susceptible organisms* — **Adults:** 200 mg P.O. q.d. as single or divided doses q 12 hr for 10 days. Don't use in children < 12 yr. ***Adjust-a-dose:*** For patients with CrCl 15 to 30 ml/min, give 50 mg P.O. q 12 hr; if < 15 ml/min, don't use.	▪ Obtain urine specimen for culture and sensitivity tests before 1st dose. ▪ Monitor CBC routinely. Sore throat, fever, pallor, and purpura may be early signs of serious blood disorders. ▪ Prolonged use at high doses may cause bone marrow suppression.
trimipramine maleate Apo-Trimip†, Surmontil *Antidepressant, anxiolytic* Pregnancy Risk Category: C	*Depression* — **Adults:** 75 to 100 mg P.O. q.d. in divided doses, increased to 200 to 300 mg/day. Doses ≤ 300 mg/day in hospitalized patients; ≤ 200 mg in outpatients. Total dose requirement may be given h.s. **Elderly and adolescent patients:** initially, 50 mg/day, gradually increased to 100 mg/day.	▪ Gradually stop several days before surgery. ▪ If signs of psychosis occur or increase, expect to reduce dose. Monitor for suicidal tendencies and allow only minimum drug supply. ▪ Tell patient to relieve dry mouth with sugarless hard candy or gum.
trovafloxacin mesylate Trovan Tablets **alatrofloxacin**	*Nosocomial pneumonia; gynecologic, pelvic and complicated intra-abdominal infections, including postsurgical infection*— **Adults:** 300 mg I.V. q.d.; then 200 mg P.O. q.d. for 7 to 14	▪ ***ALERT*** Use cautiously in patients with CNS disorders and in those at increased risk for seizures. Drug may cause neurologic complications, such as seizures, psy-

mesylate
Trovan I.V.
Antibiotic
Pregnancy Risk Category: C

days (10 to 14 days for pneumonia).
Community-acquired pneumonia; complicated skin infections — **Adults:** 200 mg P.O. or I.V. q.d.; then 200 mg P.O. q.d. for 7 to 14 days (10 to 14 days for skin infections).
Adjust-a-dose: For patients with mild to moderate cirrhosis, reduce 300-mg I.V. dose to 200 mg I.V. and 200-mg I.V. or P.O. dose to 100 mg I.V. or P.O.

chosis, or increased intracranial pressure. Monitor patient with preexisting condition closely.
- Assess liver function carefully.
- May cause moderate to severe phototoxicity reactions if patient exposed to direct sunlight.
- No dosage adjustment necessary when switching from I.V. to P.O. form.
- May be used to treat diabetic foot infections but not osteomyelitis.

---

urokinase
Abbokinase, Abbokinase Open-Cath, Ukidan‡
Thrombolytic enzyme
Pregnancy Risk Category: B

Lysis of acute massive pulmonary embolism (PE) or PE with unstable hemodynamics — **Adults:** for I.V. infusion *only* by infusion pump. Priming dose: 4,400 IU/kg with 0.9% NaCl or D_5W admixture over 10 min. Then 4,400 IU/kg/hr for 12 hr.
Coronary artery thrombosis — **Adults:** after bolus dose of heparin, infuse 6,000 IU/min of urokinase into occluded artery for up to 2 hr. Average total dose 500,000 IU. Initiate within 6 hr of symptoms.
Venous catheter occlusion — **Adults:** 5,000 IU/ml solution into occluded line; after 5 min, aspirate. Repeat aspiration attempts q 5 min for 30 min. If not patent, cap line and leave for 30 to 60 min before aspirating again. May require second instillation.

- ***I.V. use:*** Reconstitute according to manufacturer's directions. Don't mix with other drugs. Give through separate line.
- Be prepared with RBCs, whole blood, plasma expanders other than dextran, and aminocaproic acid to treat bleeding, and corticosteroids, epinephrine, and antihistamines to treat allergic reactions.
- I.M. injections and other invasive procedures contraindicated during therapy.
- Monitor for excessive bleeding q 15 min for 1st hr; q 30 min for 2nd through 8th hr; then q 4 hr.
- Monitor pulses, color, and sensation of extremities q hr
- Monitor vital signs and neurologic status.

DRUG & CLASS	INDICATIONS & DOSAGES	NURSING CONSIDERATIONS
valacyclovir hydrochloride Valtrex *Antiviral* Pregnancy Risk Category: B	*Herpes zoster infection (shingles) in patients with normal immune system* — **Adults:** 1 g P.O. t.i.d. for 7 days. Adjust for impaired renal function based on CrCl. *First episode of genital herpes in patients with normal immune system* — **Adults:** 1 g P.O. b.i.d. for 10 days. ***Adjust-a-dose:*** If CrCl $\geq$ 30 ml/min, 1 g P.O. q 12 hr; for 10 to 29 ml/min, 1 g P.O. q 24 hr; for < 10 ml/min, 500 mg P.O. q 24 hr. *Recurrent genital herpes in patients with normal immune system* — **Adults:** 500 mg P.O. b.i.d. for 5 days, given at 1st sign.	▪ Use cautiously in renal impairment, elderly patients, immunocompromised patients, and those receiving other nephrotoxic drugs. ▪ Alert doctor if patient is breast-feeding. ▪ Inform patient that drug may be taken without regard to meals. ▪ Teach patient signs and symptoms of herpes infection and tell him to notify doctor if they occur. Treatment should begin within 48 hr.
valproate sodium Depakene Syrup, Epilim‡ **valproic acid** Depakene **divalproex sodium** Depakote, Depakote ER, Depakote Sprinkle, Epival† *Anticonvulsant* Pregnancy Risk Category: D	*Simple and complex absence seizures, mixed seizure types* — **Adults and children:** 15 mg/kg P.O. daily, divided b.i.d. or t.i.d.; increase by 5 to 10 mg/kg daily q wk, to maximum 60 mg/kg/day. *Mania (delayed-release capsules)* — **Adults and children:** 750 mg q.d. in divided doses. Adjust per response; maximum 60 mg/kg/day. *Migraine prevention (Depakote only)* — **Adults:** initially, 250 mg P.O. b.i.d. Some patients may need up to 1,000 mg/day. For delayed-release tablets, 500 mg P.O. q.i.d. for 1 wk; then 1,000 mg P.O. q.i.d. ***Adust-a-dose:*** When using Depakote delayed-release tablets in elderly, initiate at	▪ ***ALERT*** Serious or fatal hepatotoxicity may follow nonspecific symptoms. Notify doctor; drug must be stopped if hepatic dysfunction suspected. ▪ Give with food or milk. ▪ Don't give syrup to patients on sodium restriction. ▪ Never withdraw suddenly. Call doctor if adverse reactions develop. ▪ Therapeutic serum levels 50 to 100 mcg/ml for most patients.

	lower dosage and increase dosage more slowly. Monitor for fluid and nutritional intake, dehydration, somnolence, and other adverse effects.	
valsartan Diovan *Antihypertensive* Pregnancy Risk Category: C (1st trimester); D (2nd and 3rd trimesters)	*Hypertension* — **Adults:** initially, 80 mg P.O. q.d. Expect BP reduction in 2 to 4 wk. For additional effect, increase to 160 or 320 mg q.d., or add diuretic. (Adding diuretic has greater effect than increases beyond 80 mg.) Usual dosage range: 80 to 320 mg q.d.	▪ Correct volume and salt depletions before starting. Monitor for hypotension. ▪ Advise patient to notify doctor if pregnancy occurs; drug must be discontinued. ▪ May be taken with or without food.
vancomycin hydrochloride Lyphocin, Vancocin, Vancoled *Antibiotic* Pregnancy Risk Category: C	*Serious infections* — **Adults**: 1 to 1.5 g I.V. q 12 hr. **Children:** 10 mg/kg I.V. q 6 hr. **Neonates, young infants:** 15 mg/kg I.V. loading dose; then 10 mg/kg I.V. q 12 hr if < 1 wk, and 10 mg/kg I.V. q 8 hr if > 1 wk but < 1 mo. *Pseudomembranous and staphylococcal enterocolitis from antibiotics* — **Adults:** 125 to 500 mg P.O. q 6 hr for 7 to 10 days. **Children:** 40 mg/kg P.O. q.d., in divided doses q 6 hr for 7 to 10 days. Maximum 2 g/day. *Endocarditis prophylaxis for dental procedures* — **Adults:** 1 g I.V. slowly over 1 hr, starting 1 hr before procedure. **Children:** > 27 kg (60 lb), adult dose; < 27 kg, 20 mg/kg. ***Adjust-a-dose:*** Adjust dosage in patients with renal insufficiency.	▪ Check daily for phlebitis and irritation. Report pain at infusion site. Avoid extravasation. ▪ Refrigerate I.V. solution after reconstitution; use within 96 hr. ▪ Monitor for red-neck syndrome (maculopapular rash on face, neck, trunk, and upper arms). If present, stop infusion and report to doctor. Reaction usually stimulated by too rapid I.V. infusion rate. ▪ May need to reduce I.V. dose in renally impaired patients; monitor for changes in serum creatinine.
vasopressin (ADH) Pitressin *Antidiuretic hormone,*	*Nonnephrogenic, nonpsychogenic diabetes insipidus* — **Adults:** 5 to 10 U I.M. or S.C. b.i.d. to q.i.d., p.r.n.; or intranasally in indi-	▪ Never inject during 1st stage of labor. ▪ Monitor for signs of water intoxication. ▪ Monitor BP if patient taking

(continued)

†Canadian ‡Australian

DRUG & CLASS	INDICATIONS & DOSAGES	NURSING CONSIDERATIONS
vasopressin (ADH) *(continued)* *hemostatic agent* Pregnancy Risk Category: C	vidualized doses, based on response. **Children:** 2.5 to 10 U I.M. or S.C. b.i.d. to q.i.d., p.r.n.; or intranasally in individualized doses.	b.i.d. Watch for elevated BP or lack of response. ▪ Monitor daily weight, urine specific gravity, and fluid I&O.
venlafaxine hydrochloride Effexor, Effexor XR *Antidepressant* Pregnancy Risk Category: C	*Depression* — **Adults:** initially, 75 mg P.O. q.d., in 2 or 3 divided doses with food. Increase, p.r.n., by 75 mg/day at intervals of ≥ 4 days. For moderate depression, maximum 225 mg/day; for severe depression, 375 mg/day.	▪ Closely monitor BP. ▪ If patient has received drug for ≥ 6 wk, taper over 2 wk, as ordered. ▪ Warn patient to avoid hazardous activities until CNS effects known.
verapamil Apo-Verap†, Calan, Isoptin, Novo-Veramil†, Nu-Verap† **verapamil hydrochloride** Calan, Calan SR, Covera HS, Isoptin, Isoptin SR, Verelan, Verelan PM *Antianginal, antihypertensive, antiarrhythmic* Pregnancy Risk Category: C	*Vasospastic angina and classic chronic, stable angina pectoris; chronic atrial fibrillation* — **Adults:** 80 to 120 mg P.O. t.i.d. Increase, q wk, p.r.n. Maximum 480 mg/day. *Supraventricular arrhythmias* — **Adults:** 0.075 to 0.15 mg/kg by I.V. push over 2 min. 0.15 mg/kg in 30 min if no response. **Children 1 to 15 yr:** 0.1 to 0.3 mg/kg I.V. over 2 min. May repeat in 30 min. **Children < 1 yr:** 0.1 to 0.2 mg/kg I.V. over 2 min. *Hypertension* — **Adults:** 80 mg P.O. t.i.d. Maximum 480 mg/day. Or, 120 to 240 mg extended-release tablets P.O. q.d. in morning. May add ½ tablet q.d.	▪ ***I.V. use:*** Give by direct injection into vein or into tubing of free-flowing, compatible I.V. solution. Give over ≥ 3 min to minimize adverse reactions. ▪ Monitor BP and ECG during and after I.V. administration. ▪ Assist with ambulation. ▪ Monitor R-R interval for I.V. use. All patients should be on a cardiac monitor.
vinblastine sulfate (VLB) Velban, Velbe†‡	*Breast or testicular cancer; Hodgkin's disease; malignant lymphoma* — **Adults:** 3.7 mg/m^2 I.V. q 1 to 2 wk. Maximum	▪ Give antiemetic first. ▪ ***I.V. use:*** Inject directly into vein or tubing of running I.V. line over 1 min. If extrava-

Antineoplastic Pregnancy Risk Category: D	18.5 mg/m^2 I.V. q wk per response. Don't repeat if WBC < 4,000/mm^3. **Children:** 2.5 mg/m^2 I.V. q wk. Increase by 1.25 mg/m^2 until WBC < 3,000/mm^3 or tumor response seen. Maximum 12.5 mg/m^2 I.V. q wk. ***Adjust-a-dose:*** In patients with direct serum bilirubin > 3 mg/dl, can reduce dose by 50%.	sation occurs, stop infusion and notify doctor. ▪ Don't give into arm or leg that has compromised circulation. ▪ Monitor for acute bronchospasm. ▪ Assess hands and feet for numbness and tingling. Assess gait for footdrop.
vincristine sulfate (VCR) Oncovin, Vincasar PFS *Antineoplastic* Pregnancy Risk Category: D	*Acute lymphoblastic and other leukemias; Hodgkin's disease* — **Adults:** 1.4 mg/m^2 I.V. q wk. Maximum 2 mg q wk. **Children > 10 kg (22 lb):** 2 mg/m^2 I.V. q wk. **Children ≤ 10 kg or with body surface area < 1 m^2:** initially, 0.05 mg/kg I.V. q wk.	▪ ***I.V. use:*** Inject into vein or tubing of running I.V. line over 1 min. If extravasation occurs, stop and notify doctor. ▪ Watch for acute bronchospasm and hyperuricemia. Maintain adequate hydration. ▪ Assess gait for footdrop.
vinorelbine tartrate Navelbine *Antineoplastic* Pregnancy Risk Category: D	*Alone or with cisplatin for first-line treatment of ambulatory patients with nonresectable advanced non–small-cell lung cancer (NSCLC); alone or with cisplatin in stage IV of NSCLC; with cisplatin in stage III of NSCLC* — **Adults:** 30 mg/m^2 I.V. q wk. ***Adjust-a-dose:*** Modify dosage if serum bilirubin > 2 mg/dl.	▪ ***ALERT*** Check granulocyte count. If < 1,000 cells/mm^3, withhold and notify doctor. ▪ Dilute before giving. ▪ If extravasation occurs, stop and inject remaining dose into different vein. ▪ Monitor deep tendon reflexes.
warfarin sodium Coumadin, Warfilone Sodium† *Anticoagulant* Pregnancy Risk Category: X	*Pulmonary embolism with deep vein thrombosis; MI; rheumatic heart disease with heart valve damage; prosthetic heart valves; chronic atrial fibrillation* — **Adults:** 2 to 5 mg P.O. q.d. for 2 to 4 days, then dosage based on daily PT and INR. Usual maintenance dose 2 to 10 mg P.O. q.d.	▪ Monitor PT and INR. ▪ Assess patient for bleeding. ▪ Withhold drug and call doctor if fever or rash occurs. ▪ Anticoagulant can be neutralized by vitamin K injections.

†Canadian ‡Australian

DRUG & CLASS	INDICATIONS & DOSAGES	NURSING CONSIDERATIONS
xylometazoline hydrochloride 4-Way Long Acting, Neo-Synephrine II, Otrivin *Decongestant, vasoconstrictor* Pregnancy Risk Category: NR	*Nasal congestion* — **Adults and children ≥ 12 yr:** 2 to 3 drops or sprays 0.1% solution in each nostril q 8 to 10 hr. **Children 2 to 12 yr:** 2 to 3 drops 0.05% solution in each nostril q 8 to 10 hr. **Children 6 mo to 2 yr:** 1 drop 0.05% solution in each nostril q 6 hr, p.r.n., under doctor supervision.	▪ Have patient hold head upright to minimize swallowing drug, then sniff spray briskly. ▪ Product should be used by only one person. ▪ Instruct patient to report insomnia, dizziness, weakness, tremor, or irregular heartbeat. ▪ Use p.r.n., no longer than 5 days.
zafirlukast Accolate *Anti-inflammatory* Pregnancy Risk Category: B	*Prophylaxis and treatment of chronic asthma* — **Adults and children ≥ 12 yr:** 20 mg P.O. b.i.d. 1 hr before or 2 hr after meals. **Children ages 7 to 11:** 10 mg P.O. b.i.d.	▪ ***ALERT*** Don't use to reverse bronchospasm in acute asthma attacks. ▪ Advise patient to keep taking even if symptoms disappear. ▪ Give 1 hr before or 2 hr after meals.
zalcitabine (dideoxycytidine, ddC) Hivid *Antiviral* Pregnancy Risk Category: C	*Monotherapy for advanced HIV disease in patients who can't tolerate zidovudine or whose disease progresses while on zidovudine* — **Adults and children ≥ 13 yr:** 0.75 mg P.O. q 8 hr. *Combination therapy for advanced HIV disease* — **Adults and children ≥ 13 yr:** 0.75 mg P.O. q 8 hr given with zidovudine 200 mg P.O. q 8 hr. ***Adjust-a-dose:*** In patients with CrCl 10 to 40 ml/min, give 0.75 mg P.O. q 12 hr; if < 10 ml/min, give 0.75 mg P.O. q 24 hr.	▪ Don't give with food. ▪ ***ALERT*** Assess for peripheral neuropathy; can progress to sharp shooting pain or severe continuous burning pain. May not be reversible. ▪ Monitor patient for signs of pancreatitis, such as increased serum amylase.
zaleplon Sonata	*Short-term treatment for insomnia* — **Adults:** 10 mg P.O. q.d. immediately before	▪ Use cautiously in elderly and debilitated patients, in those with compromised respi-

Hypnotic
Controlled Substance Schedule: IV
Pregnancy Risk Category: C

h.s.; may increase dose to 20 mg p.r.n. Low-weight adults may respond to 5-mg dose. ***Adjust-a-dose:* Elderly and debilitated patients:** 5 mg P.O. q.d. immediately before h.s.; maximum 10 mg. **For patients with mild to moderate hepatic failure or receiving cimetidine concomitantly:** 5 mg P.O. q.d. immediately before h.s.

ratory function, and in those with signs and symptoms of depression.

- Because drug works rapidly, it should be ingested only right before h.s. or after patient has gone to bed and has experienced difficulty falling asleep.
- Don't give drug during or after a high-fat or heavy meal.
- Limit use to 7 to 10 days. Reevaluate patient if hypnotics must be taken for 2 to 3 wk.
- Potential for drug abuse and dependence exists. Don't give drug in quantities greater than a 1-mo supply.

---

zanamivir
Relenza
Antiviral
Pregnancy Risk Category: B

Uncomplicated acute illness from influenza A and B virus in patients who have been symptomatic for $\leq$ *2 days* — **Adults and children** $\geq$ **7 yr:** 2 inhalations q 12 hr for 5 days. Two doses should be taken on the 1st day of treatment, leaving $\geq$ 2 hr between doses.

Uncomplicated acute illness from influenza A and B virus in patients symptomatic for $\leq$ *2 days* — **Adults and children ages 7 and older:** 2 inhalations q 12 hr for 5 days.

- Use cautiously in patients with severe or decompensated chronic obstructive pulmonary disease, asthma, or other underlying respiratory disease.
- Patients with underlying respiratory disease should have fast-acting bronchodilator available in case of wheezing while taking drug. Patients scheduled to use an inhaled bronchodilator for asthma should use their bronchodilator before taking zanamivir.
- Safety and efficacy of drug not supported in patients who begin treatment after 48 hr of symptoms.
- Lymphopenia, neutropenia, and elevated liver enzyme and *(continued)*

†Canadian ‡Australian

DRUG & CLASS	INDICATIONS & DOSAGES	NURSING CONSIDERATIONS
zanamivir *(continued)*		creatine kinase levels may occur during treatment. ▪ Monitor patient for bronchospasm and drop in lung function. Stop the drug if these effects occur.
zidovudine (azidothymidine, AZT) Apo-Zidovudine†, Novo-AZT†, Retrovir *Antiviral* Pregnancy Risk Category: C	*Symptomatic HIV infection, including AIDS* — **Adults and children ≥ 12 yr:** 100 mg P.O. q 4 hr or 300 mg P.O. q 12 hr; I.V. infusion 1 mg/kg (over 1 hr) q 4 hr to 6 mg/kg/day. **3 mo to 12 yr:** 180 mg/m^2 P.O. q 6 hr (720 mg/m^2/day), ≤ 200 mg q 6 hr. *Asymptomatic HIV infection* — **Adults and children ≥ 12 yr:** 100 mg P.O. q 4 hr while awake; I.V. infusion 1 mg/kg (over 1 hr) q 4 hr while awake to 5 mg/kg/day. **Children 3 mo to 12 yr:** 180 mg/m^2 P.O. q 6 hr (720 mg/m^2/day), maximum 200 mg q 6 hr. *To reduce risk of HIV transmission from mother with $CD4^+$ lymphocyte count > 200 cells/mm^3 to newborn* — **Adults:** 100 mg P.O. 5 times q.d. between 14 and 34 wks' gestation and continued through pregnancy. During labor, loading dose of 2 mg/kg I.V. over 1 hr, followed by continuous I.V. infusion of 1 mg/kg/hr until umbilical cord clamped. **Neonates:** 2 mg/kg P.O. (syrup) q 6 hr for 6 wk, starting within 12 hr of birth. Or, 1.5 mg/kg I.V. (infuse over 30 min) q 6 hr.	▪ ***I.V. use:*** Dilute first. Infuse at constant rate over 1 hr. Avoid rapid infusion or bolus injection. Don't add to biological or colloidal fluids. After dilution, stable for 24 hr at room temperature and 48 hr if refrigerated at 36° to 46° F (2° to 8° C). Store undiluted vials at 59° to 77° F (15° to 25° C); protect from light. ▪ Monitor blood studies q 2 wk. ▪ Give on empty stomach. Have patient sit up and drink adequate fluids. ▪ Monitor for superinfection. May cause overgrowth of nonsusceptible bacteria or fungi. ▪ Tell patient to continue to take drug as prescribed, even if he feels better.

	Adjust-a-dose: In end-stage renal disease on hemodialysis or peritoneal dialysis, give 100 mg P.O. or 1 mg/kg I.V. q 6 to 8 hr.	
zileuton Zyflo *Anti-inflammatory* Pregnancy Risk Category: C	*Prophylaxis and treatment of chronic asthma* — **Adults and children ≥ 12 yr:** 600 mg P.O. q.i.d.	▪ Drug isn't bronchodilator and shouldn't be used to treat acute asthma attack.
zolmitriptan Zomig *Antimigraine agent* Pregnancy Risk Category: C	*Acute migraine headaches* — **Adults:** ≤ 2.5 mg P.O.; increase to 5 mg/dose, p.r.n. If headache returns after initial dose, 2nd dose may be given after 2 hr. Maximum dose is 10 mg in 24-hr period. ***Adjust-a-dose:*** In patients with moderate to severe hepatic impairment, use lower dose.	▪ Not intended for prophylactic therapy or for use in hemiplegic or basilar migraines. ▪ Safety not established for cluster headaches. ▪ Monitor for pain or tightness in the chest or throat, heart throbbing, rash, skin lumps, or swelling of the face, lips, or eyelids.
zolpidem tartrate Ambien *Hypnotic* Pregnancy Risk Category: B Controlled Substance Schedule: IV	*Short-term management of insomnia* — **Adults:** 10 mg P.O. immediately before h.s. **Elderly:** 5 mg P.O. immediately before h.s. Maximum 10 mg/day. ***Adjust-a-dose:*** In patients with hepatic insufficiency, give 5 mg P.O. immediately before h.s. Maximum 10 mg/day.	▪ Give only for short-term management of insomnia, usually 7 to 10 days. ▪ ***ALERT*** Prevent hoarding or overdosing in depressed, suicidal, or drug-dependent patient or one with drug abuse history.
zonisamide Zonegran *Anticonvulsant* Pregnancy Risk Category: C	*Adjunct therapy for partial seizures* — **Adults > 16 yr:** 100 mg P.O. q.d. for 2 wk. After 2 wk, dose may be increased to 200 mg/day for ≥ 2 wk. It can be increased to 300 mg and 400 mg P.O. q.d., with dose stable for ≥ 2 wk at each level. Doses can be given once daily or b.i.d., except for the ini-	▪ Monitor patient for symptoms of hypersensitivity. Consider stopping drug in patients who develop an unexplained rash. ▪ Monitor body temperatures, especially in summer; decreased sweating causes heatstroke and dehydration (especially in patients ≤ 17 yr). *(continued)*

DRUG & CLASS	INDICATIONS & DOSAGES	NURSING CONSIDERATIONS
zonisamide *(continued)*	tial daily dose of 100 mg. ***Adjust-a-dose:*** Use cautiously in patients with hepatic and renal disease; may require slower titration and more frequent monitoring. If glomerular filtration rate < 50 ml/min, don't use.	▪ Abrupt withdrawal of drug may increase frequency of seizures or status epilepticus; reduce dose or stop drug gradually. ▪ Increase fluid intake and urine output to help prevent kidney stones, especially in patients with predisposing factors. ▪ Monitor renal function periodically. If patient develops acute renal failure or a clinically significant sustained increase in creatinine or BUN level, stop the drug.

Selected narcotic analgesic combination products

Many narcotic analgesics are combinations of two or more generic drugs. The following list shows common combination analgesics and their components.

Aceta with Codeine (CSS III)
- acetaminophen 300 mg
- codeine phosphate 30 mg

Anexia 7.5/650 (CSS III), Lorcet Plus (CSS III)
- acetaminophen 650 mg
- hydrocodone bitartrate 7.5 mg

Capital with Codeine (CSS V), Tylenol with Codeine Elixir (CSS V)
- acetaminophen 120 mg
- codeine phosphate 12 mg/5 ml

Darvocet-N 50 (CSS IV)
- acetaminophen 325 mg
- propoxyphene napsylate 50 mg

Darvocet-N 100, Propacet 100 (CSS IV)
- acetaminophen 650 mg
- propoxyphene napsylate 100 mg

Empirin with Codeine No. 3 (CSS III)
- aspirin 325 mg
- codeine phosphate 30 mg

Empirin with Codeine No. 4 (CSS III)
- aspirin 325 mg
- codeine phosphate 60 mg

Fioricet with Codeine (CSS III)
- acetaminophen 325 mg
- butalbital 50 mg
- caffeine 40 mg
- codeine phosphate 30 mg

Fiorinal with Codeine (CSS III)
- aspirin 325 mg
- butalbital 50 mg
- caffeine 40 mg
- codeine phosphate 30 mg

Lorcet 10/650 (CSS III)
- acetaminophen 650 mg
- hydrocodone bitartrate 10 mg

Lortab 2.5/500 (CSS III)
- acetaminophen 500 mg
- hydrocodone bitartrate 2.5 mg

Lortab 5/500 (CSS III), Lorcet-HD (CSS III)
- acetaminophen 500 mg
- hydrocodone bitartrate 5 mg

Lortab 7.5/500 (CSS III)
- acetaminophen 500 mg
- hydrocodone bitartrate 7.5 mg

Lortab 10/500 (CSS III)
- acetaminophen 500 mg
- hydrocodone bitartrate 10 mg

Lortab ASA, Damason-P (CSS III)
- aspirin 500 mg
- hydrocodone bitartrate 5 mg

Percocet (CSS II)
- acetaminophen 325 mg
- oxycodone hydrochloride 5 mg

Percodan-Demi (CSS II)
- aspirin 325 mg
- oxycodone hydrochloride 2.25 mg
- oxycodone terephthalate 0.19 mg

(continued)

CSS = Controlled Substance Schedule.

Percodan, Roxiprin (CSS II)
- aspirin 325 mg
- oxycodone hydrochloride 4.5 mg
- oxycodone terephthalate 0.38 mg

Phenaphen/Codeine No. 3 (CSS III)
- acetaminophen 325 mg
- codeine phosphate 30 mg

Phenaphen/Codeine No. 4 (CSS III)
- acetaminophen 325 mg
- codeine phosphate 60 mg

Propoxyphene Napsylate/
Acetaminophen (CSS IV)
- propoxyphene napsylate 100 mg
- acetaminophen 650 mg

Roxicet (CSS II)
- acetaminophen 325 mg
- oxycodone hydrochloride 5 mg

Roxicet 5/500 (CSS II), Roxilox
- acetaminophen 500 mg
- oxycodone hydrochloride 5 mg

Roxicet Oral Solution (CSS II)
- acetaminophen 325 mg
- oxycodone hydrochloride 5 mg/5 ml

Talacen (CSS IV)
- acetaminophen 650 mg
- pentazocine hydrochloride 25 mg

Talwin Compound (CSS IV)
- aspirin 325 mg
- pentazocine hydrochloride 12.5 mg

Tylenol with Codeine No. 2 (CSS III)
- acetaminophen 300 mg
- codeine phosphate 15 mg

Tylenol with Codeine No. 3 (CSS III)
- acetaminophen 300 mg
- codeine phosphate 30 mg

Tylenol with Codeine No. 4 (CSS III)
- acetaminophen 300 mg
- codeine phosphate 60 mg

Tylox (CSS II)
- acetaminophen 500 mg
- oxycodone hydrochloride 5 mg

Vicodin (CSS III)
- acetaminophen 500 mg
- hydrocodone bitartrate 5 mg

Vicodin ES (CSS III)
- acetaminophen 750 mg
- hydrocodone bitartrate 7.5 mg

Wygesic (CSS IV)
- acetaminophen 650 mg
- propoxyphene hydrochloride 65 mg

Zydone (CSS III)
- acetaminophen 400 mg
- hydrocodone bitartrate 10 mg

Drugs that shouldn't be crushed

Many drug forms (slow release, enteric coated, encapsulated beads, wax matrix, sublingual, or buccal preparations) release their active ingredient for a specified duration or at a predetermined time after administration. Crushing these drugs can dramatically affect drug absorption rate and increase the risk of adverse effects. Avoid crushing the drugs listed below for the reasons noted beside them.

Accutane (mucous membrane irritant)
Adalat CC (slow release)
Aerolate Sr., Jr., III (slow release)
Aller-Chlor (slow release)
Ammonium Chloride Enseals (enteric coated)
Ansaid (taste)
Artane Sequels (slow release)
ASA Enseals (enteric coated)
Asacol (slow release)
Atrohist LA, Sprinkle (slow release)
Bellergal-S (slow release)
Betapen-VK (taste)
Bisacodyl (enteric coated)
Bisco-Lax (enteric coated)
Brexin LA (slow release)
Bromfed (slow release)
Bromphen (slow release)
Calan SR (slow release)
Cardizem (slow release)
Cardizem CD, SR (slow release)
Ceftin (taste)
Cerespan (slow release)
Charcoal Plus (enteric coated)
Chloral Hydrate (liquid within a capsule, taste)
Chlor-Trimeton Repetabs (slow release)
Choledyl (enteric coated)
Cipro (taste)
Colace (liquid within a capsule, taste)
Compazine Spansules (slow release)
Congess SR, JR (slow release)
Contac 12-Hour, Maximum Strength (slow release)
Cotazym-S (enteric coated)
Creon (enteric coated)
Cystospaz-M (slow release)
Deconamine SR (slow release)
Deconsal, Sprinkle, II (slow release)
Depakote (enteric coated)
Desoxyn Gradumets (slow release)
Desyrel (taste)
Diamox Sequels (slow release)
Dimetapp Extentabs (slow release)
Disobrom (slow release)
Donnazyme (slow release)
Drisdol (liquid filled)
Drixoral (slow release)
Dulcolax (enteric coated)
Duotrate (slow release)
Duraquin (slow release)
Dynabac (enteric coated)
DynaCirc CR (slow release)
Ecotrin (enteric coated)
Efidac/24 (slow release)
Elixophyllin SR (slow release)
E-Mycin (enteric coated)
Endafed (slow release)
Entex LA (slow release)
Entozyme (enteric coated)
Equanil (taste)
Ergostat (sublingual)
Eryc (enteric coated)
Ery-Tab (enteric coated)
Erythrocin Stearate (enteric coated)
Erythromycin Base (enteric coated)

(continued)

Eskalith CR (slow release)
Feldene (mucous membrane irritant)
Feocyte (slow release)
Feosol (enteric coated)
Feratab (enteric coated)
Fergon (slow release)
Fero-Gradumet (slow release)
Ferralet Slow Release (slow release)
Ferro-Sequel (slow release)
Gris-PEG (crushing may cause precipitation as larger particles)
Guaifed (slow release)
Guaifed-PD (slow release)
Halfprin (enteric coated)
Humibid Sprinkle (slow release)
Hydergine LC (liquid within a capsule)
Hydergine Sublingual (sublingual)
Iberet-500 (slow release)
Ilotycin (enteric coated)
IMDUR (slow release)
Inderal LA (slow release)
Inderide LA (slow release)
Indocin SR (slow release)
Iso-Bid (slow release)
Isoptin SR (slow release)
Isordil Tembids (slow release)
Isosorbide Dinitrate SR (slow release)
Kaon-Cl (slow release)
K-Dur (slow release)
Klor-Con (slow release)
Klotrix (slow release)
K-Tab (slow release)
K + 10 (slow release)
Lithobid (slow release)
Meprospan (slow release)
Micro-K (slow release)
Micro-K Extencaps (slow release)
Motrin (taste)
MS Contin (slow release)
Naldecon (slow release)
Niac (slow release)
Nico-400 (slow release)
Nicobid (slow release)
Nitro-Bid (slow release)
Nitroglyn (slow release)
Nitrospan (slow release)
Nitrostat (sublingual)
Nolamine (slow release)
Nolex LA (slow release)
Norflex (slow release)
Norpace CR (slow release)
Novafed (slow release)
Optilets-500 (enteric coated)
Oramorph SR (slow release)
Ornade Spansules (slow release)
Oruvail (slow release)
OxyContin (slow release)
Pancrease (enteric coated)
Pavabid Plateau (slow release)
Pentasa (slow release)
Perdiem (wax coated)
Peritrate SA (slow release)
Phazyme (slow release)
Phenergan (taste)
Phyllocontin (slow release)
Plendil (slow release)
Prevacid (slow release)
Prilosec (slow release)
Pro-Banthine (taste)
Procanbid (slow release)
Procardia (delays absorption)
Procardia XL (slow release)
Pronestyl-SR (slow release)
Proventil Repetabs (slow release)
Prozac (slow release)
Quibron-T/SR Dividose (slow release)
Quinaglute Dura-Tabs (slow release)
Quinalan (slow release)
Quinidex Extentabs (slow release)
Respbid (slow release)
Ritalin-SR (slow release)
Ru-Tuss DE (slow release)
Sinemet CR (slow release)
Slo-bid Gyrocaps (slow release)
Slo-Niacin (slow release)
Slo-Phyllin GG, Gyrocaps (slow release)
Slow-Fe (slow release)

Slow-K (slow release)
Slow-Mag (slow release)
Sorbitrate SA (slow release)
Span-FF (slow release)
Sustaire (slow release)
Tavist-D (multiple compressed tablet)
Teldrin (slow release)
Tepanil Ten-Tab (slow release)
Tessalon Perles (slow release)
Theobid (slow release)
Theochron (slow release)
Theoclear LA (slow release)
Theo-Dur (slow release)
Theolair-SR (slow release)
Theo-Sav (slow release)
Theo-Time (slow release)
Theovent (slow release)
Theo-X (slow release)
Thorazine Spansule (slow release)
Toprol XL (slow release)
Tranxene-SD (slow release)
Trental (slow release)
Triaminic (slow release)
Triaminic TR (slow release)
Trinalin Repetabs (slow release)
Triptone Caplets (slow release)
Tuss-Ornade Spansules (slow release)
Verelan (slow release)
Voltaren (enteric coated)
Wyamycin S (slow release)
Wygesic (taste)
ZORprin (slow release)
Zyban (slow release)

Dangerous drug interactions

The following table lists drug interactions for selected drugs. Especially dangerous interactions are shown in *italic* type.

Drug	Interacting drugs	Possible effects
allopurinol	mercaptopurine	*Increased potential for bone marrow suppression*
atenolol	verapamil	Enhanced pharmacologic effects of beta blockers and verapamil
captopril	amiloride, spironolactone, triamterene	Possible hyperkalemia
	indomethacin	Decreased antihypertensive effect of ACE inhibitors
carbamazepine	erythromycin, isoniazid, propoxyphene	Increased risk of carbamazepine toxicity
carvedilol	MAO inhibitors, reserpine	*Severe hypotension or bradycardia*
clonidine	sotalol	Enhanced rebound hypertension following clonidine withdrawal
cyclosporine	erythromycin	Possible elevated cyclosporine concentrations and nephrotoxicity
	phenytoin	Reduced plasma levels of cyclosporine
digoxin	amiodarone, verapamil	*Elevated serum digoxin levels*
	bendroflumethiazide, chlorothiazide, hydrochlorothiazide, methyclothiazide, metolazone, quinethazone, trichloromethiazide	Increased risk of cardiac arrhythmias from hypokalemia
	quinidine	*Elevated serum digoxin levels*
enalapril	indomethacin	Decreased antihypertensive effect of ACE inhibitors
epinephrine	nadolol, pindolol, propranolol	*Increased systolic and diastolic pressures; marked decrease in heart rate*

esmolol	verapamil	Enhanced pharmacologic effects of beta blockers and verapamil
ethanol	acetohexamide, chlorpropamide, disulfiram, metronidazole, tolbutamide	*Acute alcohol intolerance reaction*
gentamicin	bumetanide, ethacrynic acid, furosemide	Possible enhanced ototoxicity
	ceftazidime, ceftizoxime, cephalothin	Possible enhanced nephrotoxicity
indinavir	benzodiazepines	Increased risk of sedation, respiratory impairment
lisinopril	indomethacin	Decreased antihypertensive effect of ACE inhibitors
lithium	bendroflumethiazide, chlorothiazide, hydrochlorothiazide, methyclothiazide, polythiazide, trichlormethiazide	*Decreased lithium excretion, which increases risk of lithium toxicity*
methotrexate	aspirin	*Increased risk of methotrexate toxicity*
	probenecid	*Decreased methotrexate elimination, increasing risk of methotrexate toxicity*
metoprolol	verapamil	Enhanced pharmacologic effects of beta blockers and verapamil
neomycin	bumetanide, ethacrynic acid, furosemide	Possible enhanced ototoxicity
	ceftazidime, ceftizoxime, cephalothin	Possible enhanced nephrotoxicity
penicillin	tetracycline	Reduced effectiveness of penicillins
potassium	amiloride, spironolactone, triamterene	*Increased risk of hyperkalemia*
propranolol	verapamil	Enhanced pharmacologic effects of beta blockers and verapamil
quinidine	amiodarone	Increased risk of quinidine toxicity
ritonavir	zolpidem	Increased sedation, respiratory impairment

(continued)

Drug	Interacting drugs	Possible effects
ritonavir *(continued)*	amiodarone, bepridil, encainide, flecainide, propafenone, quinidine	Increased risk of arrhythmias
sildenafil	nitrates	Increased risk of hypotension
tetracyclines	aluminum carbonate, aluminum hydroxide, aluminum phosphate, calcium carbonate, dihydroxyaluminum sodium carbonate, magaldrate, magnesium oxide antacids	*Decreased plasma levels and effectiveness of tetracyclines*
tobramycin	ceftazidime, ceftizoxime, cephalothin	Possible enhanced nephrotoxicity
warfarin sodium	amiodarone, aspirin, cefamandole, cefoperaxone, cefotetan, chloral hydrate, cimetidine, clofibrate, desipramine, erythromycin, glucagon, imipramine, nortriptyline, protriptyline, trimipramine	*Increased risk of bleeding*
	carbamazepine	Reduced effectiveness of warfarin
	cholestyramine	May bind with oral anticoagulants, resulting in impaired absorption
	co-trimoxazole, disulfiram, methimazole, metronidazole, propylthiouracil, sulfinpyrazone	*Increased risk of bleeding*
	griseofulvin, rifampin	*Decreased pharmacologic effect of oral anticoagulant*

Temperature conversions

Celsius degrees	Fahrenheit degrees	Celsius degrees	Fahrenheit degrees	Celsius degrees	Fahrenheit degrees	Celsius degrees	Fahrenheit degrees
41.1	106.0	38.4	101.2	35.8	96.4	33.1	91.6
41.0	105.8	38.3	101.0	35.7	96.2	33.0	91.4
40.9	105.6	38.2	100.8	35.6	96.0	32.9	91.2
40.8	105.4	38.1	100.6	35.4	95.8	32.8	91.0
40.7	105.2	38.0	100.4	35.3	95.6	32.7	90.8
40.6	105.0	37.9	100.2	35.2	95.4	32.6	90.6
40.4	104.8	37.8	100.0	35.1	95.2	32.4	90.4
40.3	104.6	37.7	99.8	35.0	95.0	32.3	90.2
40.2	104.4	37.6	99.6	34.9	94.8	32.2	90.0
40.1	104.2	37.4	99.4	34.8	94.6		
40.0	104.0	37.3	99.2	34.7	94.4		
39.9	103.8	37.2	99.0	34.6	94.2		
39.8	103.6	37.1	98.8	34.4	94.0		
39.7	103.4	37.0	98.6	34.3	93.8		
39.6	103.2	36.9	98.4	34.2	93.6		
39.4	103.0	36.8	98.2	34.1	93.4		
39.3	102.8	36.7	98.0	34.0	93.2		
39.2	102.6	36.5	97.8	33.9	93.0		
39.1	102.4	36.4	97.6	33.8	92.8		
39.0	102.2	36.3	97.4	33.7	92.6		
38.9	102.0	36.2	97.2	33.6	92.4		
38.8	101.8	36.1	97.0	33.4	92.2		
38.7	101.6	36.0	96.8	33.3	92.0		
38.6	101.4	35.9	96.6	33.2	91.8		

Infusion rates

Epinephrine infusion rates
Mix 1 mg in 250 ml (4 mcg/ml).

Dose (mcg/min)	Infusion rate (ml/hr)
1	15
2	30
3	45
4	60
5	75
6	90
7	105
8	120
9	135
10	150
15	225
20	300
25	375
30	450
35	525
40	600

Isoproterenol infusion rates
Mix 1 mg in 250 ml (4 mcg/ml).

Dose (mcg/min)	Infusion rate (ml/hr)
0.5	8
1	15
2	30
3	45
4	60
5	75
6	90
7	105
8	120
9	135
10	150
15	225
20	300
25	375
30	450

Nitroglycerin infusion rates

Determine the infusion rate in ml/hr using the ordered dose and the concentration of the drug solution.

Dose (mcg/min)	25 mg/250 ml (100 mcg/ml)	50 mg/250 ml (200 mcg/ml)	100 mg/250 ml (400 mcg/ml)
5	3	2	1
10	6	3	2
20	12	6	3
30	18	9	5
40	24	12	6
50	30	15	8
60	36	18	9
70	42	21	10
80	48	24	12
90	54	27	14
100	60	30	15
150	90	45	23
200	120	60	30

(continued)

Dobutamine infusion rates

Mix 250 mg in 250 ml of D_5W (1,000 mcg/ml). Determine the infusion rate in ml/hr using the ordered dose and the patient's weight in pounds or kilograms.

Dose (mcg/kg/min)	lb / kg	88 / 40	99 / 45	110 / 50	121 / 55	132 / 60	143 / 65	154 / 70	165 / 75	176 / 80	187 / 85	198 / 90	209 / 95	220 / 100	231 / 105	242 / 110
2.5		6	7	8	8	9	10	11	11	12	13	14	14	15	16	17
5		12	14	15	17	18	20	21	23	24	26	27	29	30	32	33
7.5		18	20	23	25	27	29	32	34	36	38	41	43	45	47	50
10		24	27	30	33	36	39	42	45	48	51	54	57	60	63	66
12.5		30	34	38	41	45	49	53	56	60	64	68	71	75	79	83
15		36	41	45	50	54	59	63	68	72	77	81	86	90	95	99
20		48	54	60	66	72	78	84	90	96	102	108	114	120	126	132
25		60	68	75	83	90	98	105	113	120	128	135	143	150	158	165
30		72	81	90	99	108	117	126	135	144	153	162	171	180	189	198
35		84	95	105	116	126	137	147	158	168	179	189	200	210	221	231
40		96	108	120	132	144	156	168	180	192	204	216	228	240	252	264

Dopamine infusion rates

Mix 400 mg in 250 ml of D_5W (1,600 mcg/ml). Determine the infusion rate in ml/hr using the ordered dose and the patient's weight in pounds or kilograms.

Dose (mcg/kg/ min)	lb 88 kg 40	99 45	110 50	121 55	132 60	143 65	154 70	165 75	176 80	187 85	198 90	209 95	220 100	231 105
2.5	4	4	5	5	6	6	7	7	8	8	8	9	9	10
5	8	8	9	10	11	12	13	14	15	16	17	18	19	20
7.5	11	13	14	15	17	18	20	21	23	24	25	27	28	30
10	15	17	19	21	23	24	26	28	30	32	34	36	38	39
12.5	19	21	23	26	28	30	33	35	38	40	42	45	47	49
15	23	25	28	31	34	37	39	42	45	48	51	53	56	59
20	30	34	38	41	45	49	53	56	60	64	68	71	75	79
25	38	42	47	52	56	61	66	70	75	80	84	89	94	98
30	45	51	56	62	67	73	79	84	90	96	101	107	113	118
35	53	59	66	72	79	85	92	98	105	112	118	125	131	138
40	60	68	75	83	90	98	105	113	120	128	135	143	150	158
45	68	76	84	93	101	110	118	127	135	143	152	160	169	177
50	75	84	94	103	113	122	131	141	150	159	169	178	188	197

(continued)

Nitroprusside infusion rates

Mix 50 mg in 250 ml of D_5W (200 mcg/ml). Determine the infusion rate in ml/hr using the ordered dose and the patient's weight in pounds or kilograms.

Dose (mcg/kg/min)	lb 88	99	110	121	132	143	154	165	176	187	198	209	220	231	242
	kg 40	45	50	55	60	65	70	75	80	85	90	95	100	105	110
0.3	4	4	5	5	5	6	6	7	7	8	8	9	9	9	10
0.5	6	7	8	8	9	10	11	11	12	13	14	14	15	16	17
1	12	14	15	17	18	20	21	23	24	26	27	29	30	32	33
1.5	18	20	23	25	27	29	32	34	36	38	41	43	45	47	50
2	24	27	30	33	36	39	42	45	48	51	54	57	60	63	66
3	36	41	45	50	54	59	63	68	72	77	81	86	90	95	99
4	48	54	60	66	72	78	84	90	96	102	108	114	120	126	132
5	60	68	75	83	90	98	105	113	120	128	135	143	150	158	165
6	72	81	90	99	108	117	126	135	144	153	162	171	180	189	198
7	84	95	105	116	126	137	147	158	168	179	189	200	210	221	231
8	96	108	120	132	144	156	168	180	192	204	216	228	240	252	264
9	108	122	135	149	162	176	189	203	216	230	243	257	270	284	297
10	120	135	150	165	180	195	210	225	240	255	270	285	300	315	330

Index

A

abacavir sulfate, 2
Abbokinase, 301
Abbokinase Open-Cath, 301
abciximab, 2
Abdominal distention, postoperative, neostigmine for, 218
Abdominal surgery patients
  dalteparin for, 81
  enoxaparin for, 106
Abortion, oxytocin for, 231
Abrasions, bacitracin for, 26
acarbose, 2
Accolate, 306
Accupril, 258
Accutane, 170
acebutolol hydrochloride, 3
Acel-Imune, 95
Aceon, 237
Acephen, 3
Aceta, 3
acetaminophen, 3
Acetaminophen toxicity, acetylcysteine for, 4
Aceta with Codeine, 311
Acetazolam, 3
acetazolamide, 3-4
acetazolamide sodium, 3-4
acetylcysteine, 4
acetylsalicylic acid, 20
Aches-N-Pain, 156
Achromycin V, 286
Acid indigestion
  aluminum carbonate for, 11
Acid indigestion *(continued)*
  aluminum hydroxide for, 11
  calcium carbonate for, 41
  magaldrate for, 189
  magnesium hydroxide for, 190
  magnesium oxide for, 191
Aciphex, 260
Aclin, 280
Acne rosacea, metronidazole for, 205
Acne vulgaris
  clindamycin for, 70
  erythromycin (topical) for, 113
  ethinyl estradiol for, 120
  isotretinoin for, 170
  tetracycline for, 286
  tretinoin for, 297
Acquired immunodeficiency syndrome. *See* Human immunodeficiency virus infection.
Acromegaly
  bromocriptine for, 35
  octreotide for, 224
ACT-3, 156
Acticort, 154
Actidose, 4
Actidose-Aqua, 4
Actilyse, 10
Actinic keratoses, fluorouracil for, 132
actinomycin D, 81
Actiprofen, 156
Activase, 10
activated charcoal, 4-5
Activella, 117
Actos, 243
Actron, 172
acyclovir, 5
acyclovir sodium, 5-6
Adalat, 220
Adalat CC, 220
Adapin, 101
Adapine, 220
Adenocard, 6
adenosine, 6
ADH, 303-304
Adipex-P, 239
Adrenalin, 108
Adrenalin Chloride, 108
adrenaline, 108
Adrenal insufficiency
  fludrocortisone for, 129
  hydrocortisone for, 153
Adrenogenital syndrome, fludrocortisone for, 129
Adriamycin, 101
Adriamycin PFS, 101
Adriamycin RDF, 101
Adrucil, 131
Adsorbocarpine, 242
Advil, 156
AeroBid, 130
AeroBid-M, 130
Aerolate, 286
Aeroseb-Dex, 87
Afrin, 230, 255
Agenerase, 19
Aggrastat, 292
Agitation, lorazepam for, 187
Agon SR, 123
Agrylin, 19
A-hydroCort, 154
AIDS. *See* Human immunodeficiency virus infection.
Airbron, 4
Akarpine, 242
AK-Chlor, 61
AK-Con, 215
AK-Dex, 87
AK-Dilate, 241
AK-Nefrin Ophthalmic, 241
Akne-Mycin, 113
AK-Pred, 249
AKTob, 293
AK-Tracin, 25
AK-Zol, 3
alatrofloxacin mesylate, 300-301
albumin 5%, 6
albumin 25%, 6
Albuminar 5, 6
Albuminar 25, 6
Albutein 5%, 6
Albutein 25%, 6
albuterol, 6-7
albuterol sulfate, 6-7
Alcoholism
  disulfiram for, 97
  ethanol-drug interactions, 317
  folic acid for, 137
  mesoridazine for, 197
  naltrexone for, 215
Alcohol withdrawal
  chlordiazepoxide for, 61
  clorazepate for, 72
  oxazepam for, 229
Alconefrin, 241
Aldactone, 277
Aldazine, 288
aldesleukin, 7
Aldomet, 201
Aldomet Ester Injection, 201
alendronate sodium, 7-8
Alepam, 229

Aleve, 216
Alexan, 79
alitretinoin, 8
Alka-Mints, 41
Alkeran, 195
Allegra, 127
Allegron, 223
Aller-Chlor L, 62
Allerdryl, 93
Allerest, 215
Allerest 12 Hr Nasal Spray, 230
Allergic rhinitis. *See also* Rhinitis.
  beclomethasone for, 28
  budesonide for, 35
  cetirizine for, 59
  cromolyn for, 76
  fexofenadine for, 127
  flunisolide for, 131
  fluticasone for, 135
  ipratropium for, 167
  loratadine for, 187
  triamcinolone for, 299
Allergies
  brompheniramine for, 35
  chlorpheniramine for, 62
  clemastine for, 69
  dexamethasone for, 86
  diphenhydramine for, 93
  epinephrine for, 108
  hydroxyzine for, 155
  ipratropium for, 167
  promethazine for, 253
allopurinol, 8
  drug interactions with, 316
Alo-Alpraz, 9
Alopecia, finasteride for, 128
Alphapress, 152
Alphatrex, 31
alprazolam, 9
alprostadil, 9-10
Altace, 261
alteplase, 10
AlternaGEL, 11
Alu-Cap, 11
aluminum carbonate, 11
aluminum hydroxide, 11
aluminum-magnesium complex, 189
Alupent, 198
Alu-tab, 11
Alzheimer's disease
  donepezil for, 100
  rivastigmine for, 267
  tacrine for, 281
amantadine hydrochloride, 11-12
Amaryl, 145
Ambien, 309
AmBisome, 17
Amebiasis, metronidazole for, 204
Amen, 193
Amenorrhea
  bromocriptine for, 35
  medroxyprogesterone for, 193
  norethindrone for, 223
  progesterone for, 252
Amerge, 216
A-methaPred, 202
amethopterin, 200
amifostine, 12
amikacin sulfate, 12-13
Amikin, 12
amiloride hydrochloride, 13
amino acid infusions, 13
Aminosyn, 13
Aminosyn II in Dextrose, 13
Aminosyn II with Electro-lytes in Dextrose, 13
Aminosyn-HBC, 13
Aminosyn-RF, 13
amiodarone hydrochloride, 15
amitriptyline hydrochloride, 15
amlodipine besylate, 15
amoxapine, 16
amoxicillin/clavulanate po-tassium, 16
amoxicillin trihydrate, 16-17
Amoxil, 16
amoxycillin/clavulanate potassium, 16
amoxycillin trihydrate, 16
Amphocin, 17
Amphojel, 11
Amphotec, 18
amphotericin B, 17
amphotericin B cholesteryl sulfate complex, 18
Amphotericin B for Injec-tion, 17
Amphotericin B Liposome for Injection, 17
ampicillin sodium/sulbactam sodium, 18
Amprace, 105
amprenavir, 19
Amyotrophic lateral sclerosis, riluzole for, 265
Anacin (aspirin free), 3
Anacobin, 77
Anafranil, 70
anagrelide hydrochloride, 19
Analgesia. *See* Pain.
Anandron, 220
Anaphylaxis, epinephrine for, 108
Anaprox, 216
Anaprox DS, 216
Anaspaz, 155
anastrozole, 19-20
Ancalixir, 239
Ancef, 48
Ancobon, 129
Ancotil, 129
Andro 100, 285
Androderm, 285
Androgen deficiency, methyltestosterone for, 203
Android, 202
Android-F, 132
Anemia
  cyanocobalamin for, 77
  epoetin alfa for, 110
  ferrous fumarate for, 125
  ferrous gluconate for, 126
  ferrous sulfate for, 126
  folic acid for, 137
  leucovorin for, 178
  sodium ferric gluconate complex for, 275
Anergan, 252
Anesthesia
  butorphanol for, 38
  droperidol for, 104
  fentanyl for, 125
  midazolam for, 206
  nalbuphine for, 214
Anexia 7.5/650, 311
Angina
  amlodipine for, 15
  aspirin for, 20
  atenolol for, 20
  bepridil for, 29
  dalteparin for, 82
  diltiazem for, 92
  enoxaparin for, 106
  eptifibatide for, 112
  isosorbide for, 170

Angina *(continued)*
metoprolol for, 204
nadolol for, 213
nicardipine for, 219
nifedipine for, 220
nitroglycerin for, 221-222
propranolol for, 254
verapamil for, 304
Anginine, 221
Angioedema, clemastine for, 69
Angioplasty
abciximab for, 2
tirofiban for, 292
Ankylosing spondylitis
diclofenac for, 89
indomethacin for, 160
naproxen for, 216
sulindac for, 280
Anorexia, dronabinol for, 103
Ansaid, 134
Antabuse, 97
Anthrax, ciprofloxacin for, 66-67
Antiemetic action. *See* Nausea and vomiting.
Antiflux, 189
Antihist-1, 69
Antiretroviral therapy. *See* Human immunodeficiency virus infection.
Antispas, 90
Anti-Tuss, 150
Antivert, 193
Antrizine, 193
Anxiety
alprazolam for, 9
buspirone for, 38
chlordiazepoxide for, 61
clorazepate for, 73
diazepam for, 88
Anxiety *(continued)*
doxepin for, 101
hydroxyzine for, 155
lorazepam for, 187
mesoridazine for, 197
oxazepam for, 229
paroxetine for, 233
prochlorperazine for, 252
thioridazine for, 288
trifluoperazine for, 299
Anzemet, 99
Apacet, 3
APAP, 3
Aparkane, 300
Apo-Amitriptyline, 15
Apo-Atenolol, 20
Apo-Benztropine, 29
Apo-Capto, 43
Apo-Carbamazepine, 44
Apo-Cephalex, 59
Apo-Chlorthalidone, 63
Apo-Clorazepate, 72
Apo-Diazepam, 88
Apo-Diltiaz, 92
Apo-Ferrous Sulfate, 126
Apo-Flurbiprofen, 134
Apo-Furosemide, 139
Apo-Haloperidol, 151
Apo-Hydralazine, 152
Apo-Hydro, 153
Apo-Hydroxyzine, 155
Apo-Imipramine, 159
Apo-Indomethacin, 160
Apo-ISDN, 170
Apo-Lorazepam, 187
Apo-Methyldopa, 201
Apo-Metoclop, 203
Apo-Metoprolol, 204
Apo-Metronidazole, 204
Apo-Minocycline, 208
Apo-Napro-Na, 216
Apo-Nifed, 220
Apo-Perphenazine, 238
Apo-Pindol, 243
Apo-Piroxicam, 245
Apo-Primidone, 250
Apo-Quinidine, 259
Apo-Ranitidine, 262
Apo-Sulfamethoxazole, 279
Apo-Sulfatrim, 75
Apo-Sulin, 280
Apo-Thioridazine, 288
Apo-Timol, 291
Apo-Triazo, 299
Apo-Trifluoperazine, 299
Apo-Trihex, 300
Apo-Trimip, 300
Apo-Verap, 304
Apo-Zidovudine, 308
Appendicitis
meropenem for, 196
piperacillin and tazobactam for, 244
Apresoline, 152
Aquachloral Supprettes, 60
AquaMEPHYTON, 242
Aquazide-H, 153
ara-C, 79
Aralen HCl, 62
Aralen Phosphate, 62
Aratac, 15
Arava, 177
Aredia, 231
Aricept, 100
Arimidex, 19
Aristocort, 298
Aromasin, 122
Arrhythmias
acebutolol for, 3
adenosine for, 6
amiodarone for, 15
atropine for, 22
bretylium for, 34
digoxin for, 90
diltiazem for, 92
disopyramide for, 96
dofetilide for, 98
esmolol for, 115
Arrhythmias *(continued)*
flecainide for, 128
ibutilide for, 156
isoproterenol for, 169
lidocaine for, 182
magnesium sulfate for, 192
mexiletine for, 205
moricizine for, 211
procainamide for, 250
propranolol for, 254
quinidine for, 259
sotalol for, 277
tocainide for, 293
verapamil for, 304
warfarin for, 305
Artane, 300
Arterial occlusion
alteplase for, 10
streptokinase for, 278
urokinase for, 301
Arthritis
aspirin for, 20
auranofin for, 23
aurothioglucose for, 23
azathioprine for, 24
capsaicin for, 43
celecoxib for, 58
choline magnesium trisalicylate for, 64
cyclosporine for, 78
diclofenac for, 89
diflunisal for, 90
etanercept for, 118
etodolac for, 121
fenoprofen for, 124
flurbiprofen for, 134
gold sodium thiomalate for, 23
ibuprofen for, 156
indomethacin for, 160
infliximab for, 161
ketoprofen for, 172
leflunomide for, 177
magnesium salicylate for, 191

Arthritis *(continued)*
nabumetone for, 213
naproxen for, 216
oxaprozin for, 229
penicillamine for, 234
piroxicam for, 245
rofecoxib for, 267
sulfasalazine for, 279-280
sulindac for, 280
A.S. Wycillin, 235
A.S.A., 20
Ascriptin, 20
Asendin, 16
Asig, 258
Asmol, 6
asparaginase, 20
Aspergillosis
amphotericin B cholesteryl sulfate complex for, 18
itraconazole for, 171
Aspergum, 20
aspirin, 20
Asthma. *See also* Bronchospasm.
aminophylline for, 14
beclomethasone for, 28
budesonide for, 36
cromolyn for, 76
epinephrine for, 108
flunisolide for, 130
fluticasone for, 134
hydroxyzine for, 155
isoproterenol for, 169
metaproterenol for, 198
montelukast for, 211
pirbuterol for, 245
salmeterol for, 269
triamcinolone for, 298
zafirlukast for, 306
zileuton for, 309
AsthmaHaler Mist, 108
Asthma-Nefrin, 108
Astramorph, 211
Astramorph PF, 211
Astrocytoma, temozolomide for, 283
Atacand, 41
Atarax, 155
Atelectasis, acetylcysteine for, 4
atenolol, 20-21
drug interactions with, 316
Atherectomy
abciximab for, 2
tirofiban for, 292
Atherosclerosis, clopidogrel for, 72
Ativan, 187
atorvastatin calcium, 21
atovaquone, 21
Atrial fibrillation or flutter
digoxin for, 90
diltiazem for, 92
dofetilide for, 98-99
esmolol for, 115
flecainide for, 128
heparin for, 152
ibutilide for, 156
quinidine for, 259
sotalol for, 277
verapamil for, 304
warfarin for, 305
Atrop, 22
atropine sulfate (ophthalmic), 22
atropine sulfate (systemic), 22
Atropisol, 22
Atrovent, 167
attapulgite, 22-23
Attention deficit disorder with hyperactivity
dextroamphetamine for, 88
methamphetamine for, 199
Attention deficit disorder with hyperactivity *(continued)*
methylphenidate for, 201
pemoline for, 234
Augmentin, 16
auranofin, 23
Auro Ear Wax Removal Aid, 44
Aurolate, 23
aurothioglucose, 23
Avandia, 268-269
Avapro, 168
Avelox, 212
Aventyl, 223
Avirax, 5
Avita, 297
Avlosulfon, 83
Avomine, 253
Avonex, 166
Axid, 222
Axid AR, 222
Ayercillin, 235
Aygestin, 223
Azactam, 25
azathioprine, 24
azidothymidine, 308-309
azithromycin, 24-25
Azmacort, 298
Azo-Standard, 239
AZT, 308-309
aztreonam, 25
Azulfidine, 279
Azulfidine EN-tab, 279

B

Baciguent, 26
Baci-IM, 26
Bacitin, 26
bacitracin (ophthalmic), 25
bacitracin (systemic), 26
bacitracin (topical), 26
baclofen, 26-27
Bacteremia. *See also* Septicemia.
cefoperazone for, 51
cefotaxime for, 51
cefoxitin for, 52
ceftazidime for, 54
ceftizoxime for, 55
ceftriaxone for, 56
linezolid for, 183, 184
Bacterial vaginosis
clindamycin for, 70
metronidazole for, 205
Bactocill, 228
Bactrim DS, 75
Bactroban, 212
Baldness, finasteride for, 128
Barbita, 239
Baridium, 239
Basal cell carcinoma, fluorouracil for, 132
Basaljel, 11
basiliximab, 27
Bayer Select Maximum Strength Backache Pain Relief Formula, 191
Bayer Timed-Release, 20
BCNU, 45-46
becaplermin, 27-28
Becloforte Inhaler, 28
beclomethasone dipropionate (nasal), 28
beclomethasone dipropionate (oral inhalant), 28
Beclovent, 28
Beconase AQ Nasal Spray, 28
Beconase Nasal Inhaler, 28
Bedoz, 77

Behavior disorders
haloperidol for, 151
mesoridazine for, 197
Bell/ans, 274
Bellaspaz, 155
Benadryl, 93
benazepril hydrochloride, 29
Benign prostatic hyperplasia
doxazosin for, 101
finasteride for, 128
tamsulosin for, 282
terazosin for, 284
Bentyl, 90
Benuryl, 250
Benzodiazepine reversal, flumazenil for, 130
benzonatate, 29
benztropine mesylate, 29
benzylpenicillin benzathine, 234-235
benzylpenicillin potassium, 235
benzylpenicillin procaine, 235
benzylpenicillin sodium, 236
Bepadin, 29
bepridil hydrochloride, 29
beractant, 30
Beriberi, thiamine for, 287
Betagan, 179
betamethasone, 30-31
betamethasone acetate and betamethasone sodium phosphate, 30-31
betamethasone dipropionate, 31
betamethasone sodium phosphate, 30-31
betamethasone valerate, 31
Betamin, 287
Betapace, 277
Betapace AF, 277
Betaseron, 166
Betatrex, 31
Beta-Val, 31
betaxolol hydrochloride (ophthalmic), 31
betaxolol hydrochloride (oral), 31
bethanechol chloride, 32
Betimol, 291
Betnesol, 30
Betnovate, 31
Betoptic, 31
Betoptic S, 31
bexarotene, 32-33
Biaxin, 69
Bicillin L-A, 235
BiCNU, 45
Biliary infection, cefazolin for, 48
Biliary obstruction, cholestyramine for, 64
Biocef, 59
Bisac-Evac, 33
bisacodyl, 33
Bisacodyl Uniserts, 33
Bismatrol, 33
bismuth subsalicylate, 33
bisoprolol fumarate, 33-34
Bladder atony
bethanechol for, 32
neostigmine for, 218
Bladder cancer
cisplatin for, 68
doxorubicin for, 101
Bladder overactivity, tolterodine for, 294
Blastomycosis, itraconazole for, 171
Blenoxane, 34
bleomycin sulfate, 34
Blocadren, 291
Blood transfusion recipients, calcium for, 40
Bonamine, 193
Bone and joint infection
cefazolin for, 48
cefonicid for, 50
cefotaxime for, 51
cefotetan for, 52
cefoxitin for, 52
ceftizoxime for, 55
ceftriaxone for, 56
cephalexin for, 58
cephradine for, 59
ciprofloxacin for, 66
imipenem and cilastatin for, 158
ticarcillin disodium/clavulanate potassium for, 290
Bone marrow transplant recipients
filgrastim for, 127
sargramostim for, 270
Bowel management, psyllium for, 255
Bowel preparation
bisacodyl for, 33
cascara sagrada for, 47
senna for, 271
Bradycardia, atropine for, 22
Brain tumor
carmustine for, 45
lomustine for, 186
temozolomide for, 283
Breast cancer
anastrozole for, 19-20
capecitabine for, 42
cyclophosphamide for, 78
Breast cancer *(continued)*
docetaxel for, 98
doxorubicin for, 101
epirubicin for, 109
esterified estrogens for, 116
estradiol for, 116
ethinyl estradiol for, 119
exemestane for, 122
fluorouracil for, 131
fluoxymesterone for, 132
goserelin for, 149
letrozole for, 177
megestrol for, 193
methyltestosterone for, 202
paclitaxel for, 231
tamoxifen for, 282
testosterone for, 285
thiotepa for, 288
toremifene for, 295
trastuzumab for, 297
vinblastine for, 304
Breast-feeding women, folic acid for, 136, 137
Breast fibrocystic disease, danazol for, 83
Brethaire, 285
Brethine, 285
Bretylate, 34
bretylium tosylate, 34
Bretylol, 34
Brevibloc, 115
Bricanyl, 285
bromocriptine mesylate, 35
Bromphen, 35
brompheniramine maleate, 35
Bronchitis
acetylcysteine for, 4

Bronchitis *(continued)*
cefdinir for, 48
cefpodoxime for, 53
ceftibuten for, 55
co-trimoxazole for, 75
dirithromycin for, 96
gatifloxacin for, 141
levofloxacin for, 180
lomefloxacin for, 185
loracarbef for, 186
moxifloxacin for, 212
salmeterol for, 269
sparfloxacin for, 277
Bronchogenic cancer. *See also* Lung cancer.
mechlorethamine for, 192
Bronchopulmonary dysplasia, respiratory syncytial virus immune globulin, intravenous, human, for, 263
Bronchospasm. *See also* Asthma.
albuterol for, 6-7
aminophylline for, 14
cromolyn for, 76
epinephrine for, 108
ipratropium for, 167
isoproterenol for, 169
levalbuterol for, 178
metaproterenol for, 198
pirbuterol for, 245
salmeterol for, 269
terbutaline for, 285
theophylline for, 286-287
Bronkaid Mist, 108
Bronkaid Mistometer, 108
Bronkaid Suspension Mist, 108
Bronkodyl, 286
Brontin Mist, 108
Brucellosis, tetracycline for, 286
budesonide (nasal), 35
budesonide (oral inhalant), 36
Bufferin, 20
BufOpto Atropine, 22
Bulimia nervosa, fluoxetine for, 132
bumetanide, 37
Bumex, 37
bupropion hydrochloride, 37
Burinex, 37
Burns
bacitracin for, 26
nitrofurazone for, 221
silver sulfadiazine for, 273
Bursitis
naproxen for, 216
sulindac for, 280
Buscopan, 270
BuSpar, 38
buspirone hydrochloride, 38
busulfan, 38
butorphanol tartrate, 38

C

Calan, 304
Calan SR, 304
Calcarb 600, 41
CalCarb-HD, 41
Calci-Chew, 41
Calcijex, 39
Calcimar, 39
calcitonin (human), 39
calcitonin (salmon), 39
Cal-citrate 250, 40
calcitriol, 39-40
calcium acetate, 40-41
calcium carbonate, 41
calcium chloride, 40-41
calcium citrate, 40-41
calcium glubionate, 40-41
calcium gluceptate, 40-41
calcium gluconate, 40-41
calcium lactate, 40-41
calcium phosphate, tribasic, 40-41
calcium polycarbophil, 41
CaldeCort, 154
Calm-X, 93
Caloric supplementation, dextrose for, 88
Caltrate 600, 41
Camptosar, 168
Cancer. *See also* specific types.
dexamethasone for, 86
filgrastim for, 127
Cancer chemotherapy adverse effects
amifostine for, 12
dolasetron for, 99
dronabinol for, 103
epoetin alfa for, 110
granisetron for, 149
leucovorin for, 177
mesna for, 197
metoclopramide for, 203
ondansetron for, 227
oprelvekin for, 227
candesartan cilexetil, 41-42
Candidal infection
amphotericin B for, 17
clotrimazole for, 73
fluconazole for, 128-129
flucytosine for, 129
itraconazole for, 171
ketoconazole for, 172
miconazole for, 206
nystatin for, 224
Candidal infection *(continued)*
terconazole for, 285
tioconazole for, 292
Canesten, 73
capecitabine, 42-43
Capital with Codeine, 311
Capoten, 43
capsaicin, 43
captopril, 43-44
drug interactions with, 316
Carafate, 279
carbamazepine, 44
drug interactions with, 316
carbamide peroxide, 44
Carbatrol, 44
Carbex, 271
Carbolith, 185
Carbon monoxide–induced parkinsonism, levodopa-carbidopa for, 179
carboplatin, 45
Carcinoid tumors, octreotide for, 224
Cardene, 219
Cardene IV, 219
Cardene SR, 219
Cardiac arrest
calcium for, 40
epinephrine for, 108
sodium bicarbonate for, 274
Cardiac glycoside adverse effects, lidocaine for, 182
Cardiac output stimulation
dobutamine for, 97
dopamine for, 100
Cardiac procedures, lidocaine for, 182

Cardiac vagal response blockade
atropine for, 22
hyoscyamine for, 155
Cardiovascular surgery
acetylcysteine for pulmonary complications of, 4
dobutamine for, 97
Cardizem, 92
Cardizem CD, 92
Cardizem SR, 92
Cardura, 101
carisoprodol, 45
carmustine, 45-46
carteolol hydrochloride (ophthalmic), 46
carteolol hydrochloride (oral), 46
Cartrol, 46
carvedilol, 46-47
drug interactions with, 316
cascara sagrada, 47
Castration, female
esterified estrogens for, 116
estradiol for, 116
estradiol/norethindrone acetate transdermal system for, 117
estrogens, conjugated, for, 118
estropipate for, 118
Cataflam, 89
Catapres, 71
Catapres-TTS, 71
Catheter occlusion
streptokinase for, 278
urokinase for, 301
Caverject, 9
CCNU, 186
CdA, 68
CDDP, 67-68
Ceclor, 47
Cedax, 55
CeeNU, 186
cefaclor, 47
cefadroxil monohydrate, 47-48
Cefanex, 59
cefazolin sodium, 48
cefdinir, 48-49
cefepime hydrochloride, 49-50
Cefizox, 55
cefmetazole sodium, 50
cefmetazone, 50
Cefobid, 51
cefonicid sodium, 50-51
cefoperazone sodium, 51
Cefotan, 52
cefotaxime sodium, 51-52
cefotetan disodium, 52
cefoxitin sodium, 52-53
cefpodoxime proxetil, 53-54
cefprozil, 54
ceftazidime, 54-55
ceftibuten, 55
Ceftin, 56
ceftizoxime sodium, 55-56
ceftriaxone sodium, 56
cefuroxime axetil, 56-58
cefuroxime sodium, 56-58
Cefzil, 54
Celebrex, 58
celecoxib, 58
Celestone, 30
Celestone Phosphate, 31
Celestone Soluspan, 30
Celexa, 68
CellCept, 213
CellCept Intravenous, 213
Celsius-Fahrenheit temperature conversions, 319
Central nervous system infection. *See also* Meningitis.
cefotaxime for, 51
ceftazidime for, 54
Cephalac, 174
cephalexin hydrochloride, 58-59
cephalexin monohydrate, 58-59
cephradine, 59
Ceptaz, 54
Cerebral edema, dexamethasone for, 86
Cerebral palsy, dantrolene for, 83
Cerebyx, 138
Cerubidine, 84
Cerumen impaction, carbamide peroxide for, 44
Cervicitis. *See also* Endocervical infection.
azithromycin for, 25
ofloxacin for, 224
C.E.S., 118
cetirizine hydrochloride, 59
cevimeline hydrochloride, 60
Charcoaid, 4
Charcocaps, 4
Cheracol Nasal, 230
Chickenpox, acyclovir sodium for, 5-6
Children's Advil, 156
Children's Kaopectate, 22
Children's Motrin, 156
Children's Sudafed, 255
Chlamydial infection
azithromycin for, 25
demeclocycline for, 85
Chlamydial infection *(continued)*
doxycycline for, 102, 103
minocycline for, 208
sulfamethoxazole for, 279
tetracycline for, 286
chloral hydrate, 60-61
chlorambucil, 61
chloramphenicol (ophthalmic), 61
chlordiazepoxide, 61
chlordiazepoxide hydrochloride, 61
2-chlorodeoxyadenosine, 68
Chloromycetin Ophthalmic, 61
Chloroptic, 61
Chloroptic S.O.P., 61
chloroquine hydrochloride, 62
chloroquine phosphate, 62
Chlorphed, 35
chlorpheniramine maleate, 62
Chlorpromanyl-5, 63
Chlorpromanyl-20, 63
Chlorpromanyl-40, 63
chlorpromazine hydrochloride, 63
Chlorquin, 62
chlorthalidone, 63
Chlor-Trimeton, 62
cholestyramine, 64
choline magnesium trisalicylate, 64
choline salicylate and magnesium salicylate, 64
Chooz, 41
Choriocarcinoma, methotrexate for, 200

Chronic granulomatous disease, interferon gamma-1b for, 166
Chronic obstructive pulmonary disease. *See also* Asthma; Bronchitis; Emphysema.
  azithromycin for, 24
  ipratropium for, 167
  isoproterenol for, 169
  salmeterol for, 269
Chronulac, 174
Cibacalcin, 39
Cibalith-S, 185
cidofovir, 64-65
Cidofovir adverse effects, probenecid for, 250
Cidomycin, 144
Cilamox, 16
cilostazol, 65
Ciloxan, 67
cimetidine, 65-66
Cipro, 66
ciprofloxacin, 66-67
ciprofloxacin hydrochloride, 67
Cipro I.V., 66
Ciproxin, 66
Cirrhosis, amino acid infusions for, 13
cisplatin, 67-68
Cisplatin adverse effects, amifostine for, 12
cisplatinum, 67-68
citalopram hydrochloride, 68
Citracal, 40
citrate of magnesia, 190
Citrocarbonate, 274
Citroma, 190
Citro-Mag, 190
Citro-Nesia, 190
citrovorum factor, 177-178
Citrucel, 201
cladribine, 68
Claforan, 51
Claratyne, 187
clarithromycin, 69
Claritin, 187
Claudication, intermittent
  cilostazol for, 65
  pentoxifylline for, 237
Clavulin, 16
Clear Eyes, 215
clemastine fumarate, 69
Cleocin HCl, 70
Cleocin Pediatric, 70
Cleocin Phosphate, 70
Cleocin T, 70
Cleocin T Gel, Lotion, Solution, 70
Cleocin Vaginal Cream, 70
Climara, 116
clindamycin hydrochloride, 70
clindamycin palmitate hydrochloride, 70
clindamycin phosphate, 70
Clinoril, 280
Clin-Quin, 259
Clofen, 26
clomipramine hydrochloride, 70-71
clonazepam, 71
clonidine, 71-72
  drug interactions with, 316
clonidine hydrochloride, 71-72
clopidogrel bisulfate, 72
Clopra, 203
clorazepate dipotassium, 72-73
clotrimazole, 73
clozapine, 73-74
Clozaril, 73
CMV-IGIV, 79-80
Coagulopathy, heparin for, 152
codeine phosphate, 74
codeine sulfate, 74
Codimal-A, 35
Codroxomin, 77
Cogentin, 29
Cognex, 281
Colace, 98
colchicine, 74
Colestid, 75
colestipol hydrochloride, 75
Colgout, 74
Cologel, 201
Colorectal cancer
  fluorouracil for, 131-132
  irinotecan for, 168
Colorectal polyps, celecoxib for, 58
Colorectal surgery patients, metronidazole for, 205
Colsalide, 74
CombiPatch, 117
Combivir, 174
Common cold, ipratropium for, 167
Compa-Z, 251
Compazine, 251
Comtan, 107
Condylomata acuminata, interferon alfa-2b, recombinant, for, 165
Conjunctivitis
  bacitracin for, 25
  chloramphenicol for, 25
  ciprofloxacin for, 67
  cromolyn for, 77
Conjunctivitis *(continued)*
  dexamethasone for, 86-87
  erythromycin (ophthalmic) for, 113
  ketorolac for, 172
Constipation
  bisacodyl for, 33
  calcium polycarbophil for, 41
  cascara sagrada for, 47
  glycerin for, 148
  lactulose for, 174
  magnesium oxide for, 191
  magnesium salts for, 190
  methylcellulose for, 201
  psyllium for, 255
  senna for, 271
  sodium phosphates for, 276
Constulose, 174
Contraception
  ethinyl estradiol for, 120
  levonorgestrel for, 181
  medroxyprogesterone for, 193
  norethindrone for, 223
  norgestrel for, 223
copolymer 1, 145
Cordarone, 15
Cordarone X, 15
Coreg, 46
Corgard, 213
Corlopam, 124
Corneal infection
  bacitracin for, 25
  chloramphenicol for, 25
Corneal inflammation, dexamethasone for, 86

Corneal injury, dexamethasone for, 86
Corneal ulcer, ciprofloxacin for, 67
Coronary artery disease
  abciximab for, 2
  dipyridamole for diagnosis of, 95
  gemfibrozil for, 143
  lovastatin for, 188
Coronary artery occlusion
  alteplase for, 10
  streptokinase for, 278
  urokinase for, 301
Coronary syndrome, acute
  eptifibatide for, 112
  tirofiban for, 292
CortaGel, 154
Cortaid, 154
Cortamed, 154
Cortef, 153, 154
Cortifoam, 153
Cortizone 5, 154
Corvert, 156
Cosmegen, 81
Cotranzine, 251
Cotrim, 75
co-trimoxazole, 75-76
Cough
  benzonatate for, 29
  codeine for, 74
  diphenhydramine for, 93
  hydromorphone for, 155
Coumadin, 305
Covera HS, 304
Cozaar, 188
Cretinism, liothyronine for, 184
Crixivan, 160
Crohn's disease
  infliximab for, 161
Crohn's disease *(continued)*
  sulfasalazine for, 279
Crolom, 76
cromolyn sodium, 76-77
Cryptococcal infection
  amphotericin B for, 17
  fluconazole for, 129
  flucytosine for, 129
crystalline zinc insulin, 163-164
Crystamine, 77
Crystapen, 236
Crysti-12, 77
Crysticillin 300, 235
Cuprimine, 234
Curretab, 193
Cutivate, 135
Cuts, bacitracin for, 26
cyanocobalamin, 77
Cyanoject, 77
Cyclidox, 103
cyclobenzaprine hydrochloride, 77
Cycloblastin, 78
Cyclomen, 83
cyclophosphamide, 78
Cycloplegic refraction
  atropine for, 22
  scopolamine for, 270
cyclosporin, 78-79
cyclosporine, 78-79
  drug interactions with, 316
Cycrin, 193
Cylert, 234
Cylert Chewable, 234
Cyomin, 77
Cyronine, 184
Cystic fibrosis
  acetylcysteine for, 4
  tobramycin for, 293
Cystinuria, penicillamine for, 234
Cystitis. *See also* Urinary tract infection.
Cystitis *(continued)*
  lomefloxacin for, 185
  mesna for, 197
  ofloxacin for, 225
Cystospaz, 155
cytarabine, 79
cytomegalovirus immune globulin (human), intravenous, 79-80
Cytomegalovirus infection
  cidofovir for, 64
  cytomegalovirus immune globulin (human), intravenous, for, 79
  fomivirsen for, 137
  foscarnet for, 138
  ganciclovir for, 140
Cytomel, 184
Cytosar, 79
Cytosar-U, 79
cytosine arabinoside, 79
Cytospaz, 155-156
Cytotec, 209
Cytovene, 140
Cytoxan, 78
Cytoxan Lyophilized, 78

D

dacarbazine, 80
daclizumab, 80-81
Dacodyl, 33
dactinomycin, 81
Dalacin C, 70
Dalalone, 86
Dalalone D.P., 86
Dalmane, 133
dalteparin sodium, 81-82
Damason-P, 311
danaparoid sodium, 82
danazol, 83
Dangerous drug interactions, 316-317
Danocrine, 83
Dantrium, 83
dantrolene sodium, 83
Dapacin, 3
dapsone, 83-84
Dapsone 100, 83
Daraprim, 257
Darvocet-N 50, 311
Darvocet-N 100, 311
Darvon, 253
Darvon-N, 253
daunorubicin hydrochloride, 84
Daypro, 229
Dazamide, 3
DDAVP, 85
ddC, 306
ddI, 90
Debrox, 44
Decaderm, 87
Decadron, 86, 87
Decadron-LA, 86
Decadron Phosphate, 86
Decadron Phosphate Ophthalmic, 86-87
Decaspray, 87
Declomycin, 85
Deep vein thrombosis. *See also* Thromboembolic disorders.
  dalteparin for, 81
  danaparoid for, 82
  enoxaparin for, 106-107
  heparin for, 151-152
  tinzaparin for, 291
  warfarin for, 305
Deficol, 33
delavirdine mesylate, 84
Delayed puberty, fluoxymesterone for, 132
Delestrogen, 116

Delirium, scopolamine for, 270
Delta-Cortef, 248
Demadex, 295
demeclocycline hydrochloride, 85
Dementia
  donepezil for, 100
  rivastigmine for, 267
  tacrine for, 281
Demerol, 195
Demulen 1/35, 120
Dental procedures
  amoxicillin for, 17
  clindamycin for, 70
  vancomycin for, 303
Depade, 215
Depakene, 302
Depakene Syrup, 302
Depakote, 302
Depakote ER, 302
Depakote Sprinkle, 302
depAndro, 285
Depen, 234
depGynogen, 116
depMedalone, 202
Depo-Estradiol, 116
Depoject, 202
Depo-Medrol, 202
Deponit, 221
Depopred, 202
Depo-Provera, 193
Depotest, 285
Depo-Testosterone, 285
Depression
  amitriptyline for, 15
  amoxapine for, 16
  bupropion for, 37
  citalopram for, 68
  desipramine for, 85
  doxepin for, 101
  fluoxetine for, 132
  imipramine for, 159
  mirtazapine for, 209
  nefazodone for, 217
  nortriptyline for, 223
Depression *(continued)*
  paroxetine for, 233
  sertraline for, 271
  thioridazine for, 288
  trazodone, 297
  trimipramine for, 300
  venlafaxine for, 304
Deptran, 101
Deralin, 254
Dermal necrosis from intravenous extravasation of norepinephrine, phentolamine for, 240
Dermatitis herpetiformis, dapsone for, 83
desipramine hydrochloride, 85
desmopressin acetate, 85-86
Desogen, 120
Desoxyn, 199
Desoxyn Gradumets, 199
Desyrel, 297
Desyrel Dividose, 297
Detensol, 254
Detrol, 294
dexamethasone acetate, 86
dexamethasone (injectable), 86
dexamethasone (ophthalmic), 86-87
dexamethasone sodium phosphate, 86-87
dexamethasone (topical), 87
Dexasone, 86
Dexasone-L.A., 86
Dexedrine, 87
Dexedrine Spansule, 87
dextroamphetamine sulfate, 87-88
dextrose, 88
Dey-Dose Isoproterenol, 169
Dey-Dose Metaproterenol, 198
Dey-Lute Metaproterenol, 198
d-glucose, 88
D.H.E. 45, 92
DiaBeta, 147
Diabetes insipidus
  desmopressin for, 85
  vasopressin for, 303
Diabetes mellitus
  acarbose for, 2
  glimepiride for, 145-146
  glipizide for, 146
  glyburide for, 147
  insulin aspart (rDNA origin) injection for, 161
  insulin for, 163
  insulin glargine (rDNA) injection for, 162
  metformin for, 198
  miglitol for, 207
  pioglitazone for, 243
  repaglinide for, 262
  rosiglitazone for, 268-269
Diabetic ketoacidosis, insulin for, 163
Diabetic neuropathy, becaplermin for, 27
Diagnostic procedures
  droperidol for, 104
  glucagon for, 147
  midazolam for, 206
Dialume, 11
Dialysis patients
  calcitriol for, 39
  epoetin alfa for, 110-111
  sodium ferric gluconate complex for, 275
Diamox, 3
Diamox Parenteral, 4
Diamox Sequels, 3
Diaqua, 153
Diarrhea
  attapulgite for, 22
  bismuth subsalicylate for, 33
  calcium polycarbophil for, 41
  diphenoxylate hydrochloride and atropine sulfate for, 94
  loperamide for, 186
  neomycin for, 217
  octreotide for, 224
  opium tincture for, 227
Diasorb, 22
diazepam, 88-89
Diazepam Intensol, 88
diazoxide, 89
Dibent, 90
Dichlotride, 153
diclofenac potassium, 89-90
diclofenac sodium, 89-90
dicyclomine hydrochloride, 90
didanosine, 90
dideoxycytidine, 306
Dietary supplementation
  calcium carbonate for, 41
  cyanocobalamin for, 77
  folic acid for, 136
  magnesium for, 190
  pyridoxine for, 257
Diflucan, 128
diflunisal, 90
Digibind, 91
Digitoxin intoxication, digoxin immune Fab (ovine) for, 91

digoxin, 90-91
  drug interactions with, 316
digoxin immune Fab (ovine), 91-92
Digoxin intoxication, digoxin immune Fab (ovine) for, 91
Dihydergot, 92
dihydroergotamine mesylate, 92
dihydromorphinone hydrochloride, 154-155
1,25-dihydroxycholecalciferol, 39-40
Dilacor-XR, 92
Dilantin, 241
Dilantin Infatabs, 241
Dilantin Kapseals, 241
Dilatrate-SR, 170
Dilaudid, 155
Dilaudid-HP, 155
diltiazem hydrochloride, 92-93
dimenhydrinate, 93
Dimetabs, 93
Dimetane, 35
Dinate, 93
Dioctocal, 98
Diovan, 303
Dipentum, 226
diphenhydramine hydrochloride, 93-94
diphenoxylate hydrochloride and atropine sulfate, 94
diphenylhydantoin, 241-242
diphtheria and tetanus toxoids and acellular pertussis vaccine, 94-95
diphtheria and tetanus toxoids and whole-cell pertussis vaccine, 95
dipivefrin, 95
Diprivan, 253
Diprolene, 31
Diprolene AF, 31
Diprosone, 31
dipyridamole, 95
dirithromycin, 96
disopyramide, 96-97
disopyramide phosphate, 96-97
Di-Spaz, 90
Disseminated intravascular coagulation, heparin for, 152
disulfiram, 97
Diuchlor, 153
divalproex sodium, 302-303
Dixarit, 71
Doan's, 191
dobutamine hydrochloride, 97-98
  infusion rates for, 322
Dobutrex, 97
docetaxel, 98
docusate calcium, 98
docusate sodium, 98
dofetilide, 98-99
dolasetron mesylate, 99-100
Dolobid, 90
Dolophine, 199
Dolorac, 43
Doloxene, 253
donepezil hydrochloride, 100
Donnagel, 22
Dopamet, 201
dopamine hydrochloride, 100-101
  infusion rates for, 323
Doryx, 103
dorzolamide hydrochloride, 101
doxazosin mesylate, 101
doxepin hydrochloride, 101
doxorubicin hydrochloride, 101-102
Doxy-Caps, 103
Doxycin, 103
doxycycline calcium, 102-103
doxycycline hyclate, 102-103
doxycycline hydrochloride, 103
doxycycline monohydrate, 103
Doxylin, 103
D-Penamine, 234
DPT, 94-95
Dramamine, 93
Dramamine Less Drowsy Formula, 193
Dristan 12 Hr Nasal, 230
Drixoral, 255
Dromitexan, 197
dronabinol, 103
droperidol, 104
Drug interactions, 316-318
Drugs that should not be crushed, 313-315
Dry mouth
  amifostine for, 12
  cevimeline for, 60
d4T, 278
DTaP, 95
DTIC, 80
DTIC-Dome, 80
DTP, 94-95
DTwP, 95
Dulcagen, 33
Dulcolax, 33
Duodenal ulcer
  cimetidine for, 65
  famotidine for, 122
  lansoprazole for, 176
  nizatidine for, 222
  omeprazole for, 226
  rabeprazole for, 260
  ranitidine for, 261-262
  sucralfate for, 279
Duphalac, 174
Duragesic, 125
Duralone, 202
Duramist Plus, 230
Duramorph, 211
Duratest, 285
Duricef, 47
Durolax, 33
Duvoid, 32
D-Vert, 193
Dymenate, 93
Dynabac, 96
Dynacin, 208
DynaCirc, 170
Dyrenium, 299
Dysbetalipoproteinemia
  atorvastatin for, 21
  simvastatin for, 273
Dyslipidemia
  atorvastatin for, 21
  cholestyramine for, 64
  fenofibrate for, 123
  fluvastatin for, 136
  gemfibrozil for, 143
  niacin for, 219
  pravastatin for, 248
  simvastatin for, 273
Dysmenorrhea
  diclofenac for, 90
  ibuprofen for, 156
  ketoprofen for, 172
  naproxen for, 216
  rofecoxib for, 267
Dyspepsia, activated charcoal for, 4

Dystonic reaction, acute, benztropine for, 29

E

Eclampsia, magnesium sulfate for, 191
Econopred Plus, 249
Ecotrin, 20
E-Cypionate, 116
Edecrin, 119
Edecrin Sodium, 119
Edema
  acetazolamide for, 4
  amiloride for, 13
  bumetanide for, 37
  chlorthalidone for, 63
  furosemide for, 139
  hydrochlorothiazide for, 153
  indapamide for, 159
  metolazone for, 203
  spironolactone for, 277
  triamterene for, 299
ED-Spoz, 156
EES, 114
efavirenz, 105
Effexor, 304
Effexor XR, 304
Efidac/24, 255
Efudex, 131
Elavil, 15
Eldepryl, 271
Electroencephalography, chloral hydrate for, 60
Ellence, 109
Embolism. *See* Thromboembolic disorders.
Emphysema
  acetylcysteine for, 4
  salmeterol for, 269
Empirin, 20
Empirin with Codeine No. 3, 311
Empirin with Codeine No. 4, 311
Empyema, bacitracin for, 26
E-Mycin, 114
enalaprilat, 105-106
enalapril maleate, 105-106
  drug interactions with, 316
Enbrel, 118
Endocarditis
  amoxicillin for, 17
  cefazolin for, 48
  cephradine for, 59
  clindamycin for, 70
  gentamicin for, 144
  imipenem and cilastatin for, 158
  vancomycin for, 303
Endocervical infection. *See also* Cervicitis.
  doxycycline for, 103
  minocycline for, 208
Endometrial ablation, goserelin for, 149
Endometrial cancer
  medroxyprogesterone for, 193
  megestrol for, 193
Endometriosis
  danazol for, 83
  goserelin for, 149
  norethindrone for, 223
Endometritis, piperacillin and tazobactam for, 244
Endoxan-Asta, 78
enoxaparin sodium, 106-107
entacapone, 107
Enterocolitis, vancomycin for, 303
Enterocutaneous fistula, infliximab for, 161
Enulose, 174
Enuresis
  desmopressin for, 85
  imipramine for, 159
Epilepsy. *See* Seizures.
Epilim, 302
Epimorph, 211
epinephrine, 108
  drug interactions with, 316
  infusion rates for, 320
epinephrine bitartrate, 108
epinephrine hydrochloride, 108
EpiPen, 108
EpiPen Jr., 108
epirubicin hydrochloride, 109-110
Epitol, 44
Epival, 302
Epivir, 174
Epivir-HBV, 174
epoetin alfa, 110-111
Epogen, 110
eprosartan mesylate, 111-112
epsom salts, 190
eptastatin, 248
eptifibatide, 112-113
Equalactin, 41
Eramycin, 114
Erectile dysfunction
  alprostadil for, 9
  sildenafil for, 272
Ergodryl Mono, 113
Ergomar, 113
ergotamine tartrate, 113
Eryc, 114
Eryc333, 114
Erycette, 113
EryDerm, 113
Erygel, 113
EryPed, 114
EryPed 200, 114
Ery-Sol, 113
Ery-Tab, 114
Erythrocin, 114
Erythrocin Stearate, 114
erythromycin, 113
erythromycin base, 114
erythromycin estolate, 114
erythromycin ethylsuccinate, 114
erythromycin lactobionate, 114
erythromycin (ophthalmic), 113-114
erythromycin stearate, 114
erythromycin (topical), 113
erythropoietin, 110-111
Esidrix, 153
Eskalith CR, 185
esmolol hydrochloride, 115
  drug interactions with, 317
Esophagitis
  lansoprazole for, 176
  omeprazole for, 226
  pantoprazole for, 232
  ranitidine for, 262
estazolam, 115
esterified estrogens, 116
Estinyl, 119
Estrace, 116
Estraderm, 116
estradiol, 116-117
estradiol cypionate, 116-117
estradiol/norethindrone acetate transdermal system, 117
estradiol valerate, 116-117
Estra-L 40, 116
Estratab, 116
estrogenic substances, conjugated, 118

estrogens, conjugated, 118
estrogens, esterified, 116
estropipate, 118
etanercept, 118-119
ethacrynate sodium, 119
ethacrynic acid, 119
ethambutol hydrochloride, 119
ethanol-drug interactions, 317
ethinyl estradiol, 119-121
Ethmozine, 211
Ethyol, 12
Etibi, 119
etodolac, 121
Etopophos, 121
etoposide, 121
etoposide phosphate, 121
Euflex, 134
Eulexin, 134
Eustachian tube congestion, pseudoephedrine for, 255
Evac-Q-Mag, 190
Evista, 261
Evoxac, 60
Ewing's sarcoma, dactinomycin for, 81
Exelon, 267
exemestane, 122
Expectorant action, guaifenesin for, 150
Extrapyramidal disorders. *See also* Parkinsonism.
  benztropine for, 29
Extravasation of norepinephrine, phentolamine for dermal necrosis from, 240
Eye infection
  bacitracin for, 25
  chloramphenicol for, 61
  ciprofloxacin for, 67
  erythromycin for, 113
  gentamicin for, 144
  polymyxin B for, 246
  tobramycin for, 293
Eye irritation and itching
  ketorolac for, 172
  naphazoline for, 215
Eyelid inflammation, dexamethasone for, 86

F

Facial wrinkles, tretinoin for, 297
Fahrenheit-Celsius temperature conversions, 319
famciclovir, 122
Familial adenomatous polyposis, celecoxib for, 58
famotidine, 122-123
Famvir, 122
Fansidar, 257
Fareston, 295
Fastin, 239
5-FC, 129
Feldene, 245
felodipine, 123
Femara, 177
Femiron, 125
Femizol, 206
Fenac, 89
fenofibrate (micronized), 123-124
fenoldopam mesylate, 124
fenoprofen calcium, 124-125
fentanyl citrate, 125
Fentanyl Oralet, 125
fentanyl transdermal system, 125
fentanyl transmucosal, 125
Feosol, 126
Feostat, 125
Fergon, 126
Ferrlecit, 275-276
ferrous fumarate, 125-126
ferrous gluconate, 126
ferrous sulfate, 126
ferrous sulfate, dried, 126
Fever
  acetaminophen for, 3
  aspirin for, 20
  choline magnesium trisalicylate for, 64
  fenoprofen for, 124
  ibuprofen for, 156
  ketoprofen for, 172
  magnesium salicylate for, 191
Feverall, 3
fexofenadine, 127
Fiberall, 41, 255
Fiber-Con, 41
Fiber-Lax, 41
FiberNorm, 41
Fibrocystic breast disease, danazol for, 83
filgrastim, 127
finasteride, 128
Fioricet with Codeine, 311
Flagyl, 204
Flagyl 375, 204
Flagyl ER, 204
Flagyl I.V. RTU, 204
Flamazine, 273
Flatulence
  activated charcoal for, 4
  simethicone for, 273
Flatulex, 273
flecainide acetate, 128
Fleet Babylax, 148
Fleet Bisacodyl, 33
Fleet Bisacodyl Prep, 33
Fleet Enema, 276
Fleet Laxative, 33
Fletcher's Castoria, 271
Flexeril, 77
Flint SSD, 273
Flomax, 282
Flonase, 135
Florinef, 129
Flovent Inhalation Aerosol, 134
Flovent Rotadisk, 134
Floxin, 224
Floxin I.V., 224
fluconazole, 128-129
flucytosine, 129
fludrocortisone acetate, 129
Fluid replacement, dextrose for, 88
Flumadine, 265
flumazenil, 130
flunisolide, 130-131
fluocinonide, 131
5-fluorocytosine, 129
Fluoroplex, 131
fluorouracil, 131-132
5-fluorouracil, 131-132
fluoxetine hydrochloride, 132
fluoxymesterone, 132-133
fluphenazine decanoate, 133
fluphenazine enanthate, 133
fluphenazine hydrochloride, 133
flurazepam hydrochloride, 133
flurbiprofen, 134
Flushing, octreotide for, 224

flutamide, 134
Flutex, 298
fluticasone propionate (inhalation), 134-135
fluticasone propionate (nasal), 135
fluticasone propionate (topical), 135
fluvastatin sodium, 136
fluvoxamine maleate, 136
Folex PFS, 200
folic acid, 136-137
Folic acid antagonist overdose, leucovorin for, 177
Folic acid deficiency, folic acid for, 137
folinic acid, 177-178
Folvite, 136
fomivirsen sodium, 137
Fortaz, 54
Fortovase, 269
Fortral, 236
Fosamax, 7
foscarnet sodium, 138
Foscavir, 138
fosinopril sodium, 138
fosphenytoin sodium, 138-139
Fowler's, 22
Fragmin, 81
FreAmine III, 13
Froben, 134
Froben SR, 134
frusemide, 139
5-FU, 131-132
Fulcin, 150
Fulvicin P/G, 150
Fulvicin-U/F, 150
Fumasorb, 125
Fumerin, 125
Fungal infection. *See also* specific infections.
Fungal infection *(continued)*
  amphotericin B cholesteryl sulfate complex for, 18
  amphotericin B for, 17
  clotrimazole for, 73
  fluconazole for, 128-129
  flucytosine for, 129
  griseofulvin for, 150
  itraconazole for, 171
  ketoconazole for, 171-172
  miconazole for, 206
  nystatin for, 224
  terbinafine for, 284
  terconazole for, 285
  tioconazole for, 292
Fungilin Oral, 17
Fungizone Intravenous, 17
Furacin, 221
Furadantin, 221
furosemide, 139

G

gabapentin, 140
Gabitril Filmtabs, 289
Galactorrhea, bromocriptine for, 35
ganciclovir, 140
Gantanol, 279
Gantrisin, 280
Gantrisin Pediatric, 280
Garamycin, 144, 145
Garamycin Ophthalmic, 144
Gastric bloating, simethicone for, 273
Gastric cancer
  doxorubicin for, 101
  fluorouracil for, 131
  mitomycin for, 210
Gastric ulcer. *See also* Peptic ulcer disease.
  cimetidine for, 66
  famotidine for, 122
  lansoprazole for, 176
  misoprostol for prevention of, 209
  nizatidine for, 222
  omeprazole for, 226
  ranitidine for, 262
Gastroesophageal reflux
  cimetidine for, 66
  famotidine for, 122
  lansoprazole for, 176
  metoclopramide for, 203
  nizatidine for, 222
  omeprazole for, 226
  pantoprazole for, 232
  rabeprazole for, 260
  ranitidine for, 262
Gastrointestinal conditions
  activated charcoal for, 4
  calcium polycarbophil for, 41
  dicyclomine for, 90
  hyoscyamine for, 155
  simethicone for, 273
Gastrointestinal infection
  amphotericin B for, 17
  cephalexin for, 58
  cephradine for, 59
Gastrointestinal procedures, gentamicin for, 144
Gas-X, 273
gatifloxacin, 141-142
GBH, 182
G-CSF, 127
gemcitabine hydrochloride, 142
gemfibrozil, 143
gemtuzumab ozogamicin, 143-144
Gemzar, 142
Genaphed, 255
Genasoft, 98
Genasol, 230
GenFiver, 255
Genital herpes
  acyclovir for, 5
  famciclovir for, 122
  valacyclovir for, 302
Genitourinary infection
  cefazolin for, 48
  cefoxitin for, 52
  cephradine for, 59
Genitourinary procedures, gentamicin for, 144
Genoptic, 144
Genora 1/35, 120
Genora 1/50, 121
Gentacidin, 144
Gentak, 144
Gentamicin Sulfate ADD-Vantage, 144
gentamicin sulfate (ophthalmic), 144
gentamicin sulfate (systemic), 144-145
  drug interactions with, 317
gentamicin sulfate (topical), 145
Gen-XENE, 72
glatiramer acetate for injection, 145
Glaucoma. *See also* Intraocular pressure elevation.
  acetazolamide for, 3-4
  betaxolol for, 31
  carteolol for, 46
  dipivefrin for, 95
  dorzolamide for, 101
  latanoprost for, 177

Glaucoma *(continued)*
levobunolol for, 179
pilocarpine for, 242
timolol for, 291
glimepiride, 145-146
glipizide, 146-147
glucagon, 147
Glucophage, 198
Glucotrol, 146
Glucotrol XL, 146
Glu-K, 247
glyburide, 147-148
glycerin, 148
glyceryl guaiacolate, 150
glyceryl trinitrate, 221-222
Glynase PresTab, 147
Glyset, 207
Glytuss, 150
GM-CSF, 270
G-Myticin, 145
Goiter, liothyronine for, 184
Gold-50, 23
gold sodium thiomalate, 23
Gonococcal infection
amoxicillin for, 17
azithromycin for, 25
ceftriaxone for, 56
erythromycin for, 114
gatifloxacin for, 141
minocycline for, 208
norfloxacin for, 223
ofloxacin for, 225
penicillin G procaine for, 235
probenecid for, 250
tetracycline for, 286
goserelin acetate, 149
Gout
allopurinol for, 8
colchicine for, 74
indomethacin for, 160
naproxen for, 216
Gout *(continued)*
probenecid for, 250
sulindac for, 280
granisetron hydrochloride, 149
granulocyte colony-stimulating factor, 127
granulocyte-macrophage colony-stimulating factor, 270
Granuloma inguinale
demeclocycline for, 85
doxycycline for, 102
Grifulvin V, 150
Grisactin, 150
Grisactin Ultra, 150
griseofulvin microsize, 150
griseofulvin ultramicrosize, 150
Griseostatin, 150
Grisovin, 150
Grisovin 500, 150
Grisovin-FP, 150
guaifenesin, 150
G-well, 182
Gynecologic infection
ampicillin/sulbactam for, 18
aztreonam for, 25
cefoperazone for, 51
cefotaxime for, 51
cefotetan for, 52
ceftazidime for, 54
ceftizoxime for, 55
ceftriaxone for, 56
imipenem and cilastatin for, 158
trovafloxacin for, 300
Gyne-Lotrimin, 73
Gynergen, 113
Gynogen L.A., 116

H

Habitrol, 220
Haemophilus influenzae infection
aztreonam for, 25
rifampin for, 265
Halcion, 299
Haldol, 151
Haldol Decanoate, 151
Haldol LA, 151
Halfprin, 20
haloperidol, 151
haloperidol decanoate, 151
haloperidol lactate, 151
Halotestin, 132
Halotussin, 150
Hansen's disease, dapsone for, 83
Headache
dihydroergotamine for, 92
ergotamine for, 113
naratriptan for, 216
rizatriptan for, 267
sumatriptan for, 281
timolol for, 291
valproate for, 302
zolmitriptan for, 309
Head and neck cancer, amifostine for, 12
Heart block, isoproterenol for, 169
Heartburn, famotidine for, 123
Heart failure
acetazolamide for, 4
amiloride for, 13
bumetanide for, 37
captopril for, 44
carvedilol for, 46-47
digoxin for, 90
dobutamine for, 97
fosinopril for, 138
inamrinone for, 159
Heart failure *(continued)*
lisinopril for, 185
metolazone for, 203
milrinone for, 208
nitroglycerin for, 222
nitroprusside for, 222
quinapril for, 258
ramipril for, 261
torsemide for, 295
trandolapril for, 296
Heart transplant recipients
cyclosporine for, 78
cytomegalovirus immune globulin (human), intravenous, for, 79
mycophenolate for, 213
Heat cramp, sodium chloride for, 275
Helicobacter pylori infection
clarithromycin for, 69
omeprazole for, 226
ranitidine for, 261
Hemolysis, folic acid for, 137
Hemophilia A, desmopressin for, 86
Hepalean, 151
Heparin overdose, protamine for, 255
heparin sodium, 151-152
Hepat-Amine, 13
Hepatic disease
amino acid infusions for, 13
bumetanide for, 37
folic acid for, 137
Hepatic encephalopathy, lactulose for, 174
Hepatitis B
interferon alfa-2b, recombinant, for, 165

Hepatitis B *(continued)*
lamivudine for, 174
Hepatitis C
interferon alfa-2b, recombinant, for, 165
interferon alfacon-1 for, 165
Herceptin, 297
Herpes simplex virus infection
acyclovir for, 5
famciclovir for, 122
foscarnet for, 138
valacyclovir for, 302
Herpes zoster
capsaicin for, 43
famciclovir for, 122
valacyclovir for, 302
Hexadrol, 86
High metabolic stress, amino acid infusions for, 13
Hip replacement surgery
dalteparin for, 81-82
danaparoid for, 82
enoxaparin for, 106
Histantil, 252
Histoplasmosis, itraconazole for, 171
Hivid, 306
Hodgkin's disease
bleomycin for, 34
carmustine for, 45
chlorambucil for, 61
cyclophosphamide for, 78
dacarbazine for, 80
doxorubicin for, 102
lomustine for, 186
mechlorethamine for, 192
procarbazine for, 251
thiotepa for, 288
vinblastine for, 304
vincristine for, 305
Hookworm infestation, mebendazole for, 192
Humalog, 163
Human immunodeficiency virus infection
abacavir for, 2
amprenavir for, 19
delavirdine for, 84
didanosine for, 90
efavirenz for, 105
indinavir for, 160
lamivudine for, 174
lamivudine/zidovudine for, 174
nelfinavir for, 217
nevirapine for, 218
ritonavir for, 266
saquinavir for, 269
stavudine for, 278
zalcitabine for, 306
zidovudine for, 308
Human immunodeficiency virus infection complications
alitretinoin for, 8
amphotericin B for, 17
azithromycin for, 25
cidofovir for, 64
clarithromycin for, 69
dronabinol for, 103
famciclovir for, 122
fomivirsen for, 137
foscarnet for, 138
ganciclovir for, 140
interferon alfa-2a, recombinant, for, 164
interferon alfa-2b, recombinant, for, 164
rifabutin for, 264
Humibid L.A., 150
Humulin 50/50, 163
Humulin 70/30, 163
Humulin L, 163
Humulin N, 163
Humulin NPH, 163
Humulin R, 163
Humulin U, 164
Hycamtin, 295
Hydatidiform mole, methotrexate for, 200
Hydeltrasol, 248
Hydeltra-T.B.A., 248
hydralazine hydrochloride, 152-153
Hydramine, 93
Hydrobexan, 77
hydrochlorothiazide, 153
Hydrocil, 255
Hydro-Cobex, 77
hydrocortisone acetate, 153-154
hydrocortisone butyrate, 154
hydrocortisone sodium phosphate, 153-154
hydrocortisone sodium succinate, 153-154
hydrocortisone (systemic), 153-154
hydrocortisone (topical), 154
hydrocortisone valerate, 154
Hydrocortone, 153
Hydrocortone Acetate, 153
Hydrocortone Phosphate, 153
Hydro-Crysti-12, 77
HydroDIURIL, 153
hydromorphone hydrochloride, 154-155
Hydrostat, 155
hydroxocobalamin, 77
hydroxyzine embonate, 155
hydroxyzine hydrochloride, 155
hydroxyzine pamoate, 155
Hygroton, 63
hyoscine butylbromide, 270
hyoscine hydrobromide, 270
hyoscine hydrobromide (systemic), 270
hyoscyamine, 155-156
hyoscyamine sulfate, 155-156
Hy-Pam, 155
Hyperbilirubinemia, albumin for, 6
Hypercalcemia
calcitonin for, 39
pamidronate for, 231
plicamycin for, 245
Hypercalciuria, plicamycin for, 245
Hypercholesterolemia
atorvastatin for, 21
cholestyramine for, 64
colestipol for, 75
fenofibrate for, 123
fluvastatin for, 136
lovastatin for, 188
niacin for, 219
pravastatin for, 248
simvastatin for, 273
Hyperglycemia. *See* Diabetes mellitus.
Hyperkalemia, sodium polystyrene sulfonate for, 276
Hyperkinesia, hydroxyzine for, 155
Hyperparathyroidism
calcitriol for, 39
paricalcitol for, 232
Hyperphosphatemia, calcium for, 41

Hyperprolactinemia, bromocriptine for, 35
Hypersecretory conditions
 famotidine for, 123
 omeprazole for, 226
 rabeprazole for, 260
 ranitidine for, 262
Hypersensitivity reactions. *See also* Allergies.
 epinephrine for, 108
Hyperstat IV, 89
Hypertension
 acebutolol for, 3
 amiloride for, 13
 amlodipine for, 15
 atenolol for, 20
 benazepril for, 29
 betaxolol for, 31
 bisoprolol for, 33
 candesartan for, 41
 captopril for, 43
 carteolol for, 46
 carvedilol for, 46
 chlorthalidone for, 63
 clonidine for, 71
 diltiazem for, 92
 doxazosin for, 101
 enalaprilat for, 105
 eprosartan for, 111
 esmolol for, 115
 felodipine for, 123
 fenoldopam for, 124
 fosinopril for, 138
 furosemide for, 139
 hydralazine for, 152
 hydrochlorothiazide for, 153
 indapamide for, 159
 irbesartan for, 168
 isradipine for, 170
 labetalol for, 173
 lisinopril for, 184
Hypertension *(continued)*
 losartan for, 188
 methyldopa for, 201
 metolazone for, 203
 metoprolol for, 204
 minoxidil for, 209
 nadolol for, 213
 nicardipine for, 219
 nifedipine for, 220
 nisoldipine for, 220
 nitroglycerin for, 222
 perindopril for, 237
 pindolol for, 243
 prazosin for, 248
 propranolol for, 254
 quinapril for, 258
 ramipril for, 261
 spironolactone for, 277
 telmisartan for, 282
 terazosin for, 284
 timolol for, 291
 torsemide for, 296
 trandolapril for, 296
 valsartan for, 303
 verapamil for, 304
Hypertensive crisis
 diazoxide for, 89
 labetalol for, 173
 methyldopa for, 201
 nitroprusside for, 222
Hyperthyroidism
 methimazole for, 199
 propylthiouracil for, 255
Hypertriglyceridemia
 atorvastatin for, 21
 fenofibrate for, 123-124
 fluvastatin for, 136
 simvastatin for, 273
Hypertrophic subaortic stenosis, propranolol for, 254
Hyperuricemia
 allopurinol for, 8
 probenecid for, 250
Hypnovel, 206
Hypocalcemia, calcitriol for, 39
Hypocalcemic emergency, calcium for, 40
Hypoglycemia, glucagon for, 147
Hypogonadism
 esterified estrogens for, 116
 estradiol for, 116
 estradiol/norethindrone acetate transdermal system for, 117
 estropipate for, 118
 ethinyl estradiol for, 119
 fluoxymesterone for, 132
 methyltestosterone for, 202
 testosterone for, 285
Hypokalemia
 potassium bicarbonate for, 246
 potassium chloride for, 246
 potassium gluconate for, 247
 spironolactone for, 278
Hypomagnesemia
 magnesium chloride for, 190
 magnesium oxide for, 191
 magnesium sulfate for, 190, 191
Hyponatremia, sodium chloride for, 275
Hypoparathyroidism, calcitriol for, 39
Hypoproteinemia, albumin for, 6
Hypoprothrombinemia, phytonadione for, 242
Hypotension
 dopamine for, 100
 fludrocortisone for, 129
 midodrine for, 207
 nitroglycerin for, 222
 norepinephrine for, 222
 phenylephrine for, 240
Hypovolemic shock, albumin for, 6
Hysterone, 132
Hytrin, 284
Hyzine-50, 155

I

ibuprofen, 156
ibutilide fumarate, 156-157
Idamycin, 157
idarubicin hydrochloride, 157
IFEX, 158
IFN-alpha 2, 164-165
ifosfamide, 158
Ifosfamide adverse effects, mesna for, 197
IL-2, 7
Ilosone, 114
Ilotycin Ophthalmic Ointment, 113
Imdur, 170
imipenem and cilastatin, 158
imipramine hydrochloride, 159
imipramine pamoate, 159
Imitrex, 281

Immunization
diphtheria and tetanus toxoids and acellular pertussis vaccine for, 94
Lyme disease vaccine (recombinant OspA) for, 189
meningococcal polysaccharide vaccine for, 195
pneumococcal 7-valent conjugate vaccine for, 245
Immunocompromised patients. *See also* Human immunodeficiency virus infection.
acyclovir for, 5
clotrimazole for, 73
ganciclovir for, 140
Immunosuppression
azathioprine for, 24
basiliximab for, 27
betamethasone for, 30
cyclosporine for, 78
daclizumab for, 80
methylprednisolone for, 202
mycophenolate for, 213
prednisolone for, 248
prednisone for, 249
triamcinolone for, 298
Imodium A-D, 186
Impacted cerumen, carbamide peroxide for, 44
Impetigo
cefuroxime for, 57
mupirocin for, 212
Impril, 159
Imuran, 24
inamrinone, 159
Inapsine, 104
indapamide, 159-160
Inderal, 254
Inderal LA, 254
indinavir sulfate, 160
drug interactions with, 317
Indochron E-R, 160
Indocid P.D.A., 160
Indocid SR, 160
Indocin, 160
Indocin I.V., 160
Indocin SR, 160
indomethacin, 160
indomethacin sodium trihydrate, 160
Infection. *See also* specific infections.
amikacin for, 12-13
amoxicillin for, 16
ceftriaxone for, 56
cefuroxime for, 56
clindamycin for, 70
demeclocycline for, 85
doxycycline for, 102
gentamicin for, 144
metronidazole for, 204
mezlocillin for, 205
minocycline for, 208
nafcillin for, 214
oxacillin for, 228
penicillin G potassium for, 235
penicillin G procaine for, 235
penicillin G sodium for, 236
piperacillin for, 244
sulfamethoxazole for, 279
sulfisoxazole for, 280
tetracycline for, 286
ticarcillin for, 289
tobramycin for, 293
vancomycin for, 303
Infergen, 165
Infertility, bromocriptine for, 35
Inflamase Forte, 249
Inflammation
aspirin for, 20
betamethasone for, 30-31
choline magnesium trisalicylate for, 64
dexamethasone for, 86-87
fluocinonide for, 131
fluticasone for, 135
hydrocortisone for, 153-154
methylprednisolone for, 202
prednisolone for, 248-249
prednisone for, 249
triamcinolone for, 298
infliximab, 161
Influenza
amantadine for, 11
oseltamivir for, 228
rimantadine for, 265
zanamivir for, 307
Infumorph 200, 211
Infusion rates, 320-324
for dobutamine, 322
for dopamine, 323
for epinephrine, 320
for isoproterenol, 320
for nitroglycerin, 321
for nitroprusside, 324
INH, 168-169
Innohep, 291-292
Inocor, 159
Insomnia
chloral hydrate for, 60
diphenhydramine for, 94
estazolam for, 115
flurazepam for, 133
lorazepam for, 187
pentobarbital for, 237
Insomnia *(continued)*
secobarbital for, 271
temazepam for, 282
triazolam for, 299
zaleplon for, 306
zolpidem for, 309
insulin aspart (rDNA origin) injection, 161-162
insulin glargine (rDNA) injection, 162
insulin injection, 163-164
insulin (lispro), 163-164
Insulin therapy replacement
glipizide for, 146
glyburide for, 148
insulin zinc suspension
extended (ultralente), 164
prompt (semilente), 163-164
insulin zinc suspension (lente), 163-164
Intal, 76
Intal Aerosol Spray, 76
Intal Nebulizer Solution, 76
Integrilin, 112
Intensive care unit patients, propofol for, 253
interferon alfa-2a, recombinant, 164
interferon alfa-2b, recombinant, 164-165
interferon alfacon-1, 165
interferon beta-1a for, 166
interferon beta-1b, recombinant, 166
interferon gamma-1b, 166
interleukin-2, 7

Intermittent claudication
cilostazol for, 65
pentoxifylline for, 237
Intestinal obstruction, folic acid for, 137
Intra-abdominal infection
ampicillin/sulbactam for, 18
aztreonam for, 25
cefepime for, 50
cefmetazole for, 50
cefoperazone for, 51
cefotaxime for, 51
cefotetan for, 52
cefoxitin for, 52
ceftazidime for, 54
ceftizoxime for, 55
ceftriaxone for, 56
imipenem and cilastatin for, 158
meropenem for, 196
trovafloxacin for, 300
Intraocular pressure elevation. *See also* Glaucoma.
betaxolol for, 31
carteolol for, 46
dipivefrin for, 95
dorzolamide for, 101
latanoprost for, 177
levobunolol for, 179
timolol for, 291
Intron A, 164
Intropin, 100
Intubated patients, propofol for, 253
Invirase, 269
Inza 250, 216
ipecac syrup, 167
ipratropium bromide, 167
ipratropium bromide nasal spray, 167
irbesartan, 168
Iridocyclitis, dexamethasone for, 86
irinotecan hydrochloride, 168
Iritis
atropine for, 22
scopolamine for, 270
Iron deficiency
ferrous fumarate for, 125
ferrous gluconate for, 126
ferrous sulfate for, 126
sodium ferric gluconate complex for, 275
Irritability, lorazepam for, 187
Irritable bowel syndrome
calcium polycarbophil for, 41
dicyclomine for, 90
ISMO, 170
Isonate, 170
isoniazid, 168-169
Isoniazid poisoning, pyridoxine for, 257
isonicotinic acid hydrazide, 168-169
isophane insulin suspension, 163-164
isophane insulin suspension with insulin injection, 163-164
isoproterenol, 169
infusion rates for, 320
isoproterenol hydrochloride, 169
isoproterenol sulfate, 169
Isoptin, 304
Isoptin SR, 304
Isopto Atropine, 22
Isopto Carpine, 242
Isopto Frin, 241
Isopto Hyoscine, 270, 271
Isorbid, 170
Isordil, 170
Isordil Tembids, 170
isosorbide dinitrate, 170
isosorbide mononitrate, 170
Isosorbide Tetradose, 170
Isotamine, 168
Isotrate, 170
isotretinoin, 170
isradipine, 170-171
Isuprel, 169
itraconazole, 171
I.V. Persantine, 95

J

Janimine, 159
Jenamicin, 144
Jenest-28, 120
Joint infection. *See* Bone and joint infection.
Joint replacement surgery
dalteparin for, 81-82
danaparoid for, 82
enoxaparin for, 106
Juvenile arthritis
choline magnesium trisalicylate for, 64
etanercept for, 118
ibuprofen for, 156
naproxen for, 216
sulfasalazine for, 280

K

K + Care ET, 246
K+10, 246
Kaluril, 13
Kaochlor 10%, 246
Kaon Liquid, 247
Kaopectate II Caplets, 186
Kaopectate Advanced Formula, 22-23
Kaposi's sarcoma
alitretinoin for, 8
interferon alfa-2a, recombinant, for, 164
interferon alfa-2b, recombinant, for, 164
Kasof, 98
Kayexalate, 276

K-Dur, 246
Keflex, 59
Keftab, 58
Kefurox, 56
Kefzol, 48
Kenalog, 298
Kenalog-10, 298
Kenalone, 298
Keppra, 178
Keratoplasty, dexamethasone for, 87
Kerlone, 31
ketoconazole, 171
ketoconazole (topical), 172
ketoprofen, 172
ketorolac tromethamine (ophthalmic), 172
ketorolac tromethamine (systemic), 173
Key-Pred-SP, 248
K-Ide, 246
Kidney transplant recipients
azathioprine for, 24
basiliximab for, 27
cyclosporine for, 78
cytomegalovirus immune globulin (human), intravenous, for, 79
daclizumab for, 80

Kidney transplant recipients (continued)
  mycophenolate for, 213
  sirolimus for, 273
Klonopin, 71
Klor-Con/EF, 246
K-Lyte, 246
K-Lyte/Cl, 246
Knee replacement surgery, enoxaparin for, 106
Konsyl, 255
Kristalose, 174
K-Tab, 246
Kwellada, 182
Kytril, 149

L

LA-12, 77
labetalol hydrochloride, 173
Labor
  oxytocin for induction of, 231
  pentazocine for, 236
Lactulax, 174
lactulose, 174
Lamictal, 175
Lamisil, 284
lamivudine, 174
lamivudine/zidovudine, 174-175
lamotrigine, 175-176
Laniazid, 168
Lanoxicaps, 90
Lanoxin, 90
lansoprazole, 176
Lantus, 162
Larodopa, 179
Larotid, 16
Lasix, 139
L-asparaginase, 20
latanoprost, 177
Laxative action. *See* Constipation.
Ledermycin, 85
leflunomide, 177
Legionnaires' disease
  dirithromycin for, 96
  gatifloxacin for, 141
Leg ulcers, becaplermin for, 27
Lennox-Gastaut syndrome
  clonazepam for, 71
  lamotrigine for, 175
Lente Insulin, 163
Leprosy, dapsone for, 83
Lescol, 136
letrozole, 177
leucovorin calcium, 177-178
Leukemia
  asparaginase for, 20
  busulfan for, 38
  chlorambucil for, 61
  cladribine for, 68
  cyclophosphamide for, 78
  cytarabine for, 79
  daunorubicin for, 84
  doxorubicin for, 102
  gemtuzumab ozogamicin for, 143
  idarubicin for, 157
  interferon alfa-2a, recombinant, for, 164
  interferon alfa-2b, recombinant, for, 164
  mechlorethamine for, 192
  mercaptopurine for, 196
  methotrexate for, 200
  pegaspargase for, 233
  tretinoin for, 298
  vincristine for, 305
Leukeran, 61
Leukine, 270
levalbuterol, 178
Levaquin, 180
Levbid, 156
levetiracetam, 178-179
levobunolol hydrochloride, 179
levodopa, 179
levodopa-carbidopa, 179-180
levofloxacin, 180-181
levonorgestrel, 181
Levophed, 222
levothyroxine sodium, 181-182
Levsin, 156
Levsin Drops, 156
Levsin S/L, 156
Libritabs, 61
Librium, 61
Lidex, 131
Lidex-E, 131
lidocaine hydrochloride, 182
LidoPen Auto-Injector, 182
lignocaine hydrochloride, 182
lindane, 182-183
linezolid, 183-184
Lioresal, 26
Lioresal Intrathecal, 26
liothyronine sodium, 184
Lipex, 273
Lipidil, 123
Lipitor, 21
Liquaemin Sodium, 151
Liqui-Char, 4
Liquid Pred, 249
lisinopril, 184-185
  drug interactions with, 317
Lithane, 185
Lithicarb, 185
lithium carbonate, 185
  drug interactions with, 317
lithium citrate, 185
Lithobid, 185
Lithonate, 185
Lithotabs, 185
Liver transplant recipients
  cyclosporine for, 78
  cytomegalovirus immune globulin (human), intravenous, for, 79
  mycophenolate for, 213
  tacrolimus for, 281
LoCholest, 64
Locoid, 154
Lodine, 121
Loestrin 21 1/20, 120
Loestrin Fe 1/20, 120
lomefloxacin hydrochloride, 185-186
Lomocot, 94
Lomotil, 94
lomustine, 186
Loniten, 209
Lonox, 94
loperamide, 186
Lopid, 143
Lopresor SR, 204
Lopressor, 204
Lopurin, 8
Lorabid, 186
loracarbef, 186-187
loratadine, 187
lorazepam, 187-188
Lorazepam Intensol, 187
Lorcet 10/650, 311
Lorcet Plus, 311
Lortab 2.5/500, 311
Lortab 5/500, 311
Lortab 7.5/500, 311
Lortab 10/500, 311
Lortab ASA, 311

losartan potassium, 188
Losec, 226
Losopan, 189
Lotensin, 29
Lotrimin, 73
lovastatin, 188-189
Lovenox, 106
Loxapac, 189
loxapine hydrochloride, 189
loxapine succinate, 189
Loxitane, 189
Loxitane C, 189
Loxitane IM, 189
Lozide, 159
Lozol, 159
L-phenylalanine mustard, 195
L-thyroxine sodium, 181-182
Luminal Sodium, 239
Lung cancer
  amifostine for, 12
  docetaxel for, 98
  doxorubicin for, 101
  etoposide for, 121
  topotecan for, 295
  vinorelbine for, 305
Lung transplant recipients, cytomegalovirus immune globulin (human), intravenous, for, 79
Luvox, 136
Luxiq, 31
Lyme disease
  ceftriaxone for, 56
  cefuroxime for, 57-58
  doxycycline for, 102
Lyme disease vaccine (recombinant OspA), 189
LYMErix, 189
Lymphoma. *See also* Hodgkin's disease.
  bexarotene for, 32
  bleomycin for, 34
  carmustine for, 45
  chlorambucil for, 61
  cyclophosphamide for, 78
  doxorubicin for, 102
  rituximab for, 266
  thiotepa for, 288
  vinblastine for, 304
Lymphosarcoma
  bleomycin for, 34
  chlorambucil for, 61
Lyphocin, 303

M

Mac, 221
Macrobid, 221
Macrocytic anemia, folic acid for, 137
Macrodantin, 221
magaldrate, 189
Magan, 191
magnesium chloride, 190
magnesium citrate, 190
magnesium hydroxide, 190
Magnesium intoxication, calcium for, 40
magnesium oxide, 191
magnesium salicylate, 191
magnesium sulfate, 190-192
Mag-Ox, 191
Malaria
  chloroquine for, 62
  primaquine for, 249
  pyrimethamine for, 257
Male pattern baldness, finasteride for, 128
Manganese-induced parkinsonism, levodopa-carbidopa for, 179
Mania
  lithium for, 185
  olanzapine for, 225
  valproate for, 302
mannitol, 192
Maox 420, 191
Marinol, 103
Matulane, 251
Mavik, 296
Maxair, 245
Maxair Autohaler, 245
Maxalt, 267
Maxalt-MLT, 267
Maxaquin, 185
Maxidex Ophthalmic, 86-87
Maxidex Ophthalmic Suspension, 86
Maxipime, 49
Maxivate, 31
Maxolon, 203
mebendazole, 192
Mechanically ventilated patients, propofol for, 253
mechlorethamine hydrochloride, 192-193
meclizine hydrochloride, 193
Medihaler-Epi, 108
Medihaler Ergotamine, 113
Medihaler-Iso, 169
Medralone, 202
Medrol, 202
medroxyprogesterone acetate, 193
Mefoxin, 52
Megace, 193
Megacillin, 235
Megaloblastic anemia
  folic acid for, 137
  leucovorin for, 178
megestrol acetate, 193-194
Megostat, 193
Melanoma
  dacarbazine for, 80
  interferon alfa-2b, recombinant, for, 165
Melipramine, 159
Mellaril, 288
Mellaril Concentrate, 288
Mellaril-S, 288
meloxicam, 194
melphalan, 195
Menaval-20, 116
Menest, 116
Meni-D, 193
Meningitis
  amphotericin B for, 17
  ceftizoxime for, 55
  ceftriaxone for, 56
  fluconazole for, 129
  gentamicin for, 144
  meningococcal polysaccharide vaccine for prevention of, 195
  meropenem for, 196
Meningococcal carrier state
  minocycline for, 208
  rifampin for, 264
meningococcal polysaccharide vaccine, 195
Menomune-A/C/Y/W-135, 195
Menopausal symptoms
  estradiol for, 116

Menopausal symptoms *(continued)*
estradiol/norethindrone acetate transdermal system for, 117
estropipate for, 118
ethinyl estradiol for, 120
meperidine hydrochloride, 195-196
Mephyton, 242
Mepron, 21
mercaptopurine, 196
6-mercaptopurine, 196
Meridia, 272
meropenem, 196-197
Merrem IV, 196
mesalamine, 197
mesna, 197
Mesnex, 197
mesoridazine besylate, 197-198
Mestinon, 256
Mestinon-SR, 256
Mestinon Timespans, 256
mestranol, 121
Metabolic acidosis, sodium bicarbonate for, 275
Metabolic bone disease, calcitriol for, 39
Metamucil, 255
Metaprel, 198
metaproterenol sulfate, 198
metformin hydrochloride, 198-199
methadone, 199
Methadose, 199
methamphetamine, 199
Methergine, 201
methimazole, 199-200
methocarbamol, 200
methotrexate, 200
drug interactions with, 317
Methotrexate adverse effects, leucovorin for, 177
methotrexate sodium, 200
methylcellulose, 201
methyldopa, 201
methyldopa hydrochloride, 201
methylergonovine maleate, 201
Methylmalonic aciduria, cyanocobalamin for, 77
methylphenidate hydrochloride, 201-202
methylprednisolone, 202
methylprednisolone acetate, 202
methylprednisolone sodium succinate, 202
methyltestosterone, 202-203
Meticorten, 249
metoclopramide hydrochloride, 203
metolazone, 203
metoprolol succinate, 204
metoprolol tartrate, 204
drug interactions with, 317
MetroGel, 205
MetroGel-Vaginal, 205
Metro I.V., 204
Metro Lotion, 205
metronidazole hydrochloride, 204-205
metronidazole (systemic), 204-205
metronidazole (topical), 205
Metrozine, 204
Mevacor, 188
mevinolin, 188-189
Mexate-AQ, 200
mexiletine hydrochloride, 205
Mexitil, 205
Mezlin, 205-206
mezlocillin sodium, 205-206
Miacalcin, 39
Miacalcin Nasal Spray, 39
Micardis, 282
Micatin, 206
miconazole nitrate, 206
Micro, 123
Micronase, 147
Micronor, 223
Microzide, 153
Midamor, 13
midazolam hydrochloride, 206
midodrine hydrochloride, 207
Midol Maximum Strength Cramp Formula, 156
miglitol, 207-208
Migraine
dihydroergotamine for, 92
ergotamine for, 113
naratriptan for, 216
rizatriptan for, 267
sumatriptan for, 281
timolol for, 291
valproate for, 302
zolmitriptan for, 309
Migranal, 92
milk of magnesia, 190
milrinone lactate, 208
Minax, 204
Minidiab, 146
Minimal change nephrotic syndrome, cyclophosphamide for, 78
Minipress, 248
Minirin, 85
Minitran, 221
Minocin, 208
Minocin IV, 208
minocycline hydrochloride, 208-209
minoxidil (oral), 209
Miocarpine, 242
Mirapex, 247
mirtazapine, 209
misoprostol, 209
Mithracin, 245
mithramycin, 245
mitomycin, 210
mitomycin-C, 210
Mitrolan, 41
Moban, 210
Mobic, 194
Mobidin, 191
modafinil, 210
Modane Bulk, 255-256
Modecate, 133
Moditen Enanthate, 133
Moditen HCl, 133
molindone hydrochloride, 210
Mol-Iron, 126
Momentum Muscular Backache Formula, 191
Monistat, 206
Monistat-Derm Cream and Lotion, 206
Monocid, 50
Monodox, 103
Monoket, 170
Monopril, 138
montelukast sodium, 211
moricizine hydrochloride, 211

Morphine H.P., 211
morphine hydrochloride, 211
morphine sulfate, 211
morphine tartrate, 211
Morphitec, 211
M.O.S., 211
Motion sickness
dimenhydrinate for, 93
diphenhydramine for, 93
meclizine for, 193
promethazine for, 252
scopolamine for, 270
Motrin, 156
Motrin-IB Caplets, 156
Motrin-IB Tablets, 156
Motrin Migraine Pain, 156
moxifloxacin hydrochloride, 212
M-Oxy, 230
6-MP, 196
MS Contin, 211
MSIP, 211
MTX, 200
Mucomyst, 4
Mucomyst 10, 4
Mucosil-10, 4
Mucosil-20, 4
Mucus secretions, acetylcysteine for, 4
Multipax, 155
Multiple myeloma
carmustine for, 45
cyclophosphamide for, 78
melphalan for, 195
pamidronate for, 232
Multiple sclerosis
baclofen for, 26
dantrolene for, 83
glatiramer acetate for injection for, 145
interferon beta-1a for, 166
Multiple sclerosis *(continued)*
interferon beta-1b, recombinant, for, 166
methylprednisolone for, 202
mupirocin, 212
Murine Ear Drops, 44
Muscle spasm. *See* Spasticity.
Musculoskeletal conditions
carisoprodol for, 45
methocarbamol for, 200
Mustargen, 192
Mutamycin, 210
Myambutol, 119
Myasthenia gravis
neostigmine for, 218
pyridostigmine for, 256
Mycelex, 73
Mycelex-7, 73
Mycelex-G, 73
Mycelex OTC, 73
Mycifradin, 217
Myciguent, 217
Mycobacterium avium complex infection
azithromycin for, 25
clarithromycin for, 69
rifabutin for, 264
Mycobutin, 264
mycophenolate mofetil, 213
mycophenolate mofetil hydrochloride, 213
Mycosis fungoides, cyclophosphamide for, 78
Mycostatin, 224
Mydfrin, 241
Mydriasis
phenylephrine for, 241
pilocarpine for, 243
My-E, 114
Mykrox, 203
Mylanta Gas, 273
Myleran, 38
Mylicon, 273
Mylotarg, 143
Myocardial infarction
alteplase for, 10
aspirin for, 20
atenolol for, 21
captopril for, 44
clopidogrel for, 72
enoxaparin for, 106
eptifibatide for, 112
heparin for, 151
lidocaine for, 182
lisinopril for, 185
metoprolol for, 204
pravastatin after, 248
propranolol for, 254
ramipril for, 261
reteplase, recombinant, for, 263
tenecteplase for, 283
timolol for, 291
warfarin for, 305
Myocardial perfusion scintigraphy, dipyridamole for, 95
Myotonachol, 32
Myrosemide, 139
Mysoline, 250
Myxedema coma
levothyroxine for, 181
liothyronine for, 184
M-Zole, 206

N

nabumetone, 213
nadolol, 213-214
Nadostine, 224
nafcillin sodium, 214
nalbuphine hydrochloride, 214
Nalfon, 124
Nalfon 200, 124
Nallpen, 214
naloxone hydrochloride, 214-215
naltrexone hydrochloride, 215
naphazoline hydrochloride (ophthalmic), 215
Naphcon, 215
Naphcon Forte, 215
Naprelan, 216
Naprogesic, 216
Naprosyn, 216
Naprosyn SR, 216
naproxen, 216
naproxen sodium, 216
naratriptan hydrochloride, 216
Narcan, 214
Narcolepsy
dextroamphetamine for, 87
methylphenidate for, 202
modafinil for, 210
Narcotic analgesic combination products, 311-312
Narcotic depression, postoperative, naloxone for, 215
Narcotic-induced respiratory depression, naloxone for, 214
Narcotic withdrawal syndrome, methadone for, 199
Nasacort, 299
Nasal congestion
oxymetazoline for, 230
phenylephrine for, 241

Nasal congestion *(continued)*
pseudoephedrine for, 255
xylometazoline for, 306
Nasalcrom, 76
Nasalide, 130
Nasal polyps, beclomethasone for, 28
Natrilix, 159
Natulan, 251
natural lung surfactant, 30
Nausea and vomiting. *See also* Motion sickness.
chlorpromazine for, 63
dolasetron for, 99-100
dronabinol for, 103
granisetron for, 149
hydroxyzine for, 155
metoclopramide for, 203
ondansetron for, 227
perphenazine for, 238
prochlorperazine for, 251
promethazine for, 252
Navane, 288, 289
Navelbine, 305
Nebcin, 293
NebuPent, 236
nefazodone hydrochloride, 217
nelfinavir mesylate, 217
Nembutal, 237
Nembutal Sodium, 237
Neo-Calglucon, 40
NeoEstrone, 116
Neo-fradin, 217
Neo-Metric, 204
neomycin sulfate (oral), 217
drug interactions with, 317
neomycin sulfate (topical), 217
Neopap, 3
Neoquess, 156
Neoral, 78
Neosar, 78
Neo-Spec, 150
neostigmine bromide, 218
neostigmine methylsulfate, 218
Neosulf, 217
Neo-Synephrine, 240, 241
Neo-Synephrine II, 306
Neo-Synephrine 12-Hr Nasal Spray, 230
Neo-Tabs, 217
Nephritis, magnesium sulfate for, 191
Nephrotic syndrome, cyclophosphamide for, 78
Nephrox, 11
Nestrex, 257
Neumega, 227
Neupogen, 127
Neuralgia, capsaicin for, 43
Neuroblastoma
cyclophosphamide for, 78
doxorubicin for, 102
Neuromuscular blockade reversal
neostigmine for, 218
pyridostigmine for, 256
Neurontin, 140
Neurosurgery patients, fosphenytoin for, 139
Neutropenic patients
cefepime for, 50
filgrastim for, 127
nevirapine, 218
Niac, 219
niacin, 219
niacinamide, 219
Niacor, 219
nicardipine, 219
Nico-400, 219
Nicobid, 219
Nicoderm, 220
Nicolar, 219
Nicorette, 219
Nicorette DS, 219
nicotinamide, 219
nicotine polacrilex, 219
nicotine resin complex, 219
nicotine transdermal system, 220
Nicotine withdrawal
nicotine polacrilex for, 219
nicotine transdermal system for, 220
nicotinic acid, 219
Nicotrol, 220
Nicotrol NS, 219
nifedipine, 220
Nilandron, 220
Nilstat, 224
nilutamide, 220
nisoldipine, 220-221
Nitro-Bid, 221
Nitrocine, 221
Nitrodisc, 221
Nitro-Dur, 221
nitrofurantoin macrocrystals, 221
nitrofurantoin microcrystals, 221
nitrofurazone, 221
Nitrogard, 221
nitrogen mustard, 192-193
nitroglycerin, 221-222
infusion rates for, 321
Nitroglyn, 221
Nitrol, 221
Nitrolingual, 221
Nitropress, 222
nitroprusside, 222
infusion rates for, 324
Nitrostat, 221
nizatidine, 222
Nizoral, 171, 172
Noctec, 60
Nolvadex, 282
Nolvadex-D, 282
Nordette, 120
norepinephrine bitartrate, 222-223
Norepinephrine extravasation, phentolamine for dermal necrosis from, 240
norethindrone, 223
norethindrone acetate, 223
norfloxacin, 223
Norfranil, 159
norgestrel, 223
Norisodrine Aerotrol, 169
Noritate, 205
Norlu, 223
Normodyne, 173
Noroferrogluc, 126
Norpace, 96
Norpace CR, 96
Norplant System, 181
Norpramin, 85
Nor-Pred T.B.A., 248-249
Nor-Q.D., 223
nortriptyline hydrochloride, 223
Norvasc, 15
Norvir, 266
Nostrilla Long-Acting Spray, 230
Noten, 20
Novamine, 13
Nova Rectal, 237

Novo-Alprazol, 9
Novo-AZT, 308
Novo-Captoril, 43
Novo-Carbamaz, 44
Novo-Chlorhydrate, 60
Novoclopate, 72
Novocolchicine, 74
Novodigoxin, 90
Novo-Doxepin, 101
Novoflupam, 133
Novofolacid, 136
Novofumar, 125
Novohexidyl, 300
Novo-Hydrazide, 153
Novo-Hylazin, 152
Novolin 70/30, 163
Novolin L, 163
Novolin N, 163
Novolin R, 163
NovoLog, 161
Novo-Lorazem, 187
Novomedopa, 201
Novo-Methacin, 160
Novo-Naprox, 216
Novonidazol, 204
Novo-Peridol, 151
Novo-Pirocam, 245
Novo-Poxide, 61
Novopranol, 254
Novo-Ridazine, 288
Novosecobarb, 271
Novosemide, 139
Novo-Soxazole, 280
Novo-Spiroton, 277
Novo-Sundac, 280
Novo-Thalidone, 63
Novo-Veramil, 304
NPH, 163-164
NPH Insulin, 163
Nu-Alpraz, 9
Nu-Atenol, 20
Nubain, 214
Nu-Hydral, 152
Nu-Ibuprofen, 156
Nu-Loraz, 187
Nu-Nifed, 220
Nuprin Caplets, 156
Nuprin Tablets, 156
Nutritional support
  amino acid infusions for, 13
  dextrose for, 88
Nu-Verap, 304
Nydrazid, 168
nystatin, 224
Nystex, 224
Nytol Maximum Strength, 93

O

Obe-Nix, 239
Obesity
  dextroamphetamine for, 87
  methamphetamine for, 199
  orlistat for, 228
  phentermine for, 239
  sibutramine for, 272
Obsessive-compulsive disorder
  clomipramine for, 70
  fluoxetine for, 132
  fluvoxamine for, 136
  paroxetine for, 233
  sertraline for, 271-272
Obstetric patients
  bisacodyl for, 33
  folic acid for, 136-137
  magnesium sulfate for, 191
  oxytocin for, 231
  pentazocine for, 236
  scopolamine for, 270
  zidovudine for, 308
Obstructive airway disease. *See also* Asthma; Chronic obstructive pulmonary disease.
  albuterol for, 6-7
  levalbuterol for, 178
Obstructive airway disease *(continued)*
  salmeterol for, 269
  terbutaline for, 285
Octamide, 203
octreotide acetate, 224
Ocular congestion, naphazoline for, 215
Ocular hypertension. See Intraocular pressure elevation.
Ocu-Mycin, 144
Ocupress Ophthalmic Solution, 1%, 46
Ocusert Pilo, 242
oestradiol valerate, 116-117
oestrogens, conjugated, 118
ofloxacin, 224-225
Ogen, 118
olanzapine, 225
Oliguria, mannitol for, 192
olsalazine sodium, 226
omeprazole, 226-227
Omnicef, 48
Oncaspar, 233
Oncovin, 305
ondansetron hydrochloride, 227
Onychomycosis
  itraconazole for, 171
  terbinafine for, 284
Ophthalmia neonatorum, erythromycin for, 114
Opioid-detoxified patients, naltrexone for, 215
opium tincture, 227
  camphorated, 227
oprelvekin, 227-228
Optazine, 215
Oral lesions, triamcinolone for, 298
Oramorph SR, 211
Orap, 243
Oretic, 153
Oreton Methyl, 202
Organic mental syndrome, mesoridazine for, 197
Organ rejection. *See also* Transplant recipients.
  basiliximab for, 27
  cyclosporine for, 78
  daclizumab for, 80
  mycophenolate for, 213
  sirolimus for, 273
  tacrolimus for, 281
Orgaran, 82
orlistat, 228
Ormazine, 63
Ortho-Cyclen, 120
OrthoEST, 118
Ortho-Novum 7/7/7, 120
Orthostatic hypotension
  fludrocortisone for, 129
  midodrine for, 207
Ortho Tri-Cyclen, 120
Orudis, 172
Os-Cal 500, 41
oseltamivir phosphate, 228
Osmitrol, 192
Osteitis deformans. *See* Paget's disease of bone.
Osteoarthritis
  capsaicin for, 43
  celecoxib for, 58
  diclofenac for, 89
  diflunisal for, 90
  etodolac for, 121
  fenoprofen for, 124
  flurbiprofen for, 134

Osteoarthritis *(continued)*
- ibuprofen for, 156
- indomethacin for, 160
- ketoprofen for, 172
- meloxicam for, 194
- nabumetone for, 213
- naproxen for, 216
- oxaprozin for, 229
- piroxicam for, 245
- rofecoxib for, 267
- sulindac for, 280

Osteocalcin, 39
Osteopetrosis, interferon gamma-1b for, 166
Osteoporosis
- alendronate for, 7-8
- calcitonin for, 39
- esterified estrogens for, 116
- estradiol for, 117
- estradiol/norethindrone acetate transdermal system for, 117
- estrogens, conjugated, for, 118
- estropipate for, 118
- raloxifene for, 261

Osteosarcoma, doxorubicin for, 101
Otitis media
- amoxicillin/clavulanate potassium, 16
- azithromycin for, 24
- cefaclor for, 47
- cefdinir for, 48
- cefpodoxime for, 53
- cefprozil for, 54
- ceftibuten for, 55
- ceftriaxone for, 56
- cefuroxime for, 56, 57
- cephalexin for, 58
- cephradine for, 59

Otitis media *(continued)*
- loracarbef for, 187

Otrivin, 306
Ovarian cancer
- amifostine for, 12
- carboplatin for, 45
- cisplatin for, 67
- cyclophosphamide for, 78
- doxorubicin for, 101
- melphalan for, 195
- paclitaxel for, 231
- thiotepa for, 288
- topotecan for, 295

Ovarian failure
- esterified estrogens for, 116
- estradiol for, 116
- estradiol/norethindrone acetate transdermal system for, 117
- estrogens, conjugated, for, 118
- estropipate for, 118

Ovral, 120
Ovrette, 223
oxacillin sodium, 228-229
oxaprozin, 229
oxazepam, 229
oxcarbazepine, 229-230
oxycodone hydrochloride, 230
oxycodone pectinate, 230
OxyContin, 230
Oxyfast, 230
Oxy IR, 230
oxymetazoline hydrochloride (nasal), 230-231
oxytocin, synthetic injection, 231

P

Pacerone, 15
paclitaxel, 231
Paget's disease of bone, 290
- alendronate for, 8
- calcitonin for, 39
- pamidronate for, 232

Pain
- acetaminophen for, 3
- aspirin for, 20
- butorphanol for, 38
- capsaicin for, 43
- choline magnesium trisalicylate for, 64
- codeine for, 74
- diclofenac for, 90
- diflunisal for, 90
- etodolac for, 121
- fenoprofen for, 124
- fentanyl for, 125
- hydromorphone for, 154
- ibuprofen for, 156
- ketoprofen for, 172
- ketorolac for, 173
- magnesium salicylate for, 191
- meperidine for, 195
- methadone for, 199
- morphine for, 211
- nalbuphine for, 214
- naproxen for, 216
- narcotic analgesic combination products for, 311-312
- oxycodone for, 230
- pentazocine for, 236
- propoxyphene for, 253
- rofecoxib for, 267
- tramadol for, 296

Palafer, 125
Pamelor, 223
pamidronate disodium, 231-232
Panadol, 3
Panasol, 249
Pancreas transplant recipients, cytomegalovirus immune globulin (human), intravenous, for, 79
Pancreatic cancer
- fluorouracil for, 131
- gemcitabine for, 142
- mitomycin for, 210
- streptozocin for, 279

Panic disorder
- alprazolam for, 9
- paroxetine for, 233
- sertraline for, 272

Panmycin P, 286
Panretin, 8
pantoprazole, 232
paracetamol, 3
Parapectolin, 23
Paraplatin, 45
Paraplatin-AQ, 45
Parasitic infestation, lindane for, 182
paregoric, 227
paricalcitol, 232
Parkinsonism
- amantadine for, 12
- benztropine for, 29
- bromocriptine for, 35
- diphenhydramine for, 93
- entacapone for, 107
- levodopa for, 179
- levodopa-carbidopa for, 179
- pergolide for, 237
- pramipexole for, 247
- ropinirole for, 268
- selegiline for, 271
- tolcapone for, 294
- trihexyphenidyl for, 300

Parlodel, 35

Parotid gland cancer, amifostine for, 12
paroxetine hydrochloride, 233
Paroxysmal atrial tachycardia
magnesium sulfate for, 192
quinidine for, 259
Paroxysmal supraventricular tachycardia
adenosine for, 6
digoxin for, 90
diltiazem for, 92
flecainide for, 128
quinidine for, 259
Paroxysmal ventricular tachycardia, quinidine for, 259
Patent ductus arteriosus, alprostadil for, 10
Paveral, 74
Paxil, 233
PCE, 114
Pedia Care Infant's Decongestant, 255
Pedia Profen, 156
Pediculosis, lindane for, 182
pegaspargase, 233
PEG-L-asparaginase, 233
Pellagra
niacin for, 219
riboflavin for, 264
Pelvic infection, trovafloxacin for, 300
Pelvic inflammatory disease
clindamycin for, 70
doxycycline for, 103
erythromycin for, 114
ofloxacin for, 225
Pelvic inflammatory disease *(continued)*
piperacillin and tazobactam for, 244
pemoline, 234
penicillamine, 234
penicillin, drug interactions with, 317
penicillin G benzathine, 234-235
penicillin G potassium, 235
penicillin G procaine, 235
penicillin G sodium, 236
Pentacarinat, 236
Pentam 300, 236
pentamidine isethionate, 236
pentazocine hydrochloride, 236
pentazocine hydrochloride and naloxone hydrochloride, 236
pentazocine lactate, 236
pentobarbital, 237
pentobarbital sodium, 237
pentoxifylline, 237
Pepcid, 122
Pepcid AC, 122
Pepcidine, 122
Peptic ulcer disease
cimetidine for, 65-66
famotidine for, 122-123
hyoscyamine for, 155
lansoprazole for, 176
misoprostol for prevention of, 209
nizatidine for, 222
omeprazole for, 226
rabeprazole for, 260
ranitidine for, 261-262
sucralfate for, 279
Pepto-Bismol, 33
Percocet, 311
Percodan, 312
Percodan-Demi, 311
Percolone, 230
Percutaneous transluminal coronary angioplasty
abciximab for, 2
tirofiban for, 292
pergolide mesylate, 237
Peridol, 151
perindopril erbumine, 237-238
Perioperative prophylaxis
cefazolin for, 48
cefonicid for, 50
cefotaxime for, 51
cefotetan for, 52
cefoxitin for, 52-53
cefuroxime for, 56
cephradine for, 59
neomycin for, 217
piperacillin for, 244
Peripheral arterial disease, clopidogrel for, 72
Peritonitis, meropenem for, 196
Permapen, 235
Permax, 237
Permitil Concentrate, 133
Pernicious anemia, cyanocobalamin for, 77
perphenazine, 238
Persantin, 95
Persantine, 95
Pertofran, 85
Pertofrane, 85
pethidine hydrochloride, 195-196
Pfizerpen, 235
Pharyngitis
azithromycin for, 24
cefadroxil for, 47
cefdinir for, 49
cefpodoxime for, 54
cefprozil for, 54
ceftibuten for, 55
cefuroxime for, 56, 57
clarithromycin for, 69
loracarbef for, 186
Phazyme, 273
Phenaphen/Codeine No. 3, 312
Phenaphen/Codeine No. 4, 312
Phenazine, 252
Phenazo, 239
phenazopyridine hydrochloride, 239
Phencen, 252
Phenergan, 252
Phenergan Fortis, 252
Phenergan Syrup Plain, 252
phenobarbital, 239
phenobarbital sodium, 239
phenobarbitone, 239
phenobarbitone sodium, 239
Phenoject, 252
Phentercot, 239
phentermine hydrochloride, 239-240
phentolamine mesylate, 240
Phentride, 239
phenylazo diamino pyridine hydrochloride, 239
phenylephrine hydrochloride (nasal), 241
phenylephrine hydrochloride (ophthalmic), 241

phenylephrine hydrochloride (systemic), 240-241
Phenytex, 241
phenytoin, 241-242
phenytoin sodium, 241-242
phenytoin sodium (extended), 241-242
Pheochromocytoma
  phentolamine for diagnosis of, 240
  propranolol for, 254
Pheochromocytomectomy, phentolamine for, 240
Phillips' Milk of Magnesia, 190
Phos-Lo, 40
phosphonoformic acid, 138
Phyllocontin, 14
Physeptone, 199
phytonadione, 242
Pilagan, 242
Pilocar, 242
pilocarpine, 242-243
pilocarpine hydrochloride, 242-243
pilocarpine nitrate, 242-243
Pilopt, 242
Pima, 247
pimozide, 243
pindolol, 243
Pink Bismuth, 33
Pinworm infestation, mebendazole for, 192
pioglitazone hydrochloride, 243-244
piperacillin sodium, 244
piperacillin sodium and tazobactam sodium, 244
piperazine estrone sulfate, 118
Pipracil, 244
Pipril, 244
pirbuterol acetate, 245
piroxicam, 245
Pitocin, 231
Pitressin, 303
Pituitary trauma, desmopressin for, 85
Platamine, 67
Platelet adhesion, dipyridamole for inhibition of, 95
Platelet transfusions, oprelvekin to reduce need for, 227
Platinol, 67
Platinol AQ, 67
Plavix, 72
Plendil, 123
Plendil ER, 123
Pletal, 65
Pleural effusions, bleomycin for, 34
plicamycin, 245
PMS-Benztropine, 29
PMS Isoniazid, 168
PMS-Methylphenidate, 201
PMS Metronidazole, 204
PMS Perphenazine, 238
PMS Primidone, 250
PMS Prochlorperazine, 251
PMS-Promethazine, 253
PMS Thioridazine, 288
pneumococcal 7-valent conjugate vaccine (diphtheria CRM197 protein), 245-246
Pneumocystis carinii pneumonia
  atovaquone for, 21
  co-trimoxazole for, 75
Pneumocystis carinii pneumonia *(continued)*
  pentamidine for, 236
Pneumonia
  acetylcysteine for, 4
  atovaquone for, 21
  azithromycin for, 24
  bacitracin for, 26
  cefdinir for, 48
  cefepime for, 49
  cefpodoxime for, 53
  co-trimoxazole for, 75
  dirithromycin for, 96
  gatifloxacin for, 141
  levofloxacin for, 180
  linezolid for, 183, 184
  moxifloxacin for, 212
  penicillin G procaine for, 235
  piperacillin and tazobactam for, 244
  sparfloxacin for, 277
  trovafloxacin for, 300, 301
Poisoning
  activated charcoal for, 4-5
  ipecac syrup for, 167
Polydipsia, desmopressin for, 85
Polymox, 16
polymyxin B sulfate, 246
Polyuria, desmopressin for, 85
Postmenopausal women
  alendronate for, 7-8
  anastrozole for, 19-20
  calcitonin for, 39
  esterified estrogens for, 116
  estradiol for, 117
  estradiol/norethindrone acetate transdermal system for, 117
Postmenopausal women *(continued)*
  estrogens, conjugated, for, 118
  raloxifene for, 261
Postpartum bleeding
  methylergonovine for, 201
  oxytocin for, 231
Posttraumatic stress disorder, sertraline for, 272
Posture, 40
potassium, drug interactions with, 317
potassium bicarbonate, 246
potassium chloride, 246
potassium gluconate, 247
potassium iodide, 247
  saturated solution, 247
pramipexole dihydrochloride, 247
Prandin, 262
Pravachol, 248
pravastatin sodium, 248
prazosin hydrochloride, 248
Precose, 2
Pred-Forte, 249
Prednicen-M, 249
prednisolone, 248-249
prednisolone acetate (suspension), 249
prednisolone sodium phosphate, 248-249
prednisolone tebutate, 248-249
prednisone, 249
Prednisone Intensol, 249
Preeclampsia, magnesium sulfate for, 191

Prefrin Liquifilm Relief, 241
Pregnancy prevention. *See* Contraception.
Premarin, 118
Premarin Intravenous, 118
Premature atrial contractions, quinidine for, 259
Premature infants
 beractant for, 30
 respiratory syncytial virus immune globulin, intravenous, human, for, 263
Premature ventricular contractions
 mexiletine for, 205
 quinidine for, 259
Premenstrual dysphoric disorder, fluoxetine for, 132
Premyxedema coma, liothyronine for, 184
Preoperative prophylaxis. *See* Perioperative prophylaxis.
Preoperative sedation
 chloral hydrate for, 60
 droperidol for, 104
 hydroxyzine for, 155
 lorazepam for, 188
 midazolam for, 206
 pentobarbital for, 237
 phenobarbital for, 239
 promethazine for, 253
 scopolamine for, 270
 secobarbital for, 271
Presolol, 173
Prevacid, 176
Prevalite, 64
Prevnar, 245
Priftin, 265
Prilosec, 226
Primacor, 208
primaquine phosphate, 249
Primatene Mist, 108
Primaxin IM, 158
Primaxin IV, 158
primidone, 250
Prinivil, 184
ProAmatine, 207
probenecid, 250
procainamide hydrochloride, 250-251
Procanbid, 250
procarbazine hydrochloride, 251
Procardia, 220
Procardia XL, 220
prochlorperazine, 251-252
prochlorperazine edisylate, 251-252
prochlorperazine maleate, 251-252
Procrit, 110
Proctitis
 hydrocortisone for, 154
 mesalamine for, 197
Proctosigmoiditis, mesalamine for, 197
Procytox, 78
Prodium, 239
progesterone, 252
Prograf, 281
Proleukin, 7
Prolixin, 133
Prolixin Concentrate, 133
Prolixin Decanoate, 133
Prolixin Enanthate, 133
Proloprim, 300
promethazine hydrochloride, 252-253
promethazine theoclate, 253
Prometrium, 252
Pronestyl, 250
Pronestyl-SR, 250
Propacet 100, 311
Propecia, 128
Propine, 95
propofol, 253
propoxyphene hydrochloride, 253
propoxyphene napsylate, 253
Propoxyphene Napsylate/Acetaminophen, 312
propranolol hydrochloride, 254
 drug interactions with, 317
propylthiouracil, 255
Propyl-Thyracil, 255
Prorazin, 251
Proscar, 128
ProSom, 115
Prostate biopsy, transrectal, lomefloxacin for, 186
Prostate cancer
 esterified estrogens for, 116
 estradiol for, 117
 ethinyl estradiol for, 120
 flutamide for, 134
 goserelin for, 149
 nilutamide for, 220
Prostatic hyperplasia, benign
 doxazosin for, 101
 finasteride for, 128
 tamsulosin for, 282
 terazosin for, 284
Prostatitis
 ciprofloxacin for, 66, 67
Prostatitis *(continued)*
 co-trimoxazole for, 75
 ofloxacin for, 225
ProStep, 220
Prosthetic heart valve patients
 dipyridamole for, 95
 warfarin for, 305
Prostigmin, 218
Prostin VR Pediatric, 10
protamine sulfate, 255
protamine zinc suspension, 164
Prothazine, 253
Protonix, 232
Protostat, 204
Proventil, 6, 7
Proventil Repetabs, 7
Provera, 193
Provigil, 210
Prozac, 132
Prozac 20, 132
Pruritus
 cholestyramine for, 64
 fluticasone for, 135
 hydroxyzine for, 155
pseudoephedrine hydrochloride, 255
pseudoephedrine sulfate, 255
Pseudohypoparathyroidism, calcitriol for, 39
Psittacosis
 demeclocycline for, 85
 doxycycline for, 102
Psoriasis, cyclosporine for, 78
Psychosis
 chlorpromazine for, 63
 clozapine for, 73
 fluphenazine for, 133
 haloperidol for, 151
 loxapine for, 189
 mesoridazine for, 197
 molindone for, 210

Psychosis *(continued)*
olanzapine for, 225
perphenazine for, 238
prochlorperazine for, 252
quetiapine for, 258
risperidone for, 265
thioridazine for, 288
thiothixene for, 288
trifluoperazine for, 299
psyllium, 255-256
PTU, 255
Puberty, delayed, fluoxymesterone for, 132
Pulmicort Respules, 36
Pulmicort Turbuhaler, 36
Pulmonary edema
ethacrynate for, 119
furosemide for, 139
Pulmonary embolism. *See also* Thromboembolic disorders.
alteplase for, 10
enoxaparin for, 106
heparin for, 151-152
streptokinase for, 278
tinzaparin for, 291
urokinase for, 301
warfarin for, 305
Purinethol, 196
Purinol, 8
P.V. Carpine Liquifilm, 242
Pyelonephritis. *See also* Urinary tract infection.
gatifloxacin for, 141
levofloxacin for, 180
pyrazinamide, 256
Pyridiate, 239
Pyridium, 239
pyridostigmine bromide, 256
pyridoxine hydrochloride, 257
pyrimethamine, 257-258
pyrimethamine with sulfadoxine, 257-258
PZI, 164

Q

Questran, 64
Questran Light, 64
quetiapine fumarate, 258
Quinaglute Dura-Tabs, 259
Quinalan, 259
quinapril hydrochloride, 258
Quinate, 259
Quinidex Extentabs, 259
quinidine gluconate, 259
drug interactions with, 317
quinidine sulfate, 259
quinupristin/dalfopristin, 259-260

R

rabeprazole sodium, 260
Racepinephrine, 108
Radiation protection for thyroid, potassium iodide for, 247
Radiation therapy adverse effects
amifostine for, 12
granisetron for, 149
ondansetron for, 227
Radiologic examination
glucagon for, 147
metoclopramide for, 203
raloxifene hydrochloride, 261
Ramace, 261
ramipril, 261
ranitidine bismuth citrate, 261
ranitidine hydrochloride, 262
Rapamune, 273
Reclomide, 203
Rectal examination
bisacodyl for, 33
cascara sagrada for, 47
senna for, 271
Rectal infection
doxycycline for, 103
gatifloxacin for, 141
minocycline for, 208
Regitine, 240
Reglan, 203
Regonol, 256
Regranex Gel, 27
Regular (Conc.) Iletin II, 163
regular insulin, 163-164
Reguloid, 256
Rehaban Maximum Strength, 23
Relafen, 213
Relenza, 307
Remeron, 209
Remicade, 161
Renal cancer
aldesleukin for, 7
medroxyprogesterone for, 193
Renal disease
bumetanide for, 37
metolazone for, 203
piperacillin and tazobactam for, 244
Renal failure
amino acid infusions for, 13
calcitriol for, 40
epoetin alfa for, 110-111
mannitol for, 192
paricalcitol for, 232
probenecid for prevention of, 250
torsemide for, 296
Renedil, 123
Renitec, 105
Renova, 297
ReoPro, 2
repaglinide, 262-263
Requip, 268
Rescriptor, 84
Respid, 286
RespiGam, 263
Respiratory depression, narcotic-induced, naloxone for, 214
Respiratory distress syndrome, beractant for, 30
respiratory syncytial virus immune globulin, intravenous, human, 263
Respiratory syncytial virus infection
respiratory syncytial virus immune globulin, intravenous, human, for, 263
ribavirin for, 263
Respiratory tract infection. *See also* specific infections.
amantadine for, 11
amoxicillin/clavulanate potassium, 16
aztreonam for, 25
cefaclor for, 47
cefazolin for, 48
cefmetazole for, 50
cefonicid for, 50
cefoperazone for, 51
cefotaxime for, 51
cefotetan for, 52
cefoxitin for, 52
ceftazidime for, 54
ceftizoxime for, 55
ceftriaxone for, 56
cefuroxime for, 56

Respiratory tract infection (continued)
cephalexin for, 58
cephradine for, 59
co-trimoxazole for, 75
erythromycin for, 114
imipenem and cilastatin for, 158
ofloxacin for, 224
penicillin G benzathine for, 234-235
ticarcillin disodium/clavulanate potassium for, 290
Respolin Inhaler, 7
Respolin Respirator Solution, 7
Restoril, 282
Retavase, 263
reteplase, recombinant, 263
Reticulum cell carcinoma, bleomycin for, 34
Retin-A, 297
Retinitis, cytomegalovirus
cidofovir for, 64
fomivirsen for, 137
foscarnet for, 138
ganciclovir for, 140
Retinoblastoma, cyclophosphamide for, 78
retinoic acid, 297
Retrovir, 308
ReVia, 215
Revimine, 100
Rhabdomyosarcoma, dactinomycin for, 81
Rheumacin, 160
Rheumatic fever, penicillin G benzathine for, 235
Rheumatic heart disease, warfarin for, 305
Rheumatoid arthritis
aspirin for, 20
auranofin for, 23
aurothioglucose for, 23
azathioprine for, 24
capsaicin for, 43
celecoxib for, 58
choline magnesium trisalicylate for, 64
cyclosporine for, 78
diclofenac for, 89
diflunisal for, 90
etanercept for, 118-119
etodolac for, 121
fenoprofen for, 124
flurbiprofen for, 134
gold sodium thiomalate for, 23
ibuprofen for, 156
indomethacin for, 160
infliximab for, 161
ketoprofen for, 172
leflunomide for, 177
nabumetone for, 213
naproxen for, 216
oxaprozin for, 229
penicillamine for, 234
piroxicam for, 245
sulfasalazine for, 279
sulindac for, 280
Rheumatrex, 200
Rhinitis
beclomethasone for, 28
brompheniramine for, 35
budesonide for, 35
cetirizine for, 59
chlorpheniramine for, 62
clemastine for, 69
cromolyn for, 76
Rhinitis (continued)
diphenhydramine for, 93
fexofenadine for, 127
flunisolide for, 131
fluticasone for, 135
ipratropium for, 167
loratadine for, 187
promethazine for, 253
triamcinolone for, 299
Rhinocort, 35
Rhinorrhea, ipratropium for, 167
ribavirin, 263-264
riboflavin, 264
Riboflavin deficiency, riboflavin for, 264
Rickettsial infection
demeclocycline for, 85
doxycycline for, 102
Ridaura, 23
rifabutin, 264
Rifadin, 264
Rifadin IV, 264
rifampicin, 264-265
rifampin, 264-265
rifapentine, 265
rIFN-A, 164
Rilutek, 265
riluzole, 265
Rimactane, 264
rimantadine hydrochloride, 265
Rimycin, 264
Ringworm infestation, griseofulvin for, 150
Riopan, 189
Risperdal, 265
risperidone, 265-266
ritonavir, 266
drug interactions with, 317-318
Rituxan, 266
rituximab, 266
rivastigmine tartrate, 267
rizatriptan benzoate, 267
RMS Roxanol, 211
Roaccutane, 170
Robaxin, 200
Robimycin, 114
Robitet, 286
Robitussin, 150
Rocaltrol, 39
Rocephin, 56
Rodex, 257
Rofact, 264
rofecoxib, 267-268
Roferon-A, 164
Rogitine, 240
Rolaids Calcium Rich, 41
Romazicon, 130
ropinirole hydrochloride, 268
Rosacea, metronidazole for, 205
rosiglitazone maleate, 268-269
Roundworm infestation, mebendazole for, 192
Rowasa, 197
Roxicet, 312
Roxicet 5/500, 312
Roxicet Oral Solution, 312
Roxicodone, 230
Roxicodone Intensol, 230
Roxiprin, 312
RSV-IGIV, 263
Rubesol-1000, 77
Rubex, 102
Rythmodan, 96
Rythmodan-LA, 96

S

salazosulfapyridine, 279-280
salbutamol, 6-7
salbutamol sulfate, 6-7
salmeterol xinafoate, 269
Salmonine, 39
Salt depletion, sodium chloride for, 275
Sandimmun, 78
Sandimmune, 78
Sandostatin, 224
Sandostatin LAR, 224
Sani-Supp, 148
saquinavir, 269
saquinavir mesylate, 269
Sarafem, 132
Sarcoma
  alitretinoin for, 8
  bleomycin for, 34
  chlorambucil for, 61
  cyclophosphamide for, 78
  dactinomycin for, 81
  doxorubicin for, 101-102
  interferon alfa-2a, recombinant, for, 164
  interferon alfa-2b, recombinant, for, 164
sargramostim, 270
Scabene, 182
Scabies, lindane for, 182
SCF, 279
Schizophrenia. *See also* Psychosis.
  clozapine for, 73
  mesoridazine for, 197
  olanzapine for, 225
  trifluoperazine for, 299
Scopace, 270
scopolamine, 270
scopolamine butylbromide, 270
scopolamine hydrobromide (ophthalmic), 270-271
scopolamine hydrobromide (systemic), 270
Seasonal rhinitis. *See* Allergic rhinitis.
Seborrheic dermatitis
  hydrocortisone for, 154
  ketoconazole for, 172
secobarbital sodium, 271
Seconal Sodium, 271
Secretions, preoperative diminishing of
  atropine for, 22
  hyoscyamine for, 155
Sectral, 3
Sedation
  chloral hydrate for, 60
  diphenhydramine for, 93
  hydroxyzine for, 155
  lorazepam for, 188
  midazolam for, 206
  pentobarbital for, 237
  phenobarbital for, 239
  promethazine for, 253
  propofol for, 253
  scopolamine for, 270
  secobarbital for, 271
Seizures
  carbamazepine for, 44
  clonazepam for, 71
  clorazepate for, 72
  diazepam for, 89
  fosphenytoin for, 138-139
  gabapentin for, 140
  lamotrigine for, 175
  levetiracetam for, 178
Seizures *(continued)*
  magnesium sulfate for, 191
  oxcarbazepine for, 229-230
  phenobarbital for, 239
  phenytoin for, 241
  primidone for, 250
  pyridoxine for, 257
  secobarbital for, 271
  tiagabine for, 289
  topiramate for, 294
  valproate for, 302
  zonisamide for, 309
selegiline hydrochloride, 271
Semilente, 163
Senexon, 271
senna, 271
Senokot, 271
Septicemia. *See also* Bacteremia.
  aztreonam for, 25
  cefazolin for, 48
  cefonicid for, 50
  cefoperazone for, 51
  cefotaxime for, 51
  ceftazidime for, 54
  ceftizoxime for, 55
  ceftriaxone for, 56
  cephradine for, 59
  imipenem and cilastatin for, 158
  ticarcillin disodium/clavulanate potassium for, 290
Septra, 75
Serax, 229
Serenace, 151
Serentil, 197
Serentil Concentrate, 197
Serevent, 269
Serevent Diskus, 269
Seroquel, 258
Sertan, 250
sertraline hydrochloride, 271-272
Serutan Concentrated Powder, 256
Serzone, 217
Shigellosis, co-trimoxazole for, 75
Shingles
  capsaicin for, 43
  famciclovir for, 122
  valacyclovir for, 302
Shock
  albumin for, 6
  dexamethasone for, 86
  dopamine for, 100
  hydrocortisone for, 153
  isoproterenol for, 169
  methylprednisolone for, 202
  phenylephrine for, 240
sibutramine hydrochloride monohydrate, 272
sildenafil citrate, 272
  drug interactions with, 318
Silvadene, 273
silver sulfadiazine, 273
simethicone, 273
Simron, 126
Simulect, 27
simvastatin, 273
Sinemet, 179
Sinemet CR, 179
Sinequan, 101
Sinex, 241
Singulair, 211
Sinusitis
  amoxicillin/clavulanate potassium for, 16
  cefdinir for, 48
  cefpodoxime for, 53
  cefprozil for, 54
  cefuroxime for, 58
  ciprofloxacin for, 66

Sinusitis *(continued)*
clarithromycin for, 69
gatifloxacin for, 141
levofloxacin for, 180
loracarbef for, 186
moxifloxacin for, 212
sirolimus, 273-274
Sjögren's syndrome, cevimeline for, 60
Skelid, 290
Skin allograft rejection, nitrofurazone for, 221
Skin conditions. *See also* specific conditions.
betamethasone for, 31
dexamethasone for, 87
fluocinonide for, 131
fluticasone for, 135
hydrocortisone for, 154
triamcinolone for, 298
Skin infection. *See also* specific infections.
amoxicillin/clavulanate potassium for, 16
ampicillin/sulbactam for, 18
aztreonam for, 25
cefaclor for, 47
cefazolin for, 48
cefdinir for, 48
cefepime for, 50
cefmetazole for, 50
cefonicid for, 50
cefoperazone for, 51
cefotaxime for, 51
cefotetan for, 52
cefoxitin for, 52
cefprozil for, 54
ceftazidime for, 54
ceftizoxime for, 55
ceftriaxone for, 56
cefuroxime for, 57
cephalexin for, 58
Skin infection *(continued)*
cephradine for, 59
ciprofloxacin for, 66
dirithromycin for, 96
erythromycin for, 114
gentamicin for, 145
griseofulvin for, 150
imipenem and cilastatin for, 158
ketoconazole for, 172
levofloxacin for, 180, 181
linezolid for, 183
loracarbef for, 187
miconazole for, 206
neomycin for, 217
ofloxacin for, 225
piperacillin and tazobactam for, 244
quinupristin/dalfopristin for, 259
terbinafine for, 284
ticarcillin disodium/clavulanate potassium for, 290
trovafloxacin for, 301
Slo-Phyllin, 286
Slow-K, 246
Slow-Mag, 190
Small-bowel intubation, metoclopramide for, 203
Smoking cessation
bupropion for, 37
nicotine polacrilex for, 219
nicotine transdermal system for, 220
So-bid Gyrocaps, 286-287
Social anxiety disorder, paroxetine for, 233
Soda Mint, 274
sodium bicarbonate, 274-275
sodium chloride, 275
sodium cromoglycate, 76-77
sodium ferric gluconate complex, 275-276
sodium phosphates, 276
sodium polystyrene sulfonate, 276
Soft-tissue infection
cefaclor for, 47
cefadroxil for, 47
cefazolin for, 48
cefoxitin for, 52
cephalexin for, 58
cephradine for, 59
erythromycin for, 114
imipenem and cilastatin for, 158
Soft-tissue sarcoma, doxorubicin for, 101-102
Solazine, 299
Solfoton, 239
Solganal, 23
Solu-Cortef, 154
Solu-Medrol, 202
Soma, 45
Sominex, 93
Somnal, 133
Sonata, 306
Sorbitrate, 170
Sotacor, 277
sotalol, 277
Spancap #1, 87
sparfloxacin, 277
Spasmoban, 90
Spasticity
baclofen for, 26
cyclobenzaprine for, 77
dantrolene for, 83
diazepam for, 88
scopolamine for, 270
Spinal cord–injured patients
baclofen for, 26
dantrolene for, 83
spironolactone, 277-278
Sporanox, 171
SPS, 276
Squamous cell carcinoma, bleomycin for, 34
Squibb-HC, 154
Sris-PEG, 150
SSKI, 247
Stadol, 38
Stadol NS, 38
Status epilepticus. *See also* Seizures.
diazepam for, 89
fosphenytoin for, 138
phenobarbital for, 239
phenytoin for, 242
secobarbital for, 271
stavudine, 278
Stelazine, 299
Stemetil, 251
StieVA-A, 297
Stimate, 85
Stool softening, docusate for, 98
Streptase, 278
streptokinase, 278
streptozocin, 279
Stroke
alteplase for, 10
clopidogrel for, 72
dantrolene for, 83
pravastatin to reduce risk of, 248
ramipril for, 261
ticlopidine for, 290
strong iodine solution, 247
Subaortic stenosis, hypertrophic, propranolol for, 254
Sublimaze, 125

sucralfate, 279
Sudafed, 255
Sular, 220
Sulcrate, 279
sulfamethoxazole, 279
sulfasalazine, 279-280
Sulfatrim, 75
sulfisoxazole, 280
sulfisoxazole acetyl, 280
sulindac, 280
sulphasalazine, 279-280
sumatriptan succinate, 281
Sumycin, 286
Supeudol, 230
Supraventricular arrhythmias
  adenosine for, 6
  digoxin for, 90
  diltiazem for, 92
  esmolol for, 115
  flecainide for, 128
  propranolol for, 254
  quinidine for, 259
  verapamil for, 304
Surfactant deficiency, beractant for, 30
Surfak, 98
Surgical infection
  aztreonam for, 25
  trovafloxacin for, 300
Surmontil, 300
Survanta, 30
Sus-Phrine, 108
Sustiva, 105
Symadine, 11
Symmetrel, 11
Synercid, 259
Synflex, 216
Syntocinon, 231
synvinolin, 273
Syphilis
  minocycline for, 208
  penicillin G benzathine for, 234, 235

T

T_3, 184
T_4, 181-182
Tachycardia
  adenosine for, 6
Tachycardia *(continued)*
  amiodarone for, 15
  bretylium for, 34
  digoxin for, 90
  diltiazem for, 92
  disopyramide for, 96
  esmolol for, 115
  flecainide for, 128
  magnesium sulfate for, 192
  mexiletine for, 205
  propranolol for, 254
  quinidine for, 259
tacrine hydrochloride, 281
tacrolimus, 281
Tagamet, 65
Tagamet HB, 65
Talacen, 312
Talwin, 236
Talwin Compound, 312
Talwin-Nx, 236
Tambocor, 128
Tamiflu, 228
tamoxifen citrate, 282
tamsulosin hydrochloride, 282
Tapazole, 199
Targretin, 32
Tasmar, 294
Tavist, 69
Tavist-1, 69
Taxol, 231
Taxotere, 98
Tazac, 222
Tazicef, 54
Tazidime, 54
Tebrazid, 256
Tegretol, 44
Teldrin, 62
telmisartan, 282
temazepam, 282
Temodar, 283
temozolomide, 283
Temperature conversions, 319
Tempra, 3
Tendinitis
  naproxen for, 216
  sulindac for, 280
tenecteplase, 283-284
Tenormin, 20
Tension. *See also* Anxiety.
  hydroxyzine for, 155
Tequin, 141
Terazol 3 Vaginal Ovules, 285
Terazol 7 Vaginal Ovules, 285
terazosin hydrochloride, 284
terbinafine hydrochloride (oral), 284
terbinafine hydrochloride (topical), 284
terbutaline sulfate, 285
terconazole, 285
Terfluzine, 299
TESPA, 288
Tessalon, 29
Testamone 100, 285
Testicular cancer
  bleomycin for, 34
  cisplatin for, 67
  dactinomycin for, 81
  etoposide for, 121
  ifosfamide for, 158
  plicamycin for, 245
  vinblastine for, 304
Testicular deficiency, fluoxymesterone for, 132
Testoderm, 285
Testoderm TTS, 286
testosterone, 285-286
testosterone cypionate, 285-286
testosterone propionate, 285-286
testosterone transdermal system, 285-286
Testred, 202
Tetanus, methocarbamol for, 200
Tetany, calcium for, 40
tetracycline hydrochloride (oral), 286
  drug interactions with, 318
Tetracyn, 286
Teveten, 111
Thalitone, 63
Thallium myocardial perfusion scintigraphy, dipyridamole for, 95
Theo-24, 287
Theo-Dur, 286
Theolair, 286
theophylline, 286-287
theophylline ethylenediamine, 14
theophylline sodium glycinate, 287
Theralax, 33
Thermazene, 273
thiamine hydrochloride, 287-288
Thioplex, 288
Thioprine, 24
thioridazine hydrochloride, 288
thiotepa, 288
thiothixene, 288-289
thiothixene hydrochloride, 288-289
Thoracic surgery, acetylcysteine for pulmonary complications of, 4

Thorazine, 63
Thrombocythemia, anagrelide for, 19
Thrombocytopenia, oprelvekin for prevention of, 227
Thromboembolic disorders
alteplase for, 10
dalteparin for, 81
danaparoid for, 82
enoxaparin for, 106-107
heparin for, 151-152
streptokinase for, 278
ticlopidine for, 290
tinzaparin for, 291
urokinase for, 301
warfarin for, 305
Thyro-Block, 247
Thyroid cancer, doxorubicin for, 101
Thyroidectomy, potassium iodide for, 247
Thyroid hormone replacement
levothyroxine for, 181
liothyronine for, 184
Thyrotoxic crisis
potassium iodide for, 247
propylthiouracil for, 255
tiagabine hydrochloride, 289
Tiamate, 92
Tiazac, 92
Ticar, 289
ticarcillin disodium, 289
ticarcillin disodium/clavulanate potassium, 290
Tic disorders. *See also* Tourette syndrome.
pimozide for, 243
Ticillin, 289
Ticlid, 290
ticlopidine hydrochloride, 290
Tikosyn, 98
tiludronate disodium, 290
Timentin, 290
timolol maleate (ophthalmic), 291
timolol maleate (systemic), 291
Timoptic Solution, 291
Timoptic-XE, 291
Tinea infection
griseofulvin for, 150
ketoconazole for, 172
miconazole for, 206
terbinafine for, 284
tinzaparin sodium, 291-292
tioconazole, 292
Tipramine, 159
tirofiban hydrochloride, 292
tissue plasminogen activator, recombinant, 10
TMP-SMZ, 75
TNKase, 283
TOBI, 293
tobramycin, 293
drug interactions with, 318
tobramycin sulfate, 293
Tobrex, 293
tocainide hydrochloride, 293
Tofranil, 159
Tofranil-PM, 159
tolcapone, 294
tolterodine tartrate, 294
Tonocard, 293
Tonsillitis
azithromycin for, 24
cefadroxil for, 47
Tonsillitis *(continued)*
cefdinir for, 49
cefpodoxime for, 54
cefprozil for, 54
ceftibuten for, 55
cefuroxime for, 56, 57
clarithromycin for, 69
loracarbef for, 186
topactin, 131
Topamax, 294
topiramate, 294-295
Toposar, 121
topotecan hydrochloride, 295
Toprol XL, 204
Toradol, 173
toremifene citrate, 295
torsemide, 295-296
Total parenteral nutrition
amino acid infusions for, 13
dextrose for, 88
Tourette syndrome
haloperidol for, 151
pimozide for, 243
Toxoplasmosis, pyrimethamine for, 257
t-PA, 10
Trachoma, erythromycin for, 113
tramadol hydrochloride, 296
Trandate, 173
trandolapril, 296
Transderm-Nitro, 221
Transderm-Scop, 270
Transderm-V, 270
Transiderm-Nitro, 221
Transient ischemic attack, pravastatin to reduce risk of, 248
Transplant recipients
azathioprine for, 24
basiliximab for, 27
Transplant recipients *(continued)*
cyclosporine for, 78
cytomegalovirus immune globulin (human), intravenous for, 79-80
daclizumab for, 80
filgrastim for, 127
ganciclovir for, 140
mycophenolate for, 213
sargramostim for, 270
sirolimus for, 273
tacrolimus for, 281
Tranxene, 72
Tranxene-SD, 72
Tranxene-T-Tab, 72
trastuzumab, 297
Travasol with Electrolytes, 13
trazodone hydrochloride, 297
Tremor, propranolol for, 254
Trental, 237
tretinoin (oral), 298
tretinoin (topical), 297
Triacet, 298
Triadapin, 101
triamcinolone acetonide (nasal), 299
triamcinolone acetonide (systemic), 298
triamcinolone acetonide (topical), 298
Triamonide 40, 298
triamterene, 299
triazolam, 299
Trichomoniasis, metronidazole for, 204
Tricor, 123
Tricosal, 64
Tridil, 221
triethylenethiophosphoramide, 288

trifluoperazine hydrochloride, 299
Trihexane, 300
trihexyphenidyl hydrochloride, 300
Tri-Immunol, 95
Trikacide, 204
Trilafon, 238
Trilafon Concentrate, 238
Trileptal, 229
Trilisate, 64
Trilog, 298
trimethoprim, 300
trimethoprim-sulfamethoxazole, 75-76
Trimipex, 300
trimipramine maleate, 300
Trimox, 16
Tripedia, 95
Triphasil, 120
Triprim, 300
Triptone, 93
Tritace, 261
Tritec, 261
TrophAmine, 13
Trophoblastic tumors
  dactinomycin for, 81
  methotrexate for, 200
trovafloxacin mesylate, 300-301
Trovan I.V., 301
Trovan Tablets, 300
Truphylline, 14
Trusopt, 101
TSPA, 288
Tuberculosis
  acetylcysteine for, 4
  ethambutol for, 119
  isoniazid for, 168-169
  pyrazinamide for, 256
  rifampin for, 264
  rifapentine for, 265
Tums, 41
Tylenol, 3
Tylenol with Codeine Elixir, 311
Tylenol with Codeine No. 2, 312
Tylenol with Codeine No. 3, 312
Tylenol with Codeine No. 4, 312
Tylox, 312

U

Ukidan, 301
Ulcerative colitis
  mesalamine for, 197
  olsalazine for, 226
  sulfasalazine for, 279
Ultralente Insulin, 164
Ultram, 296
Ultrazine-10, 251
Unasyn, 18
Uniparin, 151
Unipen, 214
Urecholine, 32
Urethral infection
  doxycycline for, 103
  minocycline for, 208
Urethritis
  azithromycin for, 25
  ofloxacin for, 224
Urex, 139
Uridon, 63
Urinary frequency/urgency, tolterodine for, 294
Urinary retention
  bethanechol for, 32
  finasteride for, 128
Urinary stones, aluminum carbonate for, 11
Urinary tract infection
  amikacin for, 13
  amoxicillin/clavulanate potassium for, 16
  amoxicillin for, 16
Urinary tract infection *(continued)*
  aztreonam for, 25
  cefaclor for, 47
  cefadroxil for, 47
  cefepime for, 49
  cefmetazole for, 50
  cefonicid for, 50
  cefotaxime for, 51
  cefotetan for, 52
  cefpodoxime for, 53
  ceftazidime for, 54
  ceftizoxime for, 55
  ceftriaxone for, 56
  cefuroxime for, 56
  ciprofloxacin for, 66
  co-trimoxazole for, 75, 76
  gatifloxacin for, 141, 142
  imipenem and cilastatin for, 158
  levofloxacin for, 180
  lomefloxacin for, 185-186
  nitrofurantoin for, 221
  norfloxacin for, 223
  ofloxacin for, 225
  phenazopyridine for, 239
  sulfamethoxazole for, 279
  sulfisoxazole for, 280
  ticarcillin disodium/clavulanate potassium for, 290
  ticarcillin for, 289
  trimethoprim for, 300
Urocarb Tablets, 32
Urogesic, 239
urokinase, 301
Uro-Mag, 191
Urticaria
  cetirizine for, 59
  clemastine for, 69
  fexofenadine for, 127
Urticaria *(continued)*
  loratadine for, 187
Uterine atony or subinvolution, methylergonovine for, 201
Uterine bleeding
  estrogens, conjugated, for, 118
  medroxyprogesterone for, 193
  norethindrone for, 223
  progesterone for, 252
UTI Relief, 239
Uveitis
  atropine for, 22
  dexamethasone for, 86
  scopolamine for, 270

V

Vaginal atrophy, estradiol/norethindrone acetate transdermal system for, 117
Vagistat-1, 292
valacyclovir hydrochloride, 302
Valergen, 116
Valisone, 31
Valium, 88
valproate sodium, 302-303
valproic acid, 302-303
valsartan, 303
Valtrex, 302
Vamate, 155
Vancenase AQ Double Strength, 28
Vancenase AQ Nasal Spray, 28
Vancenase Nasal Inhaler, 28
Vanceril, 28
Vanceril Double Strength, 28